Concise Pathology
for
Medical Students

In Question–Answer Form

SECOND EDITION

Contributors

Gopal Kumar

DCH (MAMC, Delhi)
DNB (Paediatrics PG, DDU Hospital, Delhi)

Yatendra Agrawal

DCH (LHMC, Delhi)
DNB (Paediatrics)
DDU Hospital, Delhi

Concise Pathology
for
Medical Students

In Question–Answer Form

SECOND EDITION

Prashant Patel
MBBS, MD, IDCCM
University College of Medical Sciences
and associated
Guru Teg Bahadur Hospital
Delhi

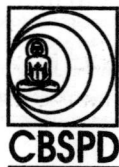

CBSPD

CBS Publishers & Distributors Pvt Ltd

New Delhi • Bengaluru • Chennai • Kochi • Kolkata • Lucknow • Mumbai
Hyderabad • Jharkhand • Nagpur • Patna • Pune • Uttarakhand

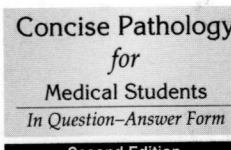

Concise Pathology
for
Medical Students
In Question–Answer Form
Second Edition

ISBN: 978-81-239-2535-6

Copyright © Author and Publisher

Second Edition: 2015
  Reprint: 2016, 2018, 2020, 2022, 2023, 2025
First Edition: 2006
  Reprint: 2006, 2007, 2008, 2009, 2011, 2012, 2013

Published by Satish Kumar Jain and produced by Varun Jain for

CBS Publishers & Distributors Pvt Ltd
4819/XI Prahlad Street, 24 Ansari Road, Daryaganj, New Delhi 110 002, India
Ph: 011-23289259, 23266838   Website: www.cbspd.com
                                    e-mail: delhi@cbspd.com
Corporate Office: 204 FIE, Industrial Area, Patparganj, Delhi 110 092
Ph: 011-4934 4934   Fax: 011-4934 4935   e-mail: publishing@cbspd.com; publicity@cbspd.com

Branches

- **Bengaluru:** Seema House 2975, 17th Cross, K.R. Road, Banasankari 2nd Stage, Bengaluru 560 070, Karnataka, India
  Ph: +91-80-26771678/79   Fax: +91-80-26771680   e-mail: bangalore@cbspd.com
- **Chennai:** 18/8B, Subbarayan Street, Shenoy Nagar, Chennai 600 030, Tamil Nadu, India
  Ph: +91-44-42032115, 26681266   e-mail: chennai@cbspd.com
- **Kochi:** 42/1325, 1326, Power House Road, Opp KSEB, Power House, Ernakulam 682 018, Kerala, India
  Ph: +91-484-4059061-65   Fax: +91-484-4059065   e-mail: kochi@cbspd.com
- **Kolkata:** 147, Hind Ceramics Compound, 1st Floor, Nilgunj Road, Belghoria, Kolkata-700056, West Bengal, India
  Ph: 033-25633055, 033-25633056   e-mail: kolkata@cbspd.com
- **Lucknow:** Basement, Khushnuma Complex, 7-Meerabai Marg (Behind Jawahar Bhawan), Lucknow 226001, India
  Ph: 0522-4000032   e-mail: tiwari.lucknow@cbspd.com
- **Mumbai:** PWD Shed. Gala no. 25/26, Ramchandra Bhatt Marg, Next to JJ Hospital Gate no. 2 Opp. Union Bank of India Noorbaug
  Mumbai-400009, Maharashtra, India
  Ph: 022-66661880/89   e-mail: mumbai@cbspd.com

Representatives

- **Hyderabad** 0-9885175004 • **Jharkhand** 0-9811541605 • **Nagpur**   0-8692091830
- **Patna**   0-9334159340 • **Pune**   0-9664372571 • **Uttarakhand** 0-9716462459

Printed at: Glorious Printers, Delhi, India

to

---

my parents
Mr Praphulla Kumar Singh and
Mrs Kumod Devi

Preface to the Second Edition

Important advances and changes in basic pathology have prompted bringing out the second edition of this book. As with the previous edition, the book written in Question–Answer form with suitable format of presentation will cater to the needs of all the MBBS and allied students in their professional examinations.

In keeping with the new concepts and changes in standard textbooks, this edition has been completely updated. A few chapters like 'Cellular Pathology', 'Diseases of Immunity', and 'Disorders of Red Blood Cells', have been extensively updated, while chapters 'Heart and Blood Vessels' and 'Urinary System' have been reorganised and rewritten.

New flowcharts, illustrations, figures and tables have been incorporated with better presentation to make this book more student-friendly. Recently asked questions have been added to the text.

I sincerely hope that this edition of the book will be appreciated by undergraduate students and it will be beneficial to them for clearing the university examinations confidently.

I have tried to make the book error-free and up-to-date; your suggestions and constructive criticism for improving this book will be appreciated.

Prashant Patel

drprashant2002@gmail.com
ppatel_med@yahoo.co.in

Preface to the First Edition

It gives me immense pleasure to bring out *Concise Pathology for Medical Students*. Now when there is an explosion in the recent advances and knowledge in pathology, undergraduate students are not able to go through the entire pathology. Even after adequate prior revision of most chapters, students find themselves almost 'handicapped', a night before 'sent-up' examination. In a single day they have to revise and remember 13 chapters, and of course reproduce them in the examination on the next day, only for looking next 13 chapters in queue to be finished in 8 hours for 2nd paper.

During that crucial time I had always missed a "book" which should be complete from our examination point of view. Such a book should contain questions asked in the last 10 years, most probable questions, and their answers in a form that can be remembered and reproduced in the examination.

With these purposes in mind I started writing this 'book' on my computer.

The questions have been selected from the last 10–15 years of Delhi University question papers (annual/supplementary); and years in which they have been asked are indicated within bracket. Questions asked repeatedly in the last 10 years are the most likely to be asked again, so indicating years in front of them may be used as tools for "self ultra-selection" of questions. But in each year some new questions appear in the paper, so I have also included other "questions marked by seniors".

Questions related to differences consume a lot of time to prepare answer, but they share substantial marks in question paper, and they are highly scoring. So maximum number of differences has been given. Even short notes can be derived from difference tables.

Hematology is becoming important in terms of its 'marks sharing' in question paper. It has been given special attention as most of us find it difficult to ascertain the type of questions that would be asked in the examination, and of course, their answers at single place. I remember that we tried to "procure and preserve" every bit of paper that has flavor of hematology. At the same time, we cannot afford to read voluminous foreign or Indian hematology textbooks without any substantial gain due to lack of time. The pathology textbooks that we read are good for learning the concept of hematology, but they are not compatible with our examination system.

Questions in each chapter are arranged in an order that is in accordance with the textbooks and are more productive when used along with these books. Some questions that are less frequently asked, have been left unanswered—to be read from the textbook.

This book should be used as 'add-on book' to which you may add some facts while reading the textbook that you would like to remember later on. This book should not be used as an alternative to the standard textbook, but is meant to be used only as an 'add-on book'. As all of us have to get PG seats through competitive examinations, we must read books that will also help us later on, in addition to overcoming the "2nd Prof. crisis".

Though years indicated in brackets are from DU question papers, but same questions have been asked in other universities also. I hope this book will help students of MBBS and allied subjects of all universities.

I have tried to be precise, up-to-date, avoid mistakes, and compile complete data/information. I request you to send your suggestions regarding correction, omission, addition or better presentation or so by e-mail to: *ppatel_med@yahoo.co.in*.

My sincere thanks to my parents, brother, sister and all family members, whose expectations and dedication made me what I am today.

Friends, seniors and juniors at hostel, in particular Abhishek Anand, Sankalp Sethi, Deepak Chahar, Arvind Jhajharia, Mukesh Jha, Anurag Singla, Kutbuddin Akbari, Prakash Jha, Umesh Mittal, Varun Singh, Kishore Chawla and others cannot be neglected for their unconditional support. Thanks to all the teachers, who have taught and guided me at various stages of my life.

My special thanks to friends Mr Arun Kumar Tiwari, Mr Siddharth Singhal and Miss Aparna Kashyap. I am very indebted and thankful to Dr Ram Nawal Rao for thorough review of this book, and for his suggestion and guidance.

I am thankful to Mr YN Arjuna, Director of CBS Publishers & Distributors, New Delhi, for his cooperation in bringing out this book in short time.

I am obliged to two friends, who have accepted to contribute one chapter each and helped in proofreading, in addition to moral and study material support.

"The Heart and Blood Vessels" by Mr Gopal Kumar, UCMS

"The Urinary System" by Mr Yatendra Agrawal, UCMS

Dec, 2005   **Prashant Patel**

UCMS, Delhi

ppatel_med@yahoo.co.in

Acknowledgments

My sincere thanks to Dr Gopal Kumar and Dr Yatendra Agrawal, for contributing chapters "Heart and Blood Vessels" and "Urinary System" respectively.

I am thankful to my parents, brother, sister-in-law and younger sister Pratibha Sinha, for their unconditional support.

I am thankful to Dr Nilesh Kumar of UCMS, Delhi, for providing recent questions and inputs to make this book better.

I am thankful to my friends, juniors, seniors, teachers and colleagues of UCMS and GTB Hospital, New Delhi, and Dr BLK Super Speciality Hospital, New Delhi.

My special thanks to Mr YN Arjuna, Senior Vice President, and other staffs of CBS Publishers & Distributors, New Delhi; for bringing out this book in a great format.

Prashant Patel

How to Use this Book

This book is an attempt to give an overview of pathology in Question–Answer format. The content is based on the latest edition of *Robbins Pathologic Basis of Disease*. However, *Textbook of Pathology* by Harsh Mohan, has also been kept in mind while preparing this book.

According to new syllabus (prescribed by Medical Council of India) only 'short note', 'difference' and 'very short note' types of questions are to be asked in university examinations. Therefore, the questions in this book are framed accordingly and the answers compiled as 'short notes' and 'differences'. Some old long questions (LQ) have also been given, because a part of LQ may appear as a 'short note' under the new examination pattern. Differences are given in a standard table form.

Readers must keep in mind that this book is intended to serve just as a supplementary to the standard textbook and not as an alternative. They should not keep this book for the last moment, it would be better to start reading this book from day one.

Steps to be followed

1. First see this book to select important questions/topics for the examination.
2. Read the entire chapter/topic (almost) from the textbook (preferably Robbins; others will also do). Now you have an idea of the topic/chapter and an overall understanding of the topic.
3. Within a day or two, you should go through the above chapter/topic from this book. This will be an easy job. As you have fresh memories of textbook, you can decide how much of textbook you can remember for examination (take care of it!). I have prepared this book based on the concept that *we cannot remember (and we don't have to) everything given in the textbook for our examination*. If you wish to add some more points to this book from textbook, you can add in each answer. This book becomes your *personalized notebook* for your examination and future for quick review.
4. Whenever you are required (for tutorial, internal exams) to read that chapter, use this personalized notebook. Revision will take very less time and you will retain more. It means more efficient study.
5. Try to revise this book many times as you can. You will remember each and every topic and chapter till the time you have your exams.
6. It will be easier to revise small and concise book that you have revised many times. You will be able to finish all chapters in short duration for 'sent-up' and prof. exams.
7. Some questions, left unsolved (less important), are to be read from the textbooks.

8. For those who believe in the last moment preparation, this is the best available book around. They will be getting best possible marks by reading this book in short duration; but memory of topics will be short-lived!

9. This book gives very short, concise and appropriate description of the practical exams. Though enough, yet you should prepare 'favorite questions' of your teachers as advised by your seniors.

10. List of gross specimens is given. You should see these specimens in the museum and prepare *Frequently Asked Questions* (given in the practical section).

Similarly, try to find out identifying features of histopathology slides from your practical classes (like clinical features/other features).

We have avoided in giving details of gross specimen and histopathology slides separately for the practical to keep the volume of the book minimum.

Contents

Preface to the Second Edition   *vii*

Preface to the First Edition   *ix*

How to Use this Book   *xiii*

Part I

1. Cellular Pathology I: Cell Injury and Cell Death   *3*
2. Cellular Pathology II: Tissue Repair   *15*
3. Acute and Chronic Inflammation   *19*
4. Hemodynamic Disorders, Thrombosis and Shock   *30*
5. Genetic Disorders   *43*
6. Diseases of Immunity   *48*
7. Neoplasia   *71*
8. Infectious Diseases, Environmental and Nutritional Pathology   *92*
9. Diseases of Infancy and Childhood   *97*
10. Disorders of Red Blood Cells   *100*
11. Bleeding Disorders   *139*
12. Disorders of White Blood Cells   *147*
13. Miscellaneous Questions for Paper I   *165*

Part II

14. Heart and Blood Vessels   *169*
15. Lung   *189*
16. Gastrointestinal Tract   *209*
17. Liver and Biliary Tract   *229*
18. Pancreas   *249*
19. Urinary System   *256*
20. Male Genital Tract   *275*
21. Female Genital Tract   *285*
22. Breast   *298*
23. Endocrine System   *307*

24. Skin   320
25. Bones and Joints   323
26. Central Nervous System and Eye   333
27. Miscellaneous Questions for Paper II   340

Part III: Practicals

28. Hematology Practical   343
29. Urine Practical   347
30. Gross Specimen   352
31. Histopathology Slides   354

Marks Distribution

Marks Distribution: UCMS, Delhi University

(Theory part has fixed marks distribution in all colleges, but practical marks are almost always redistributed in every college. So look for those changes from the concerned department.)

Theory (110)	Paper I (University examination) (Part I of this book)		40
	Paper II (University examination) (Part II of this book)		40
	Theory viva (based on gross specimens; university exam)		15
	Internal assessment (semester and other college exams)		15
Practical (40)	Spotting and case history		8
	Histopathology slides	General and systemic diseases (3 slides)	6
		Hematological slides (2 slides)	3
	'Practical'	Hematology practical	4
		Urine practical	4
	Internal assessment (semester and other college exams)		15
Total			**150**

Theory

Each theory paper has three parts:

Part I:	1. 4 differences ($2 \times 4 = 8$)	2. 3 short notes ($2 \times 3 = 6$)
Part II:	3. 2 short notes ($3 \times 2 = 6$)	4. 2 short notes ($3 \times 2 = 6$)
Part III:	5. 4 short notes ($2 \times 4 = 8$)	6. 3 short notes ($2 \times 3 = 6$)

*Each part must be solved in separate answer books.

Practical

1. *Spotting and case history*
   a. Gross specimens
   b. Histopathology slides
   c. Clinical cases
2. *Histopathology slides* that are generally asked have been included in this book. Slides are to be indentified based on the brief clinical presentation and its microscopic appearance.

Questions asked are

- Identify the parent/original tissue.
- Give two identifying features.
- What is the lesion/disease?

3. *Hematological slides include*
- DLC slide:
  - Identify the conditions like neutrophilia, eosinophilia, etc (you may require to perform counting of cells).
  - Give conditions where such DLC changes are observed.
- Second hematology slide has a good clinical history, some investigations. It is generally the slide of anemia or some hematological malignancies.

4. *Hematology practical*
- Hb estimation
- Total leukocyte count
- DLC

5. *Urine*
Chemical analysis for:
- Protein
- Sugar
- Ketone bodies
- Bile salts
- Bile pigments

Provisional diagnosis on the basis of urinary finding of the sample (a set of findings like sugar, protein and ketone bodies: Indicating uncontrolled DM and related nephropathy) provided.

PART I

1

Cellular Pathology I: Cell Injury and Cell Death

Definition: Cell injury is a condition of cell leading to deviation from normal morphologic, physiologic and functional state of cell due to any assault.

Causes

- Oxygen deprivation
- Physical agents like physical trauma, radiations, heat/cold, pressure, etc.
- Chemical agents and drugs
- Genetic derangements
- Immunologic reactions
- Infectious agents
- Nutritional imbalances

Mechanism of cell injury

a. Diminished generation of ATP: Critical mechanism
   - Depletion of ATP to < 5 to 10% of normal levels has widespread effects on many critical cellular systems:

  - Decreased activity of $Na^+/K^+/ATP$-ase
  - Intracellular influx of Ca^{2+}
  - Cell swelling, clumping of nuclear material, detachment of ribosomes from endoplasmic reticulum (decrease protein synthesis).

b. Increased intracellular calcium: Result in activation of enzymes:

   ATPase: Further ATP depletion

   Phospholipase: Membrane damage

   Proteases: Damage to membrane and cytoskeletal proteins

   Endonuclease: Damage to DNA

c. Membrane damage and defect in membrane permeability due to:
   - Mitochondrial dysfunction
   - Activation of proteases
   - Activation of phospholipase

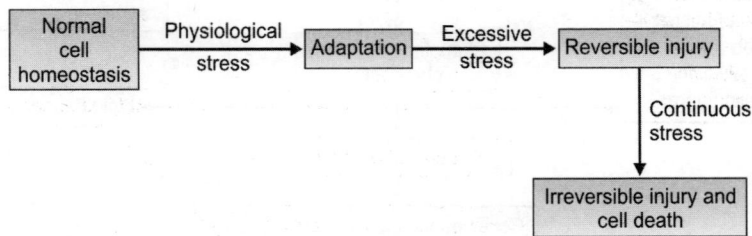

Fig. 1.1

3

- Cell membrane damage due to free radicals
d. Release of lysosomal enzymes due to membrane damage.

2. Fate of ischemic injury (2004)

3. Mechanism of ischemic/hypoxic cell injury (1993)

4. Difference between reversible and irreversible cell injuries (1999, 2003, 07)

Traits	Reversible injury	Irreversible injury
1. Definition	If the structural and functional changes induced by an injurious stimulus, can revert back to normal on removal of the same.	If the structural and functional changes induced by an injurious stimulus, cannot be reversed even after removal of stimulus.
2. Cell membrane:		
Bleb formation	Present	Absent
Defect in membrane	Absent	Present
3. Endoplasmic reticulum	Swelling	Swelling and lysis
4. Ribosomes	Dispersion	Dispersion and destroyed
5. Lysosomes	Autophagy of organelles by lysosomes, no rupture	Rupture of lysosomes and autolysis of cell
6. Nucleus	Clumping of nuclear chromatin	Pyknosis, karyolysis, or karyorrhexis
7. Mitochondria	Swelling, small densities present	Swelling, large densities present
8. Fate of cell	Stimuli, if removed, changes to normal	Permanent change—cell death
9. Calcification	Absent	Dystrophic calcification

Mechanism of Reversible Cell Injury

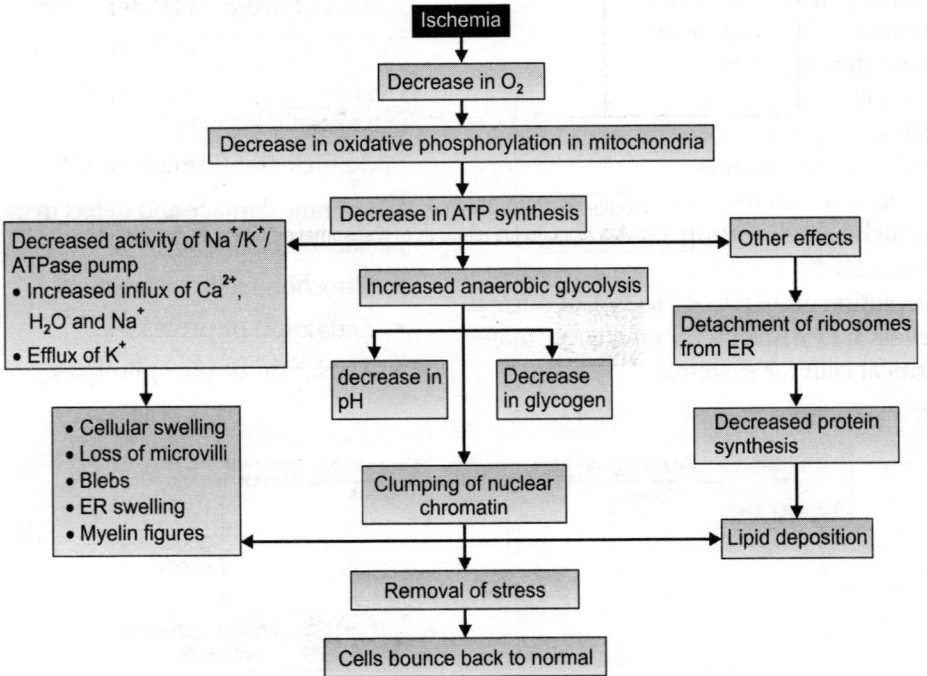

Fig. 1.2: Reversible cell injury

Mechanism of Irreversible Cell Injury

"Membrane damage is the central factor" in the pathogenesis of irreversible cell injury. It is the continuum of reversible injury.

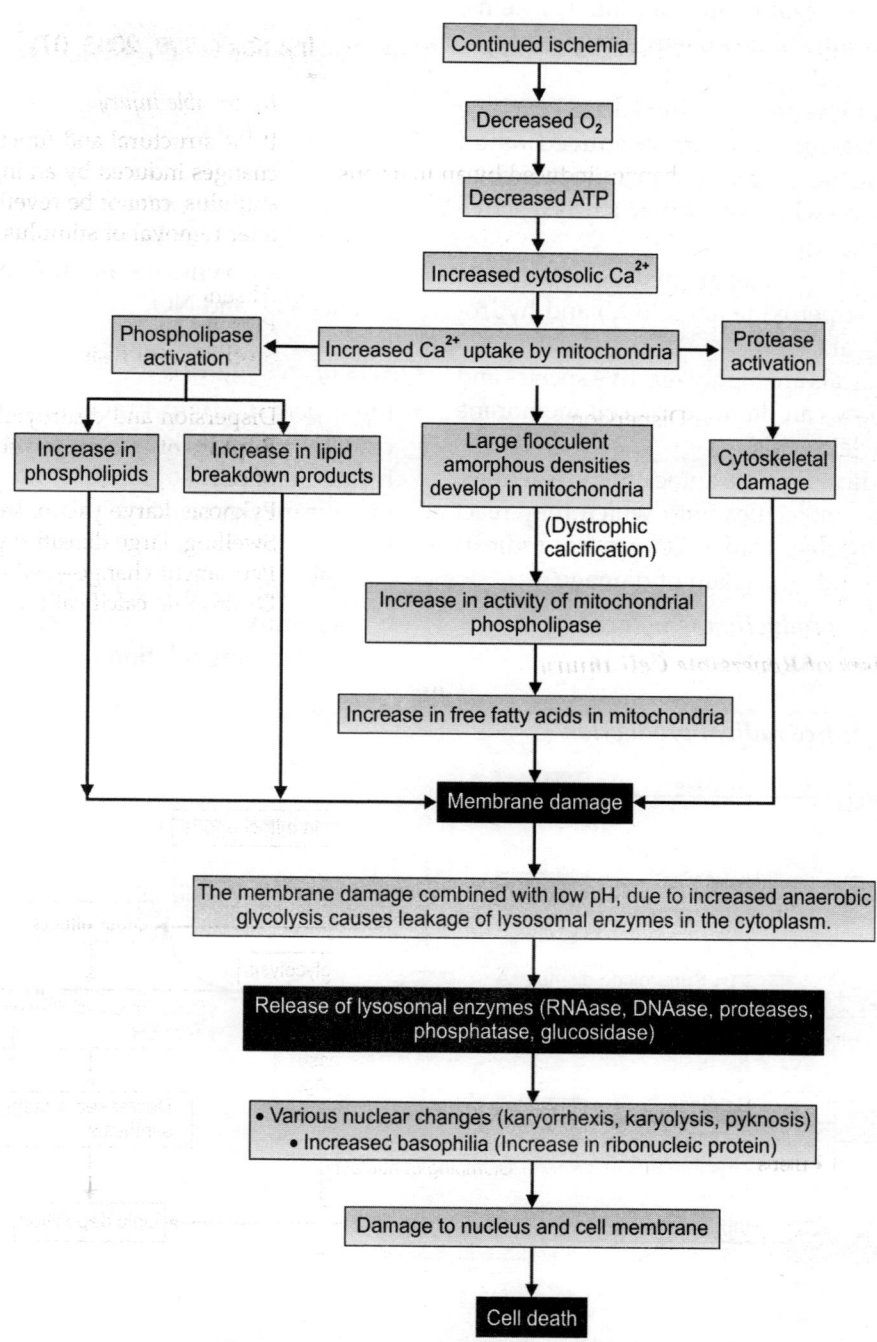

Fig. 1.3: Irreversible cell injury

5. Free radical cell injury (1993, 98)

Free radicals: These are chemical species with unpaired electrons in their outer orbit. They react with inorganic and organic (proteins, lipids, carbohydrate) chemicals mainly of membrane and nucleic acids.

- Most of these are partially reduced reactive oxygen forms that are produced as an unavoidable by-product of mitochondrial respiration which is also known as reactive oxygen species.
- The most important are hydrogen peroxide (H_2O_2), superoxide anion (O_2^-) and hydroxyl radical ($^\bullet HO$).
- Free radicals are highly reactive species and toxic, they can damage the cell membrane and nucleic acids.
- Free radicals initiate autocatalytic reactions, whereby molecules with which they react are themselves converted into free radicals to propagate the chain of damage.

Free radical production is induced by

- *Radiation:* Like UV rays, X-rays
- *Enzymatic metabolism* of exogenous chemicals/drugs: Like CCl_4 to CCl_3
- *Reduction-oxidation reaction* processes occurring during normal metabolism: Formation of superoxide anion (O_2^-), hydrogen peroxide (H_2O_2), hydroxyl ion (OH^-).
- *Reaction involving transition metals:* Like iron (Fenton reaction), copper, etc.
- *Reactions involving nitric oxide (NO):* Acts as a free radial and can be converted to a highly reactive peroxynitrite anion ($ONOO^-$) as well as NO_2 and NO_3^-.

Effects of free radicals

- *Lipid peroxidation:* Free radicals, particularly $^\bullet HO$ attack double bond of unsaturated fatty acid of plasma and organelle membranes producing peroxides (*initiation*).
  - Peroxide itself is a reactive and unstable entity, which starts a chain reaction of lipid peroxidation (*propagation*).

Pathway of free radical production

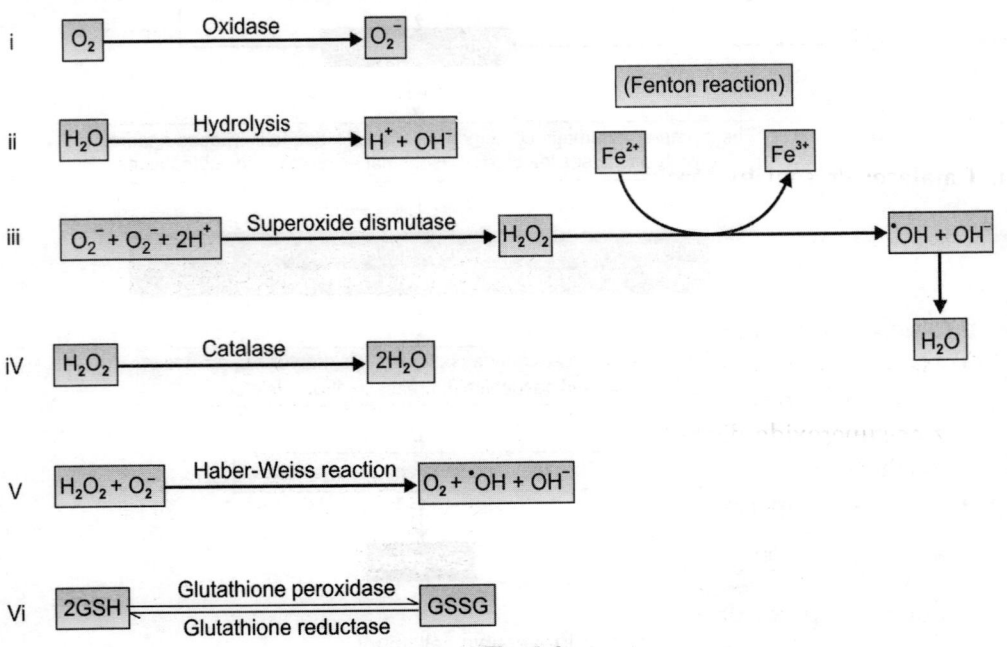

Fig. 1.4

– In some cases, chain reaction may be terminated by antioxidants.

• *Modification of proteins by oxidation*: Oxidation of amino acid residue side chain, protein-protein cross linkage, and oxidation of protein backbone resulting in protein fragmentation.

• *DNA lesion*: Attacks thymine and other nucleotides of nuclear and mitochondrial DNA to produce single-stranded breaks in DNA.

Inactivation of free radicals/antioxidant mechanism

Cells have several non-enzymatic and enzymatic systems that contribute for inactivation of free radicals, and thus minimizing damage.

a. *Non-enzymatic system*

   i. Antioxidants (vitamins C, A, E, β-carotene, glutathione and cysteine): They block the initiation of free radicals formation and inactive free radicals.

   ii. Tissue proteins (Transferrin, ferritin, lactoferrins and ceruloplasmins): These transport and storage proteins bind with copper and iron to decrease their role in production of free radicals.

b. *Enzymatic system*

   A series of enzymes act as free radicals scavenging systems and breakdown of hydrogen peroxide and superoxide anion.

   i. **Catalase:** Present in peroxisomes and decomposes H_2O_2

$$2H_2O_2 \xrightarrow{\text{catalase}} 2H_2O$$

   ii. **Superoxide dismutase (SOD)**

   • Manganese superoxide dismutase is present in mitochondria, while copper-zinc-superoxide dismutase is found in cytosol.

   • It converts superoxide to H_2O_2.

$$2O_2^- + 2H \xrightarrow{\text{SOD}} 2H_2O_2 + O_2$$

   iii. **Glutathione peroxidase**

   • Present in mitochondria and cytosol

• It catalyses free radical breakdown

$$H_2O_2 + 2GSH \longrightarrow GSSG + 2H_2O$$

$$2\,OH + 2GSH \longrightarrow GSSG + 2H_2O$$

• Intracellular ratio of oxidized glutathione (GSSG) to reduced glutathione (GSH) is a reflections of the oxidative state of the cell.

6. Mechanism of fatty liver (1993, 98, 2000, 08)

(*Also see liver*)

7. Causes of fatty liver. Injury caused by carbon tetrachloride

Causes

• Alcohol
• Starvation/Malnutrition
• Diabetes mellitus
• Obesity
• Hepatotoxins like CCl_4, ether, aflatoxins, etc.
• Certain drugs like steroids, tetracycline, Reye's syndrome in infants (aspirin)
• Hypoxia in anemia, cardiac failure
• Late pregnancy
• Chronic illness like TB (*see* next page Fig. 1.5 for injury caused by CCl_4)

8. Write briefly about necrosis

Definition: A spectrum of morphological changes that follow cell death in a living tissue. They largely result from the progressive degenerating activity of enzymes on lethally injured cells.

It should be noted that cell death is 'Not' due to necrosis rather necrosis occurs after cell death. Necrosis only represents the morphological changes that occur after cell death.

Pathogenesis: These morphological changes (necrosis) are the result of two concurrent processes:

Injury caused by carbon tetrachloride

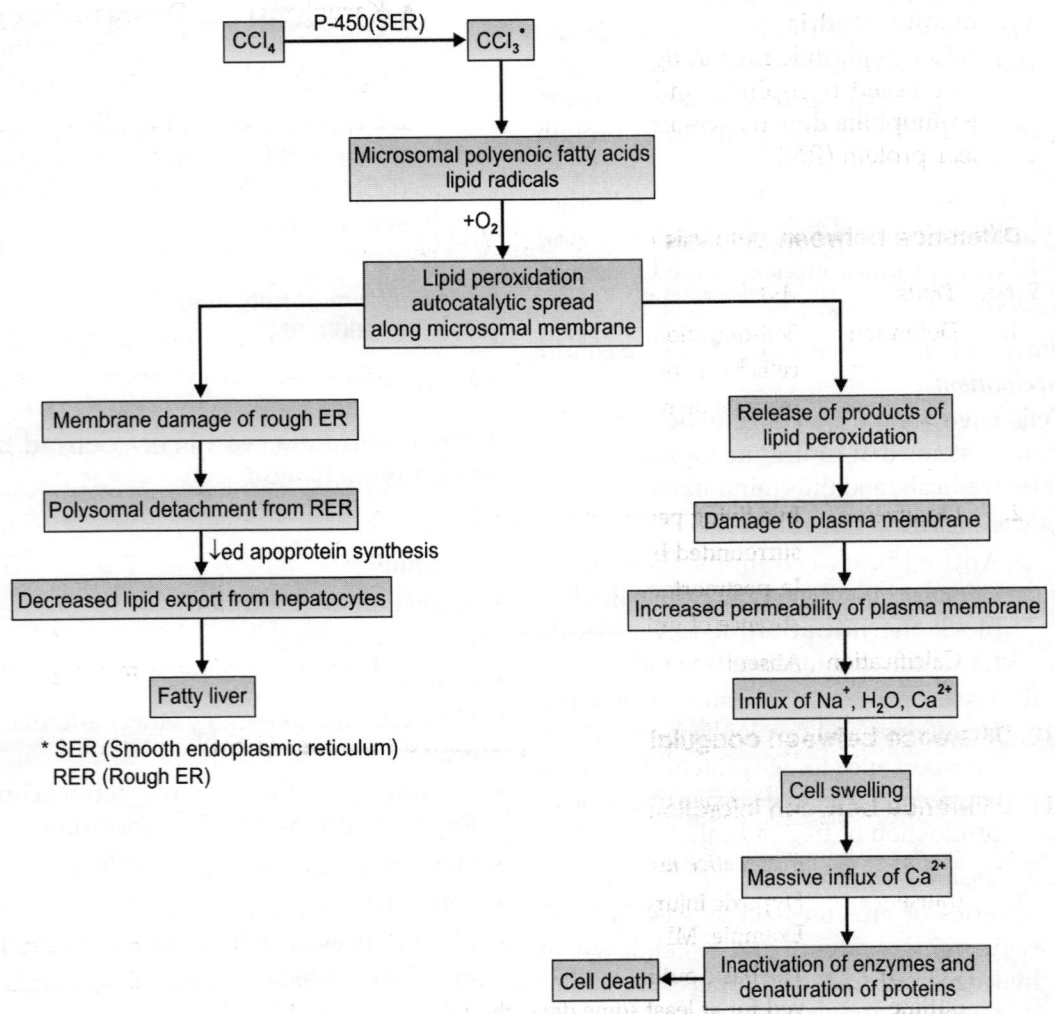

Fig. 1.5

i. Enzymatic digestion of cells:

Enzymes used in the process are derived from two sources.

- From the lysosome of dead cells themselves (autolysis).
- From the lysosome of immigrant leukocytes (heterolysis).

ii. Denaturation of cellular proteins

- These processes require hours to develop. So immediately after the cell

death there is no detectable necrotic changes.

- Necrosis usually affects a group of continuous cells.
- In necrosis, there is disruption of membrane integrity (intracellular contents leak out and elicit inflammatory changes in surrounding tissues).

Morphological changes: A necrosis follows irreversible injury, so morphological changes resemble:

- Membrane damage
- Large flocculent amorphous densities in mitochondria
- Intracytoplasmic myelin figures
- Decreased basophilia and increased eosinophilia due to decreased ribonuclear protein (RNP)

- Nuclear changes
  - Karyolysis – Decreased basophilia of chromatin
  - Pyknosis – Nuclear shrinkage
  - Karyorrhexis – Fragmentation of pyknotic nucleus

9. Difference between autolysis and necrosis (1990)

S. No.	Traits	Autolysis	Necrosis
1.	Definition	Self-digestion or disintegration of cells by its own enzyme liberated from its own lysosomes	Spectrum of morphologic changes that follow cell death in living tissue, largely resulting from the progressive degenerating action of enzymes on lethally injured cells
2.	Occurrence	In a living person, it occurs when surrounded by inflammatory cells. In postmortem cases—complete absence of inflammatory cells	Occurs only in the presence of inflammatory cells Does not take place in postmortem
3.	Calcification	Absent	Dystrophic calcification may be present.

10. Difference between coagulative and liquefactive necroses (1994)

11. Difference between infarction (coagulative) and gangrene (liquefactive)

S. No.	Traits	Coagulative necrosis	Liquefactive necrosis
1.	Cause	Hypoxic injury except in brain Example: MI	Hypoxic injury in CNS; bacterial and fungal infections induced injuries
2.	Cellular outline	The basic outline of cell is preserved for at least some days, though cytoplasmic and nuclear details are lost.	Cell outline and intracellular details are completely lost, tissue architecture is not preserved.
3.	Mechanism	Due to intracellular acidosis (due to hypoxia) structural as well as enzymatic proteins are denatured and block its proteolysis. Dead cells are removed by fragmentation and phagocytosis.	Bacteria and fungus stimulate accumulation of inflammatory cells. Hydrolytic enzymes (autolysis and heterolysis) result in complete digestion of dead cells.
4.	Gross	Firm texture	Formation of liquid viscous mass
5.	Cell features	Conversion of cells into acidophilic, coagulated and anucleated cells	No cellular architecture is recognized rather than liquid mass is seen, which in case of acute inflammation is creamy yellow (pus).

12. Difference between coagulative and caseous necroses (a distinct form of coagulative necrosis) (1997, 98, 2002, 10)

S. No.	Traits	Coagulative necrosis	Caseous necrosis
1.	Causes	Hypoxia, like MI	Tubercular infection, like TB lung
2.	Mechanism	Denaturation of cellular proteins due to acidity	Reaction between *mycobacterium* capsular antigens and inflammatory cells
3.	Gross	Affected organ is firm in texture.	White and cheesy appearance
4.	Microscopy	Cells are acidophilic, coagulated and anucleated.	Typical caseous material—amorphous granular debris (fragmented, coagulated cells and granular debris) surrounded by distinct inflammatory cells.
5.	Cellular features	Basic cell shape preserved	Not preserved
6.	Tissue architecture	Preserved	Completely obliterated
7.	Inflammation	Diffuse, no border	Within specified border—granulomatous reaction

13. Difference between caseous and gangrenous necroses

S. No.	Traits	Caseous necrosis	Gangrenous (coagulative) necrosis
1.	Definition	A distinct form of coagulative necrosis, seen in TB.	A form of coagulative necrosis which may be followed by liquefactive necrosis, when a part loses its blood supply and followed by infection.
2.	Gross	Cheesy white appearances	Affected tissue is firm in texture.
3.	Histology	(See difference table)	(See difference table)
4.	Granuloma-tous reaction	May be present	Absent

14. Difference between dry and wet gangrenes (1994)

S. No.	Traits	Dry gangrene	Wet gangrene
1.	Cause	Arterial occlusion (coagulative necrosis)	More in venous obstruction than arterial obstruction. It is followed by bacterial infection (coagulative to liquefactive necrosis).
2.	Sites	Commonly limbs	More common in bowel
3.	Gross	Organ is dry, shrunken and black.	Moist, soft, swollen, rotten, dark
4.	Line of demarcation	Present at junction between healthy and gangrenous parts	Not clear
5.	Putrefaction	Limited (no infection and less blood supply)	Marked
6.	Presence of bacteria	Absent; little or no septicemia	Overwhelming; septicemia present
7.	Affected parts	Cold, black, begins to atrophy	Initially hot and red; later cold, bluish, offensive odor
8.	Prognosis	Better	Poor

15. Difference between apoptosis and necrosis (1995, 98, 2002, 03, 04, 08, 11)

S. No.	Traits	Apoptosis	Necrosis
1.	Definition	Programed and coordinated cell death which eliminate unwanted/harmful cells or remove cells damaged beyond repair	Spectrum of morphologic changes that follow cell death in living tissues, largely resulting from the progressive degenerative action of enzymes on lethally injured cells.
2.	Causes	May be physiological or pathological	Always pathological—hypoxia, toxins
3.	Involves	Single or small group of cells	Large groups of cells
4.	Inflammation	Absent	Present
5.	Cellular change	Cell shrinkage	Cell swelling
6.	Cell membrane	Bleb formation	Membrane disruption
7.	Nucleus	Chromatin condensation followed by fragmentation	Nuclear disruption/chromatin clumping
8.	Removal of cell	Phagocytosis of apoptotic bodies by macrophages	Enzymatic digestion or phagocytosis of cell debris by macrophages
9.	Lysosomes/other organelles	Intact	Hydrolytic enzyme release due to rupture
10.	Mechanism	Genetically coordinated	Due to ATP depletion, free radicals, mitochondrial damage, etc.
11.	Electrophoresis	Step ladder DNA pattern	Diffuse DNA

16. Fat necrosis (1990, 94, 2004)

Process leading to a focal area of fat destruction, which results due to release of activated lipase enzymes.

Causes
- Acute pancreatitis (*see chapter pancreas*)
- Traumatic fat necrosis as in breast

Pathogenesis
- Released enzymes cause hydrolysis of neutral fat present in adipose tissue (of pancreas, peritoneal cavity, breast, bones) into free fatty acids and glycerol.
- These fatty acids may combine with calcium to form calcium soap (*saponification*).

Morphology
- *Gross:* Yellowish-white and firm deposits.
- *Microscopy:* The necrosed cells are cloudy in appearance, surrounded by inflammatory cells.

Calcium soap: Appears as amorphous, granular and basophilic deposits.

Non-enzymatic/traumatic fat necrosis
- It occurs due to trauma.
- It is seen in subcutaneous tissues of breast, thigh and abdomen.

17. Causes of apoptosis (2007)

18. Apoptosis (1994, 97, 98, 2001, 02, 08)

Definition: This is a form of cell death designed to eliminate unwanted host cells through activation of a coordinated and internally programed series of events effected by a set of gene products.

Occurrence
Physiological apoptosis
- Death by apoptosis is a normal phenomenon that "serves to eliminate cells that are no longer needed".

- It is important in following physiological situations:
  - The programed destruction of cells during embryogenesis including implantation, organogenesis and metamorphosis.
  - Hormonal dependent involution in adults, e.g. endometrial cell breakdown during menstrual cycle, ovarian follicular atresia in the menopause, the regression of lactating breast after weaning, and prostatic atrophy after castration.
  - Cell deletion in proliferating cell population in order to maintain a constant number, e.g. intestinal crypt epithelium.
  - Death of host cells that have served their useful purpose such as neutrophils after an acute inflammatory response, and lymphocytes at the end of an immune response.
  - Elimination of potentially harmful self-reactive lymphocytes in the thymus.
  - Cell death induced by cytotoxic T cells to eliminate virus infected and neoplastic cells. Same mechanism occurs in graft versus host disease.

Pathological apoptosis

- When cells are damaged beyond repair, especially when the damage affects cell's DNA, the irreparably damaged cells are eliminated:
  - Cell death produced by injurious stimuli—radiation and cytotoxic anticancer drugs damage DNA, and if repair mechanisms cannot cope with the injury, the cell kills itself by apoptosis. In these situations, elimination of the cell may be a better alternative than risking mutations and translocations in the damaged DNA which may result in malignant transformations.
  - Cell injury in certain viral disease—viral hepatitis.
  - Pathologic atrophy in parenchymal organs after duct obstruction such as occurs in pancreas and parotid gland.
  - Cell death in tumors

Morphological changes in apoptosis

i. Cell shrinkage
   - This is the earliest change.

- It is due to the damage of cytoskeletal proteins that provide structural support to the cell.

ii. Chromatin condensation (pyknosis)
   - It is due to the breakdown and clumping of chromatin.
   - This is the most characteristic features of apoptosis.

iii. Formation of cytoplasmic blebs and apoptosis bodies.

iv. Chromosomal DNA fragmentation due to endonuclease and caspases activity.

v. Phagocytosis of apoptotic cells and bodies by adjacent macrophages or healthy parenchymal cells without the sign of inflammation.

Biochemical features

- Protein cleavage by proteolytic enzymes
  Activation of caspases (family of cysteine proteases having a unique ability to cleave after aspartic acid residues).
  - Protein hydrolysis
    → cleavage or breakup of nuclear scaffold
    → cleavage or breakup of cytoskeletal proteins
- Protein cross-linkage
  Activation of transglutaminases
  ↓
  Cross-linking of cytoplasmic proteins leading to covalently linked shrunken cells
  ↓
  Easy breakdown in apoptotic bodies
- DNA condensation and breakdown
  DNA breakdown in large pieces (50–300 kb)
  ↓
  Internucleosomal cleavage by endonuclease forming oligonucleosomes (180– 200 kb) visualized on agarose gel electrophoresis as DNA ladders
- Recognition of dying cells by phagocytes
  Flip-flop of apoptotic cells
  ↓
  Phosphatidylserine and thrombospondin flip on the external surface from inner layer
  ↓
  Easy recognition and phagocytosis of apoptotic cells

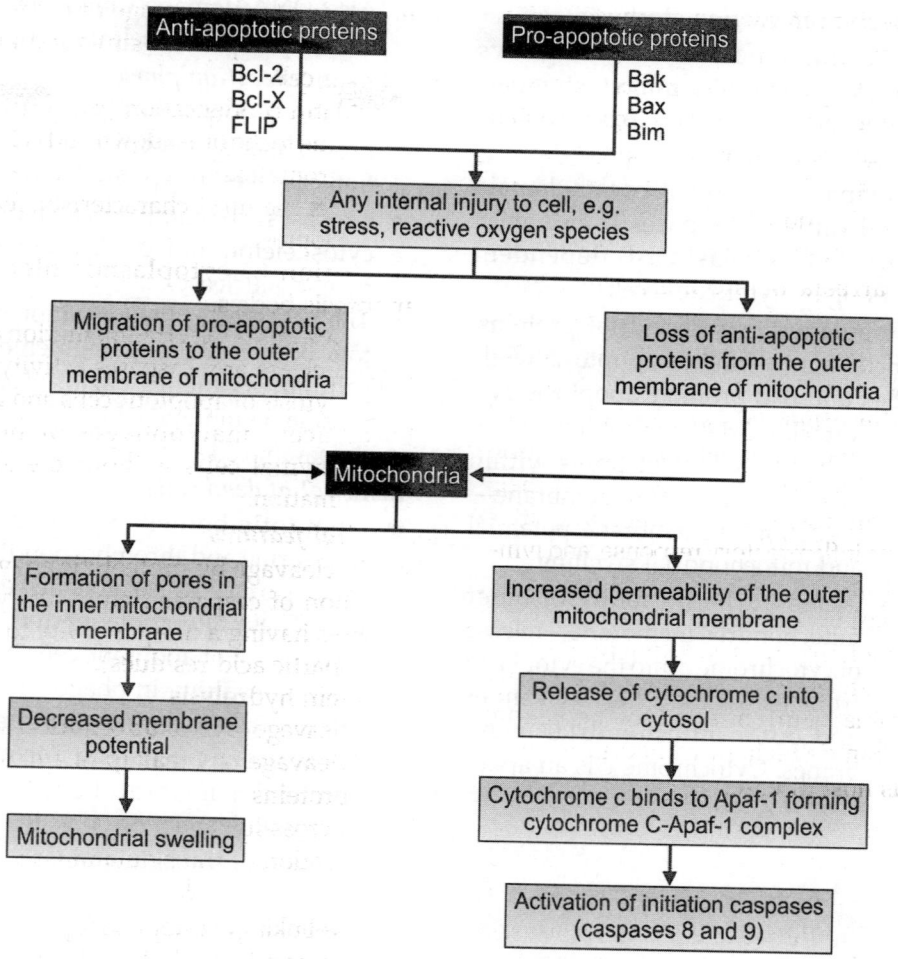

Fig. 1.6

Mechanism: Apoptosis is the end point of an energy dependent cascade of molecular events having four steps.

1. **Signaling pathways:** Initiates apoptosis
   - Intrinsic or mitochondrial pathway (*see* Fig. 1.6).
   - Extrinsic or death receptor pathway: Transmembrane signals may be positive (leading to initiation) or negative (opposing initiation).

These include:

Injuries: Radiation, toxins and free radicals. Withdrawl of growth factors, hormones and cytokines. Receptor-ligand interaction 'Fas/Fas ligand', TNF/TNF receptor.

↓

Act on intracellular regulatory molecules

or

Directly affect targets within the cells, e.g. physicochemical agents like heat, radiations, viruses and xenobiotics; and glucocorticosteroids directly bind to nuclear receptors

↓

Activation of caspases → (initiation)

2. *Control and integration stage*
   i. Intracellular positive and negative regulatory molecules inhibit, stimulate or stop apoptosis. This step is carried by two sets of proteins:
      • Adapter proteins with death domain and initiator caspases (binds with Apaf-1) like Fas/FasL dependent killing by cytotoxic T cell.
      • Regulatory mitochondrial proteins: Bcl-2 family inhibits apoptosis while Bax and Bad promote apoptosis by:
        – Mitochondrial permeability transition. Formation of pores within inner mitochondrial membrane— reduction of membrane potential and mitochondrial swelling.
        – Increased permeability of outer mitochondrial membrane—release of cytochrome c into the cytoplasm from its location between inner and outer mitochondrial membranes. Cytochrome c is an apoptotic trigger.

   ii. Also DNA damage causes p53 activation—cells direct itself for apoptosis.

3. *Common execution phase*
   • This is a common final pathway of proteolysis by enzymes called 'Execution caspases' (caspases 3 and 7).
   • Caspases activation causes catabolism of cytoskeleton and DNA fragmentation by endonuclease.
   • The net result is the formation of apoptotic body containing fragmented DNA, cellular organelles enclosed within a plasma membrane which buds off from its parent cell.

4. *Removal of dead cells*
   • Apoptotic bodies express phosphatidylserine and thrombospondin on the outer surface as phagocytic cell receptors. These alterations permit the easy recognition of apoptotic cells by macrophages resulting in phagocytosis without the release of proinflammatory cellular components (no inflammation) and leaving no trace of dead cells.

2

Cellular Pathology II: Tissue Repair

1. Endogenous pigments (2007)

These are colored substances synthesized in the body itself.

i. *Lipofuscin*
ii. *Melanin*
   - It is an endogenous, non-hemoglobin derived brown-black pigment.
   - Usually present in skin, hair, choroid, meninges, and adrenal medulla.
   - Synthesized by melanocytes and dendritic cells.

   Staining characteristic: It can be bleached with hydrogen peroxide and stained with Masson-Fontana argentaffin stain.

iii. *Hemosiderin*
   - It is a hemoglobin derived, golden-yellow to brown, granular or crystalline pigment in which form iron is stored in cells. It represents aggregates of ferritin micelles. Under normal conditions, small amount of hemosiderin is present in mononuclear phagocytes of bone marrow, spleen and liver.

iv. *Bilirubin*: It is derived from hemoglobin metabolism, but does not have iron.

2. Lipofuscin (1996, 2000)

Synonyms: Lipochrome, wear and tear pigment and aging pigment.

Solubility: Insoluble in cytoplasm.

Composition: Polymers of lipids and phospholipids complexed with protein.

It is derived from lipid peroxidation of polyunsaturated lipids of subcellular membranes.

Morphology

Light microscopy: Yellow-brown, finely granular intracytoplasmic, often perinuclear pigment.

Electron microscopy: Perinuclear electron dense having membranous structure in their midst.

Occurrence: Cells undergoing slow and regressive changes; like Kupffer cells, have lipofuscin pigment in their cytoplasm as in hepatitis (due to phagocytosis of degenerating hepatocytes).

It is present particularly in liver and heart of ageing patients or patients with severe malnutrition and cancerous cachexia.

Staining characteristics of lipofuscin
- Acid-fast (AFB positive)
- Autofluorescent
- Stains positive with fat stains
- Reduces ferricyanide to ferrocyanide (Schmorl's reaction)

Importance
- It is neither injurious to cells nor interfere with its functions.
- It is taken as a sign of ageing, wear–tear of cells, etc.

- Deposition of lipofuscin in heart is referred as "brown atrophy".

3. Dystrophic calcification (1995)

i. Formation of crystalline calcium phosphate mineral in tissue similar to hydroxyapatite of bones.
ii. *Steps:* Both steps may be intracellular as well as extracellular.

Initiatial/nucleation
- *Intracellular calcification* in mitochondria of dead or dying cells (as it accumulates calcium).
- *Extracellular calcification:* Phospholipids are present in membrane-bound vesicles.
  - Calcium is concentrated in these vesicles by membrane-facilitated calcification.
  - Ca^{++} binds to phospholipids present in vesicle membrane.

- Phosphatase associated with membrane generates PO_4^{3-} which binds to Ca^{++}.
- Such cycle is repeated, resulting in local deposits near membrane.
- Structural change in the arrangement of Ca^{++} and PO_4^{3-} groups occurs in producing microcrystals which can propagate.

Propagation: Repeated cycle of formation of microcrystal may result in large deposits.

Morphology
- *Gross:* Fine, white granules or clumps often felt as gritty deposits.
- *Microscopy (H & E):* Present at intracellular or extracellular or in both locations.
  - Seen as basophilic, amorphous, granular and sometimes clumped.
  - Psammoma bodies may be seen.

4. Difference between dystrophic and metastatic calcifications (1993, 97, 98, 99, 2000, 01, 07, 10) or pathological calcifications (2000)

S. No.	Traits	Dystrophic calcification	Metastatic calcification
1.	Definition	Deposits of calcium in dead and degenerated tissues/organ	Deposits of calcium in normal tissues
2.	Calcium metabolism	Normal	Deranged
3.	Serum calcium level	Normal	Hypercalcemia
4.	Causes	Necrosis [like caseous, liquefactive, fat, coagulative (infarct)], thrombi, hematomas, dead parasites, atheromas, Monckeberg's medial calcification (sclerosis), some tumors, cysts	Hyperparathyroidism, bony destructive lesions (multiple myeloma, metastatic carcinoma), prolonged immobilization, hypervitaminosis D, milk alkali syndrome, renal failure, retention of PO_4^{3-}: $2°$ hyperparathyroidism, hypercalcemia of infancy.
5.	Pathogenesis	It is just like mineralization of bone (hydroxyapatite) in these tissues	Mineralization sequence is same, but favored by relatively high pH at certain sites like lungs, stomach, blood vessel, cornea and kidney

5. Factors affecting wound healing (1999, 2007, 10, 11)

Local factors	Systemic factors
• Infections	• Age
• Poor blood supply	• Nutritional state, anemia
• Presence of foreign bodies	• Systemic infections
• Movement of involved joints	• Administration of drugs like glucocorticoids
• Exposure to ionizing radiations	• Association of DM
• Exposure to UV rays	• Hematological abnormality
• Lesion size, type, location, involvement of a particular organ/tissue	• Uremia
	• Genetic disorder (Marfan's syndrome, Ehlers-Danlos disease)
	• Obesity
	• Vitamin and trace metals (Zn and Cu) deficiency

6. Difference between healing by first/primary and secondary intention (1993, 96, 97, 2000, 07, 09, 11)

S. No.	Traits	Healing by primary intention	Secondary intention
1.	Site	Clean, uninfected surgical incision approximated by surgical sutures	In all natural/open wounds like infarction, inflammation, abscess, surface wound as in roadside accident, etc. Infection may be present
2.	Tissue injury	Very limited to superficial layer of epithelium and connective tissues	Extensive, causing cells death and necrosis in larger area; larger defect
3.	Inflammatory reaction	Less intense	More intense (for clearing large fibrin, necrotic debris and exudates)
4.	Granulation tissue	Small amount is formed	Larger amount has to be formed to fill large defect of wound
5.	Wound contraction	Absent	Is a characteristic of such large surface wounds due to presence of myofibroblast
6.	Scarring	Less	More
7.	Keloid	Absent	May be formed

7. Difference between granuloma and granulation tissue (1996)

S. No.	Traits	Granuloma	Granulation tissue
1.	Definition	Granuloma is circumscribed, tiny lesion composed of collection of modified macrophages (epithelioid cell) and rimmed at the periphery by lymphoid cells	Hallmark of healing, there is acute inflammatory response to clear necrotic debris; followed by angiogenesis and fibrous tissue formation
2.	Present	Chronic inflammatory reactions like TB, leprosy, syphilis, etc.	Normal physiological response after any injury

(Contd.)

7. Difference between granuloma and granulation tissue (*Contd.*)

S. No.	Traits	Granuloma	Granulation tissue
3.	Microscopic features	Collection of epithelioid cells, giant cell, histiocytes, macrophages and lymphocytes	Newly formed blood vessels embedded in loose, edematous matrix having neutrophils (mainly), monocytes and plasma cells
4.	Vascularization	No angiogenesis; not highly vascularized	Highly vascularized due to angiogenesis
5.	Fibroblast	Proliferation not marked	Marked
6.	Role	May cause damage to host	Not pathological
7.	Remodelling	Maturation and reorganization of fibrous tissue: Not seen	Seen
8.	Growth factors	Cytokines like IL-1, IL-12 and γ-IFN	Angiogenic and fibrogenic growth factors—PDGF, FGF, TNF, VEGF

8. Labile cells and stable cells (1994)

- *Labile cells/continuously dividing cells* continue to multiply throughout life under normal physiological conditions. Examples are surface epithelia, mucosal lining of all excretory ducts of glands, cells of bone marrow, hematopoietic tissues, transitional epithelium of urinary tract, columnar cells of GIT and uterus.

- *Stable/quiescent cells* have normally low level of replication but can undergo rapid division in response to external stimuli. Examples are parenchyma of all glands like liver, pancreas, kidney, etc. and some mesenchymal cells like fibroblast, smooth muscle cell, and vascular endothelial cells.

3

Acute and Chronic Inflammation

1. Define inflammation. What are the different stimuli for inflammation?

Inflammation is a series of molecular and cellular responses to eliminate foreign agents or damaged (necrotic) cells and to promote repair of damaged tissues. It is the reaction of blood vessels leading to accumulation of fluid and leukocytes in extravascular tissues. It is essentially a protective response, which may be potentially harmful at times.

Stimuli for inflammation includes
- *Physical agents*: Heat, radiation and mechanical trauma
- *Chemical agents*: Organic and inorganic poisons
- *Infectious agents*: Bacteria, virus and parasites
- *Immunological agents*: Hypersensitivity reactions

2. Difference between acute and chronic inflammation

S. No.	Traits	Acute inflammation	Chronic inflammation
1.	Onset	Rapid	Slow
2.	Duration	Short; lasting for minutes, hours, days and a few days	Longer; weeks and months
3.	Inflammatory cell type	Mainly neutrophils	Mainly lymphocytes and macrophages; plasma cells
4.	Hallmark	Exudation of fluid and plasma proteins (edema)	Proliferation of blood vessels, fibrosis and tissue necrosis
5.	Characteristics	Differ at different times/phages. Vascular changes, protein exudation, edema and neutrophilic inflammatory cells emigration seen	Phase of active inflammation, tissue destruction and attempt to repair by connective tissue replacement of damaged cells, angiogenesis, and fibrosis at same time seen.
6.	Cardinal signs of inflammation	Rubor, tumor, color, dolor, functio laesa are present	Absent

3. Vascular changes and cellular events in acute inflammation (1992, 93)

or

Describe the cellular events in acute inflammation

- Acute inflammation is a rapid response to an injurious agent that serves to deliver mediators of host defence, i.e. leukocytes and plasma proteins to the site of injury.
- Acute inflammation has two major components: Vascular response and cellular response.

Vascular response

1. *Change in vascular flow and caliber*
   - Transient vasoconstriction is followed by vasodilation, first involving arterioles.
   - This is followed by opening of new capillary beds. Increase in blood flow to that area (heat and redness).
   - There is increased permeability of microvasculature resulting in slowing of blood circulation–exudation.
   - RBCs get concentrated in vessels—increased viscosity (stasis-dilated small vessel packed with RBCs).
2. *Increased vascular permeability (vascular leakage)*
   - "Exudation is hallmark of acute inflammation".
   - There is increased hydrostatic pressure at arteriolar end (due to increased blood flow), increased hydrostatic pressure in capillaries bed [due to vasodilation (opening of new capillaries beds)], and decreased colloidal osmotic pressure (due to exudation of plasma proteins). The whole sequence leads to net outflow of fluid from vessels leading to edema.
3. Change in vascular flow (stasis)
   - The loss of fluid results in concentration of red cells and viscosity of blood → Slower blood flow → Stasis

$$\downarrow$$

Leukocytic migration or peripheral orientation of WBCs

Endothelium becomes leaky: Mechanisms proposed to explain it:
- Formation of endothelial gaps in venules
- Cytoskeleton reorganization (endothelial retraction)
- Increased transcytosis across endothelial cytoplasm
- Direct endothelial injury—endothelial cell necrosis and detachment
- Delayed prolonged leakage
- Leukocyte mediated endothelial injury
- Leakage from new blood vessels

Cellular events

Cellular events comprises extravasation, chemotaxis, leukocytic activation and phagocytosis.

Steps of extravasation are as follows:
1. Extravasation is the sequence of events in the journey of leukocytes from the vessel lumen to the interstitial tissue.

   a. In the vessel lumen:
      - As stasis develops, leukocytes principally neutrophils accumulate along the vascular endothelium: Migration
      - The rows of leukocytes move (tumble) slowly along the endothelium: Rolling
      - Finally coming to at rest, leukocytes adhere firmly to endothelium: Adhesion
      - The endothelium can be virtually lined by white cells: Pavementing

   b. Diapedesis
      - It is the process of transmigration of leukocytes across the endothelium.
      - After firm adhesion, leukocytes migrate through interendothelial junctions and assume a position between endothelial cells and basement membrane. Eventually, they pierce the basement membrane by secreting collagenase and escape into the extravascular space.
      - The processes of adhesion and transmigration are regulated by the binding of complimentary adhesion molecules

(selectin, integrins, members of immunoglobulins, mucin-like glyco-proteins) and endothelium.

2. Chemotaxis

After extravasation, leukocytes emigrate into tissues towards the site of injury.

3. Leukocyte activation by cytokines

Leukocytes acts as:

- Production of arachidonic acid metabolites (PG, LT) as a result of activation of phospholipase A_2.
- Degranulation and secretion of lysosomal enzymes and activation of oxidative burst.
- Secretion of cytokines.
- Modulation of leukocyte adhesion molecules, allowing a firm adhesion of activated neutrophils to endothelium.

4. Phagocytosis and release of enzymes by neutrophils and macrophages are responsible for eliminating the injurious agents.

4. Chemotaxis of leukocytes (1989, 99, 2000, 07, 11) and chemotactic factors (1991)

Definition: This is the process of leukocytes migration in tissues towards the site of injury after extravasation. (Locomotion oriented along a chemical gradient).

Chemotactic agents

- *Exogenous:* Bacterial products—peptides and lipid molecules
- *Endogenous*
  - Components of complement system like C5a.
  - Products of lipoxygenase pathway like LTB4—cytokines like IL-8 (chemokines)

Mechanism

(Diagram: Biochemical events in leukocytes activation from textbook is must for this question)

Movement

- Ligands (chemotactic agents) bind to specific receptors on leukocyte cell surface.
- Activation of phospholipase C-hydrolysis of PIP_2 into IP_3 and DAG (diacetyl glycerol)

- IP_3 acts as a messenger releasing calcium ion first from intracellular store, followed by import from outside (extracellular).
- Increased intracellular calcium level results in assembly of contractile elements (actin and myosin).
- Cell movement is thus possible.

Direction

Migration is a step-by-step process in response to one agonist after another. Movement of direction depends on type of receptors activated and chemokine gradients at that particular time and site. With stepwise movement and direction from so many chemotactic agents, leukocytes reach their destination site.

5. Role of opsonins in phagocytosis (2002) or phagocytosis (1993, 98, 2010)

Phagocytosis is defined as the leukocytic engulfment of microorganisms, foreign particles and cellular debris. Two types of phagocytic cells are polymorphs and circulating monocytes/macrophage.

Three steps

Recognition and attachment

- Typically, phagocytosis is initiated by recognition of microorganisms and particles by receptors expressed on the leukocyte surface.
- Mannose receptors and scavenger receptors are two important receptors that function to bind and ingest microbes.
- The process of coating a particle, such as microbes, to target it for phagocytosis is called opsonization and the substances that do this are called opsonins. Phagocytes express high affinity receptors for opsonins.
- Opsonization increases the efficacy of phagocytosis by macrophages, neutrophils or other cells.
- *Opsonins are*
  - Fc portion of IgG (naturally occurring antibodies against bacteria).

– C3b, C3bi (both, immune and non-immune mechanisms of phagocytosis).
– CHO-binding proteins like lecithin of plasma.
– Collectin binds with bacterial cell wall—mannose binding protein (innate immunity).
• *Leukocyte receptors that recognize bacteria* (coated with opsonins):
 – Fc-γ R of Fc portion of IgG
 – ClqR of collectins
 – Complement receptors (CR1, 2, 3)

Engulfment
The coated particles are recognized and engulfed with the formation of phagosomes. These phagosomes fuse with lysosome of phagocytes to form lysophagosomes.

Killing and degradation (*see textbook diagram*)
Oxygen dependent killing
• Cytoplasmic oxidase: They are normally present in their components form. During WBC activation they unite and translocate towards plasma membrane or phagocytic membrane. There, they catalyze

$$2O_2 + e^- \longrightarrow 2O_2^- + H^+$$

• Spontaneous dismutation:

$$2O_2^- + 2H^+ \longrightarrow H_2O_2 + O_2$$

• The quality of hydrogen peroxide produced in phagosome is insufficient to kill bacteria adequately. But neutrophils have myeloperoxidase (MPO) in their granule. This enzyme converts H_2O_2 to HOCl in presence of Cl^-.

• HOCl kills bacteria by covalent bonding with bacterial proteins or by oxidation of proteins and lipids.
• Dead microorganisms are then degraded by lysosomal hydrolase.

Oxygen independent mechanism
• Bacteriocidal permeability increasing proteins
• Lactoferrins
• Lysosomal hydrolase breaking muramic acid N-acetylglucosamine bond
• Major basic proteins of eosinophils
• Defensins

6. Morphological types of acute inflammation and their outcomes

i. Serous inflammation: It is characterized by collection of water, relatively protein poor fluid, derived from either the plasma or secretion of mesothelial cells (lining of peritoneal, pleural and pericardial cavities), seen in burn, viral infections, etc.

ii. Fibrinous inflammation:
 • This type of inflammation is characteristically present in body cavities like pericardium and pleura.
 • *Caused by severe injuries*, which results in high degree of vascular permeability leading to fibrinous exudation or due to some procoagulant stimulus like cancer cells in the interstitium.
 • *Histology*: Fibrin appears as eosinophilic meshwork of threads or amorphous coagulum.

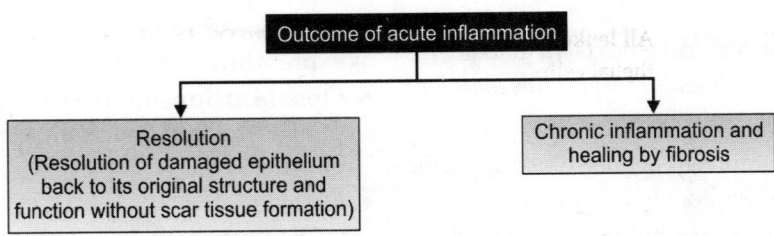

Fig. 3.1

iii. Suppurative inflammation:
  - Production of large amount of pus or purulent exudate comprising of neutrophils, necrotic cells and edema fluid.
  - Seen in association with pyogenic infection like Staphylococcus.

iv. Catarrhal (phlegmonous) inflammation
  - It is characterized by excessive production of mucus secretion.

- *Fate of fibrinous exudates*
  - *Resolution*: This fibrinous exudates may be resolved by fibrinolysis and macrophages to normal structure.
  - *Organization*: It may undergo organization to form scar tissues within the cavities. In pericardium sac, it leads either to opaque fibrous thickening of the pericardium and epicardium in the area of exudation or to the development of fibrous strands that bridge the pericardial space.

7. Chemical mediators of acute inflammation. Discuss the role of arachidonic acid metabolites as mediators of acute inflammation (1998, 2011). Role of prostaglandins in inflammation (2010)

Cell derived

Mediator	Sources	Actions
Histamin*	Mast cells, basophils and platelets	• Vasodilation • Increased permeability • Itching • Pain
Serotonin*	Platelets	Actions are like histamine, but less potent
Lysosomal enzymes*	Neutrophils and macrophages	Tissue damage
Platelet activating factor**	All leukocytes and endothelial cells	Increased vascular permeability
Leukotrienes** (slow reacting substance of anaphylaxis)	All leukocytes	LTC4, LTD4 and LTE4: • Increased vascular permeability • Smooth muscle contraction • Vasoconstriction • Bronchoconstriction LTB4: • Chemotaxis • Cell adherence
Lipoxin A4 and B4** (LXA4, LXB4)		• Chemotaxis • Vasodilation • Inhibits neutrophil • Stimulates monocyte adhesion
Prostaglandins**	All leukocytes, platelets and endothelial cells	PGD2, PGE2: • Vasodilatation • Bronchodilation • Increased vascular permeability PGF2α: • Vasodilatation • Bronchoconstriction • Platelet aggregation

(Contd.)

Cell derived (Contd.)

Mediator	Sources	Actions
		TXA2:
		• Vasoconstriction
		• Bronchoconstriction
		• Platelet aggregation
		PGI2:
		• Vasodilation
		• Bronchoconstriction
		• Inhibition of platelet aggregation
Cytokines**	Lymphocytes, macrophages and endothelial cells	• Increase in leukocyte adherence
		• Thrombosis
		• Fibroblastic proliferation
		• Acute phase reaction
		• IL8: Chemotactic for neutrophils
		• PF4: Chemotactic for neutrophils, monocytes and eosinophils
		• MCP-1: Chemotactic for monocytes
		• Eotaxin: Chemotactic for eosinophils
Nitric oxide**	Macrophages	• Vasodilation
		• Antiplatelet effect
		• Microbicidal action
Oxygen-derived free radical	Neutrophils and macrophages	• Endothelial damage
		• Increased vascular permeability

*Preformed mediators   **Newly synthesized mediation.

Plasma derived

Mediator	Sources	Actions
Fibrin split products	Clotting and fibrinolytic system	Increased vascular permeability
Kinin/bradykinin	Kinin system	Increased vascular permeability
Anaphylatoxin (C3a, C5a)	Complement system	Increased vascular permeability
C3b		
C5b–9 (membrane attack complex)		

8. Complement pathways

There are four pathways of complement system:
  i. The classical activation pathway activated by antigen/antibody immune complexes.
  ii. The mannose-binding lectin activation pathway activated by microbes with mannose terminal groups.
  iii. The alternative activating pathway activated by microbes or tumor cells.
  iv. The terminal pathway that is common to first three pathways and leads to membrane attack complex that lyse cells (*see* Fig. 3.2).

9. Role of complement in inflammation (1995, 2002)

• It contains group of 20 proteins present in greatest concentration in plasma.
• Helps in both innate and adaptive immunities.

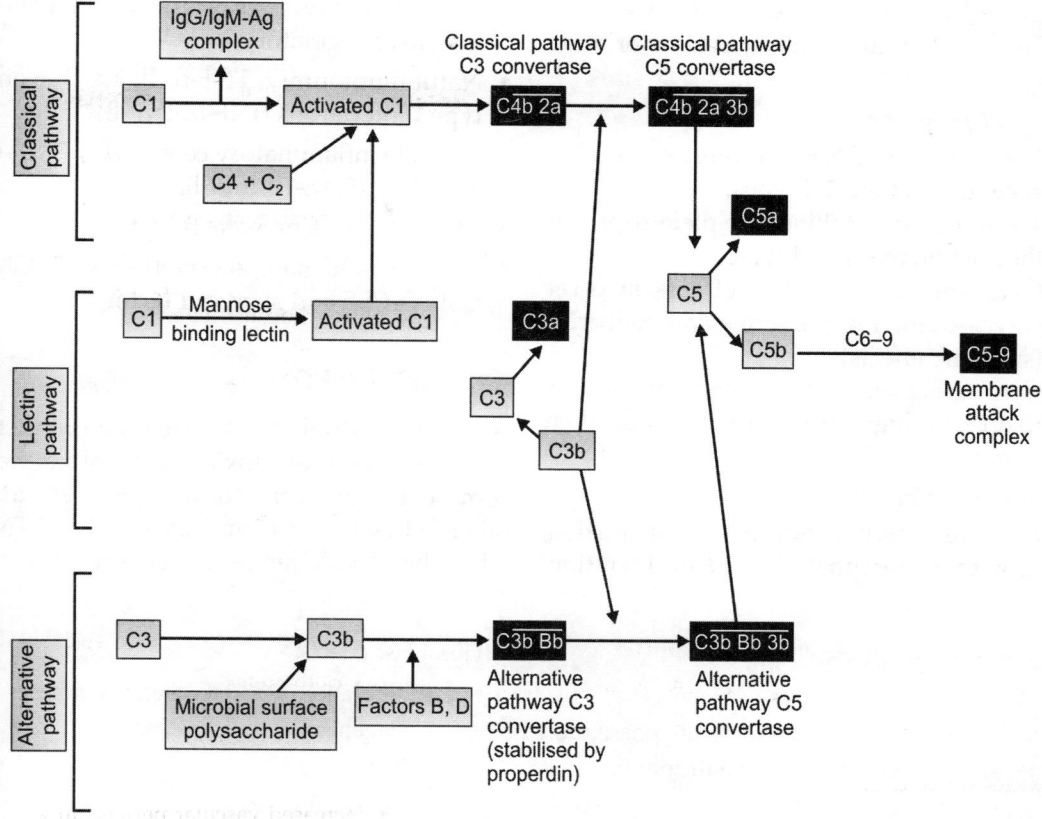

Fig. 3.2

• Formation of membrane attack complex results in lysis of cells/organisms like bacteria.

Role in acute inflammation

i. *Vascular phenomenon:* Anaphylatoxins— C3a, C5a and also C4a cause release of histamines from mast cells.

  • Increases vascular permeability and vasodilatation.

  • C5a also activates lipoxygenase pathway of arachidonic acid metabolism in neutrophils and monocytes.

ii. *Leukocyte adhesion, chemotaxis and activation:* C5a is a strong attractant for neutrophils, monocytes, eosinophils, and basophils. It also increases leukocytes adhesion to endothelium and its activation to cause movement of leukocytes.

iii. *Phagocytosis:* C3b and C3bi act as opsonin and favor phagocytosis by macrophages and neutrophils.

iv. C3 and C5 can activate several proteolytic enzymes, like plasmin, lysosomal enzymes from neutrophils present within the inflammatory exudates.

10. Coagulation pathway (*see* Chapter 11, Bleeding Disorders)

11. Lymphokines (1988, 90)

or

Cytokines (1990, 92)

Definition: Cytokines are soluble proteins; secreted by cells, primarily immune cells like macrophages, lymphocytes (other cells like endothelium, epithelium, connective tissue cells) when they are activated by some stimulus. They modulate functions of other cells.

General properties

1. Many individual cytokines are produced by several different cell types.
2. The effects of cytokines are pleiotropic, i.e. they act on many cell types.
3. Cytokines induce their effects in three ways—autocrine, paracrine and endocrine (systemic effects).
4. Cytokines mediate their effects by binding to specific high-affinity receptors on their target cells.

Summary of functions

- Regulate lymphocytic functions, activation, growth, differentiation, and proliferation:

IL-2, IL-4 (favor growth); IL-10, TFG-β (negative regulator)
- Natural immunity: TNF-α, IL-1β, IL-6 and type I interferons (INF-α, INF-β)
- Activate inflammatory cells: INF-γ, TNF-α, TNF-β, IL-5, IL-10, and IL-12
- Chemokines: Chemotactic activities
- Stimulates hematopoiesis: IL-3, IL-7, GM-CSF, G-CSF and stem cell factor

12. IL-1/TNF (1987)

A variety of stimulus like bacterial products, immune complexes, toxins physical injuries, some cytokines activate macrophages and other cells, which in turn, secrete IL-1 and TNF which have wide range of functions like:

Acute phase reactions:		Fibroblast effects:	
• Fever	• ↑ Sleep	• ↑ Proliferation	• ↑ Collagen synthesis
• ↓ Appetite	• ↑ Acute phase proteins	• ↑ Collagenase	• ↑ Protease
• Hemodynamic effects	• Neutrophilia	• ↑ PGE synthesis	

Endothelial effects:		Leukocytic effects:
• ↑ Leukocytes adherence	• ↑ PGI synthesis	• ↑ Cytokine secretions
• ↑ Procoagulant activity	• ↓ Anticoagulant activity	• Priming
• ↑ IL-1, IL-6, IL-8, PDGF		

13. Chronic inflammation: Definition and its causes

Chronic inflammation is characterized by a prolonged duration (weeks or months) in which active inflammation (mononuclear cells infiltration), tissue destruction, and attempt to repair (replacement of damaged tissues by connective tissues) are proceeding simultaneously.

Causes

- Persistent infection (TB, syphilis, delayed type hypersensitivity, etc.)
- Prolonged exposure to exogenous or endogenous toxic agents like silica, plasma lipid/fat (atherosclerosis)
- Autoimmunity, like SLE

14. Write briefly about morphological features and cells involved in chronic inflammation

Morphological features

i. Mononuclear cell infiltration (macrophages, lymphocytes and plasma cells)
   - Recruitment of monocytes from the circulation (most common)
   - Local proliferation of macrophages
   - Immobilisation of macrophages at the site of inflammation
ii. Tissue destruction due to persistent offending agents and mediators released by activated mononuclear cells.
iii. Healing and fibrosis: Attempt at healing by connective tissue replacement of

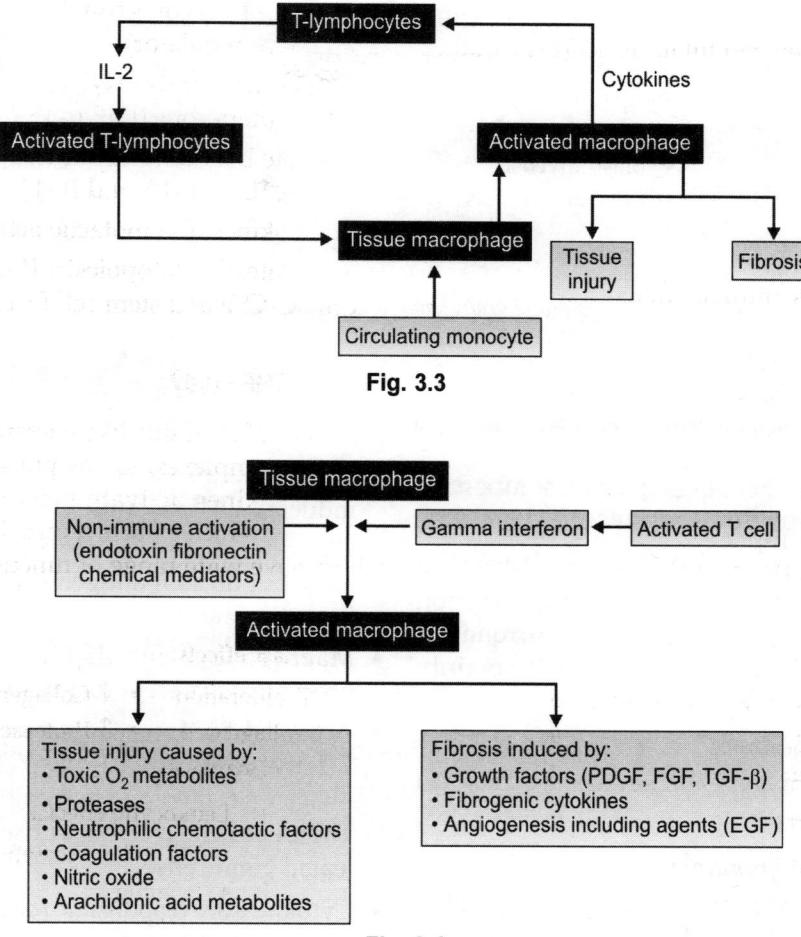

Fig. 3.3

Fig. 3.4

damaged tissue is accompanied by proliferation of new small vessels (angiogenesis) and fibrosis.

Cells involved in chronic inflammation

i. Lymphocytes: They are mobilised in the antibody mediated, cell mediated as well as non-immune inflammation (both T and B lymphocytes are involved).

ii. Macrophages: They interact with lymphocytes in chronic inflammation.

iii. Eosinophils: They are recruited from blood. Involved in IgE-mediated immune reactions and parasitic infections. Eotaxin is a chemokine for eosinophils, derived from leukocytes and epithelial cells. Major basic protein is a highly toxic protein contained in eosinophil granules and is toxic to parasites and mammalian epithelial cells.

iv. Mast cells: They are distributed in connective tissues and on degranulation they release mediators.

15. Granulomatous inflammation: Definition and its causes (1992, 95, 97, 2004, 10)

Definition: Distinctive pattern of chronic inflammatory reaction in which the predominant cell type is an activated macrophage with a modified epithelial like appearance (epithelioid). It is characterized by presence of granuloma.

Causes

Immune granuloma			
Bacteria	Fungal	Helminthic	Others
• Tuberculosis	• Histoplasma	• Schistosomiasis	• Sarcoidosis
• Leprosy	• Blastomycosis	• Trichiniasis	• Crohn's disease
• Brucellosis	• Coccidiomycosis	• Filariasis	• Wegener's
• Syphilis			granulomatosis
• Salmonellosis			• RA

Non-immune granuloma/foreign body granuloma
• Silica granulomatosis
• Foreign body type pneumonia

Caseating granuloma is seen in TB, histoplasma, syphilis and coccidiomycosis.

16. Describe the development of tubercular and foreign body granuloma (1994, 95).

Definition (granuloma): This is a focal area of inflammation having microscopic aggregation of macrophages, epithelioid cells surrounded by a collar of mononuclear WBC mainly lymphocytes and plasma cells.

Types of granuloma
• Foreign body type/non-immune granuloma
• Immune type

Foreign body granuloma
• It does not require antigen specific lymphocytes.
• Incited by relatively inert foreign bodies like talc as in intravenous drug abusers or sutures/other fibers.
• These are large enough to preclude phagocytosis by a single macrophage.
• They do not incite either immune reaction or inflammatory reaction.
• This sequence leads to formation of epithelioid cells and giant cells, which are apposed to the surface and encompass the foreign bodies.
• These foreign bodies can be identified in the center of granuloma with polarized light, as these are refractile in nature.

Immune granuloma
• It is due to lymphocytic-mediated response to an antigen.

• Incited by insoluble particles capable of inducing CMI response.
• CMI does not necessarily produce a granuloma but do so if antigen is less soluble or is particulate.
• Macrophages engulf foreign material, process and present to T helper cells.
• Activated T helper cells secrete cytokines IL-2 (activation of other T cells), TFN-γ (macrophages get converted into epithelioid cells). These epithelioid cells give rise to multinucleated giant cells.
• Cytokines are responsible for the formation and maintenance of granuloma.
• Example: TB: Non-caseating tubercle (granuloma prototypes): A focus of epithelioid cells are rimmed by fibroblasts, lymphocytes, histiocytes, and Langhans' giant cells.

Caseating tubercle: Central amorphous granular debris, no cellular details is seen, AFB is seen.

17. Write briefly about epithelioid cells, Langhans' giant cells and foreign body giant cells

Epithelioid cells: They are epithelial like appearing cells that are transformed from macrophages under the influence of cytokine TNF-γ.

Langhans' giant cells: They arise from the fusion of epithelioid cells in response to cytokines during chronic inflammation. They contain 3–5 nuclei arranged peripherally (horseshoe) in the cytoplasm.

Foreign body giant cells: These giant cells are derived either from Langhans' giant cells or directly from the fusion of macrophages. The contain 10–100 nuclei arranged haphazardly in the cytoplasm.

18. Difference between epithelioid and epithelial cells

S. No.	Traits	Epithelioid cell	Epithelial cell
1.	Origin	Macrophage	Epithelial derivative
2.	Cytoplasm	Pale, pink, granular and abundant	No granularity, less abundant
3.	Cell boundaries	Indistinct, seems to merge with each other	Distinct
4.	Nucleus	Oval or elongated Nuclear membrane folding present	Round Nuclear membrane folding absent
5.	Location	Present at the center of granuloma, a chronic inflammation	Lining of body cavities, skin and mucous membranes
6.	Function	Phagocytic activity, secrete lysosomal enzymes	Protection to underlying structures, secretion like sweat, sebum, etc.

19. Difference between tumor giant cell and Langhans' giant cell

S. No.	Traits	Tumor giant cell	Langhans' giant cell
1.	Origin	Anaplastic tumor cells—dividing nuclei of neoplastic cells	Fusion of epithelioid cells in response of some chromic inflammation
2.	Number of nucleus	Prominent nuclei—either single huge polymorphic nucleus or may have two or more nuclei	20 or more small nuclei—either around the periphery in horseshoe/ring form or clustered at two poles
3.	Character of nucleus	Nucleus hyperchromatic	Normal appearing nucleus, same as macrophage and epithelioid cells
4.	Size of nucleus	Large in relation to cells	Normal
5.	Associated features	Other features of malignancy	Absent

20. Kinin system (1998)

21. Interferon (1998)

22. Mechanism of fever

(*Refer to textbook*)

4

Hemodynamic Disorders, Thrombosis and Shock

1. Causes of edema or classification of edema (1996, 98, 2000)

Edema is defined as an abnormal and excessive accumulation of fluid in the interstitial tissue spaces. Edema fluid may be transudate or exudate.

Increased hydrostatic pressure	Reduced plasma osmotic pressure (hypoproteinemia)	Lymphatic obstruction

• Congestive heart failure
• Constrictive pericarditis
• Ascites/liver cirrhosis
• Venous obstruction/ compression
  – Thrombosis
  – External pressure
  – Lower extremity inactivity with prolonged dependency
• Arteriolar dilation
  – Heat
  – Neurohumoral dysregulation
	• Protein losing glomerulopathies (nephrotic syndrome)
	• Liver cirrhosis
	• Malnutrition (Kwashiorkor)
	• Protein losing gastroenteropathies
	Inflammation
	• Acute inflammation
	• Chronic inflammation
	• Angiogenesis
		• Inflammation
		• Neoplasm
		• Post-surgical
		• Post-irradiation
		
		Sodium retention
		• Excessive salt intake with renal insufficiency
		• Excessive tubular reabsorption
		  – Renal hypoperfusion
		  – Increased renin angiotensin aldosterone secretion

2. Difference between cardiac and renal failure edema (1993, 99)

S. No.	Traits	Cardiac edema	Renal edema
1.	Causes	CHF and right-sided heart failure	Nephrotic syndrome, nephritic syndrome and acute tubular injury
2.	Mechanism	Decreased cardiac output: Hypovolemia and resultant Na$^+$ and	Hypoalbuminemia and decreased plasma osmotic pressure in nephrotic

(Contd.)

Difference between cardiac and renal failure edema (Contd.)

S. No.	Traits	Cardiac edema	Renal edema
		water retention-back pressure hypothesis [increased venous and capillaries pressure and transudation], forward pressure hypothesis [chronic hypoxia: Increased capillary permeability]	syndrome; Na+ and water retention in nephritic syndrome (main), also plasma protein decreased
3.	Clinical features	Gravity dependent edema; changes with posture: Pedal or sacral	First around face, eyes, ankle and genitalia and then generalized
4.	Serum albumin	Normal	Decreased
5.	Protein in urine	Absent	Present

3. Difference between transudate and exudate (1994, 97, 2001, 03, 04, 08, 11)

S. No.	Traits	Transudate	Exudate
1.	Definition	It is ultrafiltrate of plasma that crosses the blood vessel without any change in vascular permeability	In response to inflammation, fluids come out of blood vessel due to change in vascular permeability
2.	Protein contents and coagulation tendency	Low (<3 g/dl), mainly albumin, low in fibrin contents so no tendency for coagulation	High (>3 g/dl). Due to high concentration of fibrinogen and other coagulation factors, coagulation tendency is present
3.	Glucose concentration	Same as blood	Low in case of association with neoplasm and infection
4.	pH	>7.3; more alkaline	<7.3; less alkaline
5.	Specific gravity	Low, <1.012	High, >1.020
6.	LDH (fluid: Serum LDH)	Low (<0.6)	High (>0.6)
7.	Microscopic features	Few cells consisting of mesothelial cells and cellular debris	Many cells—inflammatory cells and parenchymal cells
8.	Condition association/ examples	Hydrodynamic derangement; non-inflammatory; congestive heart failure	Inflammatory edema; pus (purulent exudates)

4. Sequence of events leading to cardiac (1998, 2003) and renal edema (1993, 96, 2004, 08, 09)

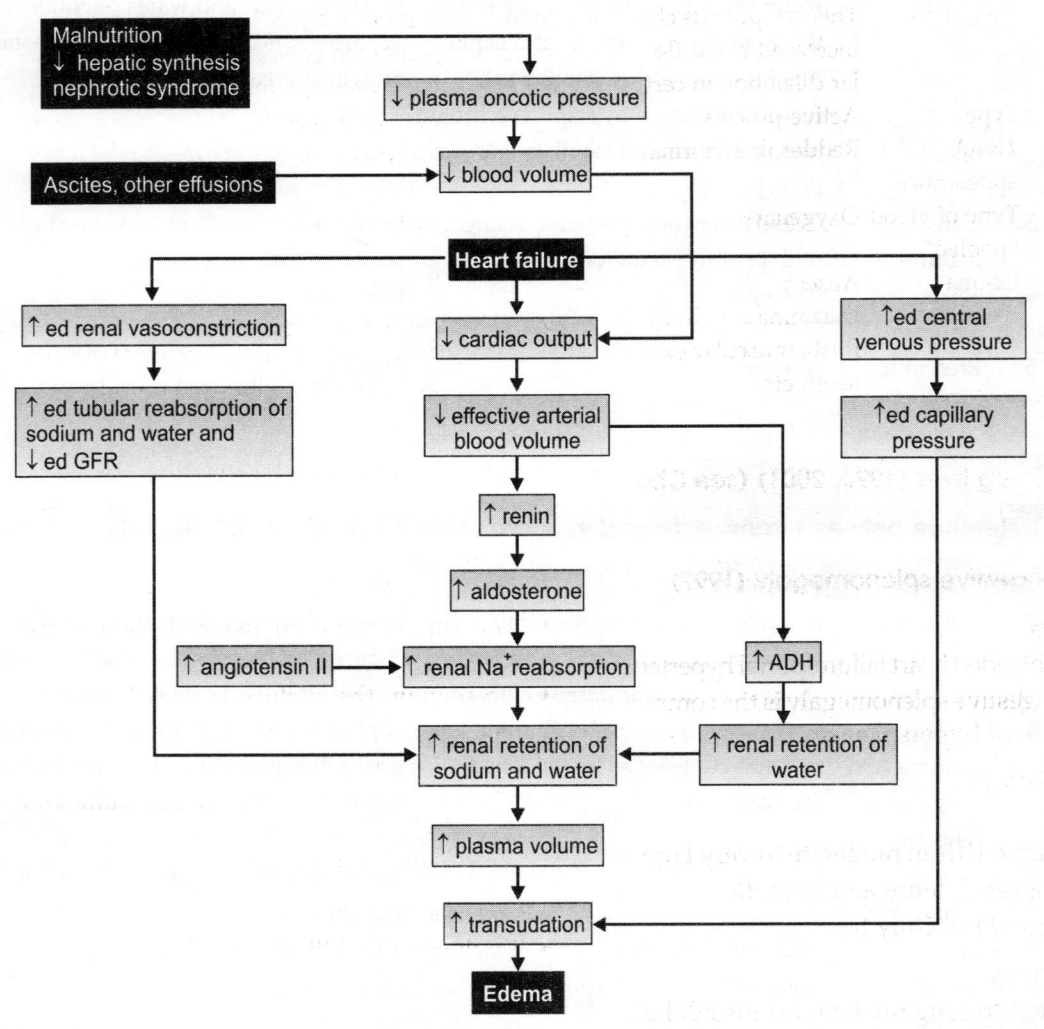

Fig. 4.1

Renal Edema

- Renal edema is seen in nephrotic syndrome glomerulonephritis and acute tubular injury, all of which are characterized by persistent and heavy proteinuria causing a reduced plasma oncotic pressure leading to generalized severe edema.
- Also, reduction in plasma volume causes activation of the renin–angiotensin aldosterone mechanism, thereby causing retention of sodium and water.
- Nephritic edema is due to the excessive reabsorption of sodium and water in renal tubule and is milder as compared to nephrotic edema.
- In acute tubular necrosis, tubules lose their capacity for selective renal concentration of the glomerular filtrate resulting in increased reabsorption and oliguria.

5. Difference between hyperemia and congestion

S. No.	Traits	Hyperemia	Congestion
1.	Definition	This is a process characterized by increased blood flow due to arteriolar dilatation in certain conditions	A process characterized by blood pooling in vessels due to impaired out flow/drainage from tissue
2.	Type	Active process	Passive process
3.	Tissue appearance	Redder than normal	Blue-red colored/cyanosed
4.	Type of blood "pooled"	Oxygenated	Deoxygenated; tissue hypoxia present
5.	Edema	Absent	Present
6.	Examples	Inflammation, blushing, menopausal flush, muscular exercise, high grade fever, etc.	Local venous congestion like portal venous obstruction in cirrhosis of liver. Systemic like right-sided heart failure

6. Nutmeg liver (1993, 2001) (see Chapter 7, Liver)

7. Congestive splenomegaly (1997)

Causes

Right-sided heart failure, portal hypertension. Congestive splenomegaly is the commonest cause of hypersplenism.

Morphology

Gross

Enlarged, from moderate to very large size
Congested, tense and cyanotic
Cut surface: Gray tan

Microscopy

Red pulp congestion and sinusoidal dilatation, area of hemorrhage
Gamna-Gandy bodies or sideroblastic nodule from organization of hemorrhage

8. Brown indurations of lung (1997) or heart failure cell

or

Chronic venous congestion (CVC) of lung

This condition is associated with long standing venous congestion due to left-sided heart failure (e.g. rheumatic mitral stenosis). It results in increased pulmonary venous pressure.

Morphology

Gross

- The lungs are firm in consistency and heavy.
- On section, the surface is dark brown in color as *brown indurations of lung*.
- Frothy, blood-tinged fluid containing mixture of air, and edematous fluid and extravasated blood/hemoglobin pigment is seen oozing out on section.

Microscopic features

- Thickening and fibrosis of alveolar septa
- Interstitial edema
- Dilatation and congestion of capillaries
- Intra-alveolar hemorrhage due to rupture of congested capillaries
- *Heart failure cells*: RBC breakdown produces hemosiderin pigments which is taken by alveolar macrophages. These hemosiderin laden machrophages are known as heart failure cells or siderophages. They are persent in alveolar lumen.

Complications

- Impaired gaseous exchange
- Predisposition to infections like pneumonia

9. Thrombus: Definition, its morphology and etiopathogenesis (1993, 99, 2002)

Definition: Thrombosis is a physiological or pathological process of forming solid plug or mass in the blood vessels from clotting factors and other components present in the blood.

Morphology: (*see difference tables* Q. 11 and 14)

Mechanism of pathological thrombosis

Relation of etiological factors resulting in pathological thrombosis is best explained by Virchow's triangle.

a. *Endothelial injury*

b. *Abnormal blood flow*: Stasis and turbulent blood flow results in:

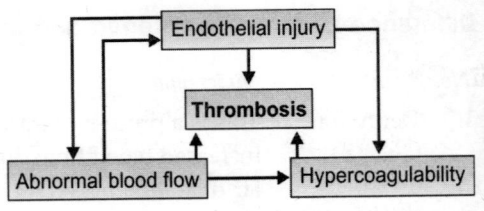

Fig. 4.2

- Disruption of laminar blood flow and platelets come in contact with endothelium
- Prevent dilution of activated clotting factors by fresh flowing blood
- Decrease the inflow of clotting factor inhibitors
- Promote endothelial cell activation

c. *Hypercoagulable state/thrombophilia* (*see* table below)

Primary/genetic thrombophilia	Secondary/acquired thrombophilia	
	High risk for thrombosis	**Low risk for thrombosis**
• Mutation in factor V	• Immobilization/prolonged bed rest	• Atrial fibrillation
• Deficiency of antithrombin III	• MI	• Cardiomyopathy
• Deficiency of protein C or S	• Tissue damage (fracture, burns, surgery)	• Nephrotic syndrome
• Defect in fibrinolytic system	• Cancer	• Hyperestrogenic states like oral contraceptive use
• Homocysteinemia	• Prosthetic cardiac valves	• Sickle cell anemia
• Allelic variation in prothrombin levels	• DIC	• Smoking
	• Heparin induced thrombocytopenia	
	• Lupus anticoagulant syndrome	

10. Role of endothelial injury in thrombosis (2000)

- Normal vascular epithelium has antiplatelet, anticoagulant, and fibrinolytic activity to prevent abnormal thrombus formation (antithrombotic).
- On the other hand, if injured, it exerts pro-coagulant action to maintain hemodynamic stability.

Antithrombotic properties

Under most circumstances, endothelial cell maintain fluidity of blood:

i. Antiplatelet effects
   - Intact endothelium prevents contact of platelets to highly thrombogenic sub endothelial ECM (collagen).
   - Endothelium secretes PGI_2 and NO (nitric oxide), both are inhibitors of platelet aggregation.

- Endothelial cells have ADPase that degrade ADP, a potent stimulator of platelets.

ii. Anticoagulant effects
- Endothelium has membrane-bound heparin-like molecule that binds with antithrombin III and inactivates factor II (thrombin, IX, X, XI, XII).
- Endothelium also produces thrombomodulin that binds to thrombin converting it from a procoagulant to anticoagulant capable of activating protein C. Protein C with the help of protein S as a cofactor, causes proteolytic cleavage of V and VIII.
- Endothelium produces tissue factor pathway inhibitor that inactivates tissue factors—factors VII and X.

iii. Fibrinolytic effect
- Endothelial cells synthesize tissue-type plasminogen activator (t-PA) that converts plasminogen to plasmin and plasmin then dissolves clot by breaking fibrin.

Prothrombotic Properties

After injury to endothelium, it becomes prothrombotic by following effects:

i. Platelet effect
- Endothelial cell injury exposes highly thrombogenic subendothelial ECM, which allows platelets to adhere to the collagen of ECM.
- This effect is due to increased production of von Willebrand factor by endothelium, an essential cofactor for platelet binding to collagen.

ii. Procoagulant effect
- Endothelial cells synthetize tissue factors (factors that activate extrinsic pathway of coagulation).

iii. Antifibrinolytic effect
- Endothelial cells secrete inhibitors of plasminogen activators (PAI) that inhibit the action of plasminogen activator → plasmin is not produced from plasminogen → No fibrinolysis.

11. Difference between antemortem thrombus and postmortem thrombus (clot) (1989, 95, 98, 2009)

S. No.	Traits	Antemortem (thrombus)	Postmortem (clot)
1.	Cause/ mechanism	In response to normal hemostatic maintenance, sometimes pathological process involves clotting pathway in living person.	In dead person—sedimentation and settling down of blood components due to gravity
2.	Gross	Dry, granular, firm, and friable. Lines of Zahn—alternate dark gray layers of platelets interspersed with lighter layers of fibrin are prominent in arterial thrombi.	Gelatinous, soft and rubbery. Two layers—currant jelly dark red appearance in the red cell rich lower and a chicken fat appearance in cell—poor upper layers
3.	Shape	May or may not fit their vascular contours	Takes the shape of vessels or its bifurcation
4.	Attachment to vessel wall	Present, strong	Very weak
5.	Location	Anywhere in the body	In dependent part in relation to the body kept after death

12. Fate of the thrombus (1986, 87, 93, 95, 99, 2007, 11)

or

Evolution of thrombus (2000, 01)

- Thrombus produces significant sign and symptoms, which may be localized to a particular organ, or it has a wide range of effects. The survived patients, after the vascular occlusion have one or a combination of changes in the thrombus in days to weeks.
- *Propagation:* More platelets can accumulate at the site of thrombus, which then capture more fibrin to form progressive enlarging thrombus.
- *Embolization:* Whole or a part of the thrombi may dislodge and may act as emboli. This is more common in case of venous thrombosis.

- *Dissolution:* Fibrinolytic activity may lyse the thrombus and remove it. This is effective in recent formed thrombus, older thrombi are resistant to lysis by t-PA, streptokinase (given therapeutically) due to extensive fibrin polymerization.
- *Organization and recanalization:* There is in-growth of endothelial cells, smooth muscle cells, and fibroblasts to form fibrin rich thrombus organization. With passage of time capillary channels may be formed which create conduits from one end to other end of thrombus, thus re-establishing blood flow to some extent.
- In some large thrombus (in aneurysm) instead of organization, the central part may undergo *enzymatic degradation*, which may be infected by bacteria (e.g. mycotic aneurysm).

13. Venous thrombosis/phlebothrombosis

14. Difference between arterial thrombosis and venous (red) thrombosis/phlebothrombosis (1992)

S. No.	Traits	Arterial thrombosis	Venous thrombosis
1.	Sites	Common in coronary, cerebral, iliac and femoral arteries; active blood flow	Superficial varicose veins, popliteal, deep veins of leg, femoral, iliac veins. Less active blood flow
2.	Pathogenesis	Endothelial injury (like atherosclerosis) or turbulent blood flow (at vessel bifurcation)	Due to venous stasis
3.	Progressions	Grow in a retrograde direction from point of attachment	Extend in the direction of blood flow
4.	Occlusion	Do not occlude lumen completely	Occlude completely
5.	Gross	Gray-white, friable, prominent lines of Zahn	Dark-red with fibrin strands, lines of Zahn less prominent or absent
6.	Microscopic	Distinct features of lines of Zahn	Not so distinct features of lines of Zahn, more of RBC and less fibrin
7.	Complications	Ischemia—infarction of brain, heart, etc.	Thromboembolism, edema, skin ulcer, etc.

15. Types of emboli (1993)

- *According to state of emboli*
  - *Solid:* Thromboemboli and atheromatous materials
  - *Liquid:* Fat and amniotic fluid emboli
  - *Gaseous:* Decompression sickness—air emboli (1999)
- *According to site of origin*
  - Cardiac emboli (left side of heart)

- Arterial emboli
- Venous emboli
- Lymphatic emboli
- *According to infectivity*
  - Sterile/bland emboli
  - Septic emboli
- *According to route followed*
  - *Paradoxical emboli/crossed emboli:* In this condition, an embolus crosses from venous circulation to arterial circulation or vice versa. Deep leg vein emboli cross to pulmonary circulation and then to systemic arterial circulation.
  - *Retrograde emboli:* Travel against the direction of blood flow.

16. Pulmonary embolism etiopathogenesis and complications (1993, 97, 2011)

This disease is one of the most common problems encountered in hospitalized patients or bed-ridden patients. It is a fatal form of thromboembolism causing occlusion of pulmonary artery and its branches.

Sources
- Thrombi from large veins of lower legs like deep vein thrombosis—most common
- Thrombi from superficial veins of leg, pelvi—less common

Pathogenesis
- Thrombus as a whole or its loosely attached tail gets detached from its origin and is carried through venous channel to right side of the heart. It enters into pulmonary circulation.
- If thrombus is large enough, it is impacted at the bifurcation of main pulmonary artery (saddle embolus) or it may even lodge in right ventricle or its outflow tract.
- Multiple, small emboli occlude smaller pulmonary vessels.
- Emboli may pass through atrial or ventricular septal defects from right side to left side of the heart to enter into arterial

circulation (paradoxical emboli) (1993, 98, 2003).

Effects of complications
- Most emboli are asymptomatic/silent and may undergo resolution.
- *Sudden death* due to right side heart failure (cor pulmonale) or cardiovascular collapse
- *Pulmonary hemorrhage* due to obstruction of terminal branches of pulmonary artery
- *Pulmonary infarction:* Obstruction of end—arteriolar pulmonary branches
- *Pulmonary hypertension* with right-sided heart failure (multiple emboli)
- Hypoxia due to impaired alveolar gas exchange

17. Fat embolism (1999)

Fat embolism results in obstruction of arterioles and capillaries by fat globules.

Causes
- Trauma to long bones—most common
- Extensive burn
- Pancreatitis
- Trauma of soft tissues
- Diabetes mellitus

Pathogenesis
- *Mechanical obstruction:* Natural fat globules occlude pulmonary or cerebral microvasculature causing platelet and RBC aggregation, thus hypoxia of that tissues/organs.
- *Biochemical injury:* Fat globules are broken down into free fatty acids causing local toxic injury to endothelium. Platelet activation and recruitment of granulocytes follow it, producing free radicals, protease and eicosanoids, thus causing vascular damage.

Clinical features
- Appears within 1–3 days of trauma
- Tachypnea, dyspnea and tachycardia (pulmonary insufficiency)
- Irritability, restlessness, delirium and coma (neurological)

- Diffuse petechial rash in non-dependent area
- Thrombocytopenia as a platelet—fat globule complex is cleared from the circulation
- Anemia due to erythrocytes aggregates and microangiopathic hemolysis

Laboratory finding
- Thrombocytopenia
- Anemia
- Hypocalcemia
- Hypoalbuminemia
- Fat microglobulinemia (not macroglobulinemia)
- Fat globules in urine
- Increased erythrocyte sedimentation rate (ESR)

18. Amniotic fluid embolism (1995, 96, 2007)

This is a grave, unpredictable and almost unpreventable cause of maternal death during labor and immediate postpartum period.
Occurrence: 1 in 50,000 deliveries
Pathogenesis: Infusion of amniotic fluids with all its contents into maternal circulation due to tear in placental membrane and rupture of uterine vessels. Actually amniotic fluid embolism is a misnomer as it is a 'hypersensitivity reaction' rather than typical embolism. Even a very small amount of amniotic fluid, that will be insignificant to cause emboli will lead to catastrophic response owing to hypersensitivity reaction to foreign particles.

Microscopic features
- Pulmonary microcirculation shows fetal skin squamous cell epithelium, lanugo hair, fat from vernix caseosa, mucin from fetal respiratory tract or GIT
- Pulmonary edema
- Diffuse alveolar damage
- Hemorrhage

Clinical findings
- Sudden respiratory distress and dyspnea

- Deep cyanosis
- Hypotensive shock
- Seizures
- Coma
- Death may occur

Causes of death
- Mechanical blockage of pulmonary circulation
- DIC
- Anaphylactic reaction to amniotic fluid
- Hemorrhage

19. Write briefly on caisson disease (decompression sickness)

Air bubble in the circulation can obstruct vascular flow and causes ischemic injury.

Pathogenesis
- Decompression sickness occurs in individuals exposed to sudden changes in atmospheric pressure, e.g. scuba and deep sea divers.
- When air is breathed at high pressure, large amount of gas particularly nitrogen, dissolves in blood and tissues.
- If the diver rapidly ascents from water (depressurizes), the nitrogen bubbles come out of tissue to blood and form gas emboli. These bubbles lodge in the blood vessels of muscles and joints causing bends, edema and hemorrhage in lungs causing respiratory distress or chokes.

20. Red infarct (2002)

21. Difference between red/hemorrhagic and white/pale/anemic infarct (1997, 2000)

An infarct is an area of ischemic necrosis caused by occlusion of arterial supply or venous drainage in a particular tissue.

Almost all infarcts are due to thromboembolic events and almost all results from arterial occlusion (*see* next page).

S. No.	Traits	Red infarct	White infarct
1.	Organs	Mostly in spongy organs like lung and gastrointestinal tract	In solid organs like heart, spleen and kidney
2.	Cause	a. Venous occlusion b. Arterial occlusion—in loose tissues that allow collection of blood (lung) or that has dual blood supply (lung and GIT)—hemorrhage into infarct from non-obstructed vessels	Arterial obstruction or solid organ that limits size of hemorrhage in necrotic area
3.	Size of hemorrhage	Large area	Small area
4.	Changes	Congested, red due to large hemorrhage; turns brown, firm with time, but nerve pale. Hemosiderin laden macrophages are present in large numbers	Small amount of hemoglobin present, is degraded into hemosiderin; it progressively becomes paler
5.	Margins	Not sharply defined hemorrhagic margins	Sharply defined
6.	Edema	Present in the organ	Absent

22. Renal infarct (see also above difference table white infarct)

Morphology

Gross

- Often multiple
- May be bilateral
- Pale infarct
- Wedge-shaped—base resting under the capsule and the apex towards medulla
- A narrow rim of preserved renal tissue under the capsule is spared due to its blood supply from capsular vessels.

Microscopic features

- Affected area shows coagulative necrosis due to hypoxia.

23. Difference between cardiac shock and septic shock (2004)

Type	Reason/cause	Mechanism
Hypovolemic	• Severe hemorrhage either external or internal • Fluid loss as vomiting, diarrhea, burns, trauma	• Decreased plasma/blood volume in the circulatory compartment
Cardiogenic	• MI • Ventricular rupture • Arrhythmia • Cardiac tamponade • Pulmonary embolism	• Myocardium fails to pump adequate amount of blood due to intrinsic damage to muscle or extrinsic pressure on it or obstruction to flow in the vessel
Septic	• Microbial infection • Endotoxin (gram-negative) • Gram-positive septicemia • Fungal sepsis • Super antigens like TSST	• Peripheral vasodilatation and pooling • Endothelial activation and injury • WBC induced damage • DIC • Activation of cytokine cascades
Neurogenic	• Anesthetic accident • Spinal injury • Severe pain	• Vasodilatation and peripheral pooling of blood
Anaphylactic	• Type I hypersensitivity (like penicillin)	• Systemic vasodilatation and increased vascular permeability

24. Types of shock and their examples (1998, 2000)

25. Pathogenesis of hypovolemic shock (2001)

26. Etiopathogenesis of shock (2008)

27. Septic shock (1996, 98, 2000, 07, 09, 11)

- This is a kind of severe bacterial infection of blood resulting in hemodynamic instability, hemostatic derangements and malfunctions of various organ system.

- Currently septic shock is most frequently triggered by gram-positive bacterial infections, followed by gram-negative bacteria and fungi.

Pathology of septic shock

- There is systemic vasodilation, pooling of blood in periphery resulting in decreased tissue perfusion despite increase in cardiac output. Prolonged tissue hypoxia causes multiorgan dysfunction.

- Hemostatic mechanism is impaired resulting in hypercoagulable state followed by DIC and bleeding.

Pathogenesis

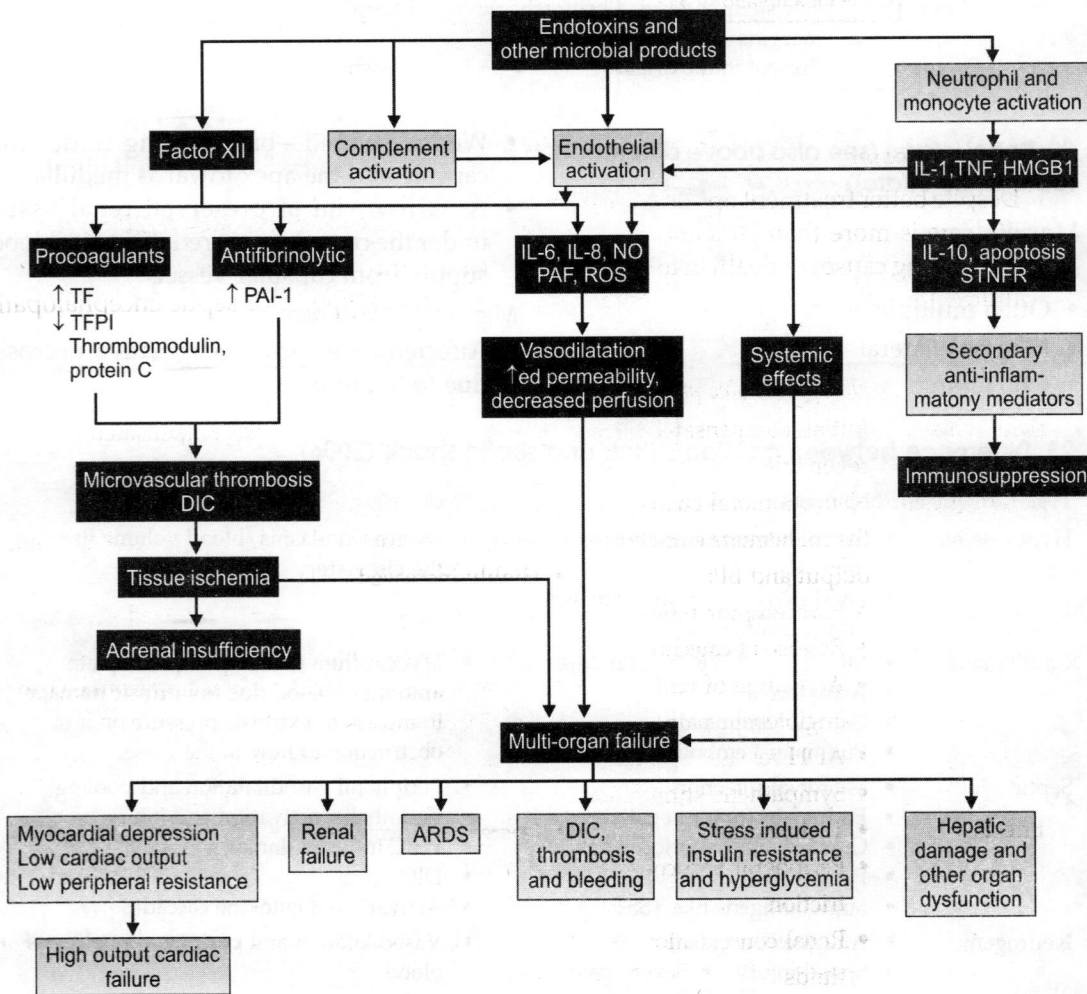

Fig. 4.3: Pathogenesis of septic shock

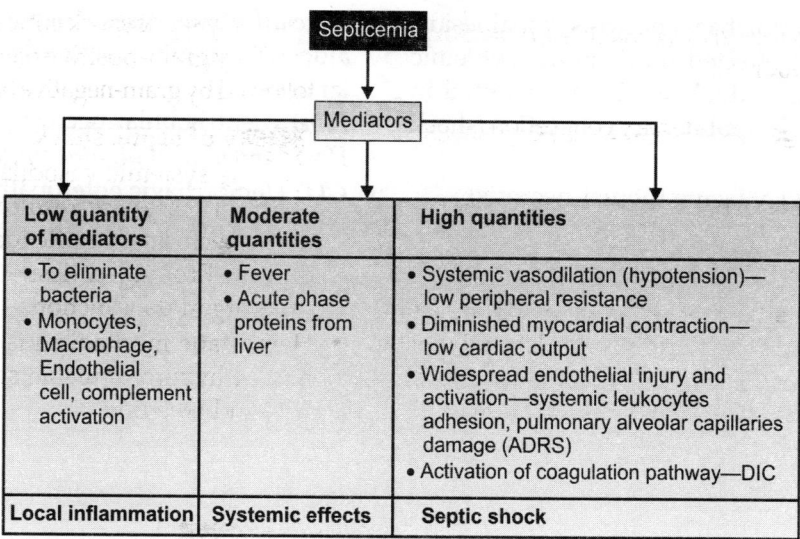

Fig. 4.4

Clinical outcome

- Despite better treatment options, the mortality rate is more than 20% and it is one of the leading causes of death in intensive care unit.

28. Stages of shock

29. Stages of septic shock (2004)

Complications of shock

- **Brain:** Hypoxic or septic encephalopathy

	Non-progressive phase	*Progressive phase*	*Irreversible phase*
Synonyms	Initial/compensated reversible	Progressive decompensated	Decompensated
Pathogenesis	Neurohumoral change for the maintenance of cardiac output and BP: • Baroreceptor reflex • Release of catecholamines • Activation of renin–angiotensin pathway • ADH release • Sympathetic stimulation	• Decreased intracellular aerobic respiration • Highly increased anaerobic glycolysis • Lactic acidosis • Decreased pH • Decreased vasomotor reflex	• Ischemia: Cardiac, brain, renal, bowel and other organs • Decreased myocardial contractility • Bacteria from GIT to circulation—septic shock • Lysosomal enzyme release
Effects	• Tachycardia • Peripheral vasoconstriction • Renal conservation of fluids	• Decreased in cardiac output • DIC • Mental confusion • Decreased urine output	• Hypotension • Weak rapid pulse • Tachypnea • Cool-clammy*, cyanotic skin

*Due to vasodilatation skin is warm in septic shock.

- *Heart:* Hemorrhage, necrosis, zonal lesion
- *Lung:* Not affected much in hypovolemic shock due to dual supply, but affected in septic shock—pulmonary congestion (shock lung).
- *Kidney:* ATN (acute tubular necrosis)
- *Adrenal gland:* Stress response to secrete aldosterone, glucocorticoids and catecholamines.
- *Liver:* Centrilobular necrosis
- *Heart and almost all other organs:* Ischemia
- *GIT:* Hemorrhagic enteropathy

5

Genetic Disorders

1. Fluorescence *in situ* hybridization (FISH)

- This is a method of visualizing or identifying the chromosome or its parts by the use of specific probes that bind to specific DNA sequence (which is its complementary) of a particular chromosome.
- It is more useful than traditional karyotyping as cells even in interphase can be visualized; even those cells that are not dividing and cannot be induced to divide can be mapped.
- The probes are attached with fluorescent dyes and are visualized under fluorescent microscope.

- *Applications*
  - Karyotyping of cells/chromosomes in interphase
  - Using a specific complementary DNA sequence, one can look for specific region on a chromosome.
  - Detection of microdeletions and complex translocations that are not readily visualized by karyotyping.
  - Mapping/localization of newly isolated genes of clinical importance
  - *Chromosome painting:* Whole part of the chromosome can be visualized using different fluorescent dyes.
  - *Spectral karyotyping:* Using computer generated signals, despite limited

number of fluorescent dyes, all chromosomes (entire human genome) can be "painted" and visualized simultaneously.

2. Down syndrome (1990, 92, 93, 94, 95, 97, 99, 2003, 07, 08, 10)

- *Incidence:* 1 in 700 live births
- *Genetic abnormalities:* The child gets an extra-somatic chromosome; the child has total of 47 chromosomes instead of 46 chromosomes.
  - Most common and important—trisomy of the chromosome 21 (47, XX; +21)
  - Extra chromosome as robertsonian translocation of the long arm of chromosome 21 to another acrocentric chromosome like 22 or 14 [46, XX/XY; der(14; 21) (q10; q10); + 21]
  - Least common—*mosaic pattern* having some cells with 46 chromosomes and some with 47 chromosomes due to mitotic non-disjunction of chromosome 21 during early stage of embryogenesis (46, XX/XY and 47, XX/XY; + 21).
- Trisomy of the chromosome 21 is influenced by mother's age—after 30 yr of maternal age chance increases much (1 in 1,550 live births at 20 yr maternal age to 1 in 25 over 45 yr).

– The extra chromosome is derived from non-disjunction of chromosome 21 during 1st meiotic division in ovum (95%; only in 5% cases from father).

Clinical features

The extragenetic material causes the physical and cognitive delays.

General	Limbs	Other congenital anomalies
• Neonatal hypotonia • Mental retardation (IQ = 25–40) • Short stature	• Fifth finger clinodactyly • Single palmar crease (simian crease) • Wide gap between first and second toes	• Intestinal (duodenal) stenosis • Umbilical hernia • Anal atresia
Craniofacial deformity	*Congenital heart defects (40%)*	*Increased incidence of leukemia (1%)*
• Mongolism/Mongolian idiocy with flat facial profile, epicanthic folds, oblique palpebral fissure • Brachycephaly • Protruding tongue • Small ears • Strabismus/Nystagmus • Brushfield spots in iris • Abundant neck skin	• Atrial septal defect • Endocardial cushion defect • Atrioventricular malformation • Ventricular septal defect (major cause of death in early life)	Neuropathological (like Alzheimer's disease) changes after the age of 40 Abnormal immune response (serious infection) and autoimmune diseases

3. Klinefelter's syndrome (1986, 88, 89, 91, 97, 2001, 09, 11)

- It is characterized by male hypogonadism due to presence of two or more X chromosomes and one or more Y chromosomes.
- *Incidence:* 1 in 850 live male births.
- *Genetic abnormalities*
  - Classical type 47, XXY karyotype (82% cases)
  - Other variants: 46, XY/47, XXY; 47, XXY/48, XXXY; may have more number of X chromosomes.
  - Maternal non-disjunction is slightly more common than paternal non-disjunction of sex chromosomes; increases with increase in parental age.

Pathogenesis

- Addition of more than one extra X or Y chromosomes to a male karyotype results in variable physical and cognitive abnormalities.

In general, extent of phenotypic abnormalities, expressive and receptive language and coordination as well as mental retardation is directly related to the number of supernumerary X chromosomes.

Clinical features

- *Sex:* Because of an additional X chromosome on an XY background, this condition is seen in males only.

- *Age:* Most males born with this syndrome go through life without being diagnosed. Diagnosis, when made, usually occurs in adulthood. The most common indication for karyotyping is hypogonadism and infertility.

- *Growth:* Infants and children have normal heights, weights and head circumferences. About 25% have clinodactyly. Affected individuals usually have disproportionately long arms and legs.

- *Sexual characteristics:* Patients lack secondary sexual characteristics because of a decrease in androgen production. This results in sparse facial/body/sexual hair, a high pitched voice. They have "eunuchoid body habitus" with long legs having increased length between the soles and the pubic bone. Gynecomastia and testicular atrophy/dysgenesis are present.
- One of the most common causes of male infertility
- *Central nervous system:* Most have normal intelligence, but mean IQ lower than normal
- *Cardiac and circulatory problems:* Mitral valve prolapsed occurs in 55% patients. Varicose veins occur in 20–40% patients. The prevalence of venous ulcers is 10–20 times higher, risk of deep vein thrombosis and pulmonary embolism is increased.
- The risk of breast carcinoma is at least 20 times higher than normal. The patient may have increased frequency of extragonadal germ cell tumors such as embryonal carcinoma, teratoma and primary mediastinal germ cell tumor.

Hormone levels
- Serum FSH: ↑ed
- Serum estradiol: ↑ed
- Serum testosterone: ↓ed

Microscopic features of testes
- Testicular atrophy/dysgenesis
- Atrophy of seminiferous tubules replaced by fibrous tissues.

4. Chromosomal anomalies and clinical features of Turner's syndrome (1987, 92, 94, 96, 98, 2001, 02, 04, 11)

- Complete or partial monosomy of X chromosome resulting in hypogonadism in female phenotype.
- **Incidence:** 1 in 3,000 female births
- *Genetic abnormalities*
  Classic type (57%): Entire X chromosome is missing (45, X).

Structural abnormality of second X chromosome (14%):
- Deletion of small arm—46, X, i (X) (q10)
- Deletion of a portion of short and long arms—46, X, r(X)
- Deletion of a portion of short or long arm—46, X, del(Xq) or 46X, del(Xp)

Mosaic pattern (29%):
- 45, X/46, XX
- 45, X/47, XXX
- 45, X/46, XY
- 45, X/46, X, i(X) (q10)

- *Pathogenesis*
  - During embryogenic development of ovaries, both X chromosomes are required. Fetal ovaries develop normally early in embryogenesis, but absence of second X chromosome leads to an accelerated loss of oocytes against a slow loss in normal female. By the age of two years, all the oocytes are destroyed and "menopause occurs before menarche".
  - Ovaries are replaced by fibrous strands, devoid of ova and follicles (*streak ovaries*).

- *Clinical features of Turner's syndrome in children*
  - Infants present with peripheral edema (lymph stasis) of the dorsum of hand and foot, and may have swelling of nape of neck (distended lymphatic channel).
  - With age, swelling is replaced by bilateral neck webbing and loose skin on the back of neck.
  - Lower posterior hairline.
  - Congenital heart diseases like coarctation of aorta and bicuspid aortic valve (most common cause of death)

- *Clinical features in adolescents and adults*
  - At puberty there is failure to develop normal secondary sex characteristics.
  - The genitalia remain infantile, breast development is inadequate and there is little pubic hair.

– Chest is broad and nipples are widely placed.
– Streak ovaries, infertility, *amenorrhea* (single most important cause of primary amenorrhea)
– Pigmented nevi and cubitus valgus
– *Short stature*
– Autoimmune diseases leading to hypothyroidism and other conditions.
– Glucose intolerance, obesity and insulin resistance
– Turner's syndrome is the single most important cause of primary amenorrhea accounting for approximately 1/3rd of cases.
– Mental status of these patients are usually normal.

5. Lyon hypothesis (1987, 99, 2000, 07)

6. *Barr body (1990, 94)

Lyon hypothesis

1. Only one of the X chromosomes is generally active.
2. The other X chromosome of either maternal or paternal origin undergoes hyperpyknosis and is rendered as inactive.
3. Inactivation of either the maternal or paternal X chromosome occurs at random among all the cells of the blastocyst on or about the 16th day of embryonic life.
4. Inactivation of the same X chromosome persists in all the cells derived from each precursor cell.
   • The inactivated X chromosome is selectively reactivated in germ cells before first meiotic division, as both

X chromosomes are required for normal oogenesis.

*The inactive X chromosome can be seen in the interphase nucleus as the darkly staining small mass in contact with the nuclear membrane known as Barr body or X chromatin. It is present in all cells of normal female. For its demonstration buccal squamous epithelium cells are taken.

Number of Barr bodies = Number of X chromosomes – 1

• Barr body is used as a test of genetic femaleness—it is possible to determine the genetic sex of an individual according to whether there is a Barr body present or not.
• Barr body is found in females, but:
  – Klinefelter's syndrome in males with Barr body.
  – Turner's syndrome in females without Barr body.

7. Hermaphroditism (1993)

8. Gaucher's disease (1998)

9. Glycogen storage disease (1987, 88, 97)

Glycogen storage disease (GSD, also **glycogenosis** and **dextrinosis)** is the result of defects in the processing of glycogen synthesis or breakdown within muscle, liver and other cell types. GSD has two classes of cause: genetic and acquired. Genetic GSD is caused by any inborn error of metabolism (genetically defective enzymes) involved in these processes. There are eleven (11) distinct diseases that are commonly considered to be glycogen storage diseases.

Glycogen storage disease			
	Hepatic type	*Myopathic type*	*Miscellaneous type*
Specific type	Hepatorenal (von Gierke's disease)	McArdle's disease (type V)	Generalised glycogenosis, Pompe disease (type II)
Enzyme deficiency	Glucose 6-phosphatase	Muscle phospnorylase	Lysosomal glucosidase (acid maltase)

(Contd.)

Glycogen storage disease (*Contd.*)

	Hepatic type	*Myopathic type*	*Miscellaneous type*
Morphological changes	Hepatomegaly and renomegaly (intracytoplasmic accumulation of glycogen)	Skeletal muscle-accumulation of glycogen in sarcolemmal location	Mild hepatomegaly, cardiomegaly. Deposits in skeletal muscle
Clinical features	Failure to thrive, stunted growth, hepatorenal megaly, hypoglycemia, hyperlipidemia, hyperuricemia, bleeding tendency	Painful cramps, myoglobinuria, no increase in lactic acid with exercise	Massive cardiomegaly, muscle hypotonia, cardiorespiratory failure within two years of life. Milder adult form—only skeletal muscle involvement (chronic myopathy)

10. Hypercholesterolemia (1993, 96)

Fredrickson classification of hypercholesterolemia

	Type I	*Type IIa*	*Type IIb*	*Type III*	*Type IV*	*Type V*
Synonyms	Familial lipoprotein lipase deficiency	Familial hypercholesterolemia	Familial combined hyperlipidemia	Familial dysbetalipoproteinemia	Familial hypertriglyceridemia	Endogenous hypertriglyceridemia
Problems	Decreased lipoprotein lipase or Apo C-II	LDL receptor deficiency	↓ LDL receptor, ↑ Apo B-100	Defect in Apo-E	↑ VLDL production and ↓ elimination (Apo V deficiency)	Same as in IV, more severe
Lipoproteins	Elevated chylomicrons	↑ LDL	↑ VLDL, ↑ LDL	↑chylomicron remnants and IDL	↑ VLDL	↑ VLDL and chylomicrons
Cholesterol	↑↑	↑↑↑	↑↑	↑↑	N	↑↑↑
Triglycerides	↑↑↑↑	N	↑↑	↑↑	↑↑	↑↑↑
Xanthomas	Eruptive	Tendon, tuberous	None	Palmer, tuberoeruptive	None	Eruptive
Pancreatitis	+++	0	0	0	0/+	+++
Coronary atherosclerosis	0	+++	+++	+++	0/+	0/+
Peripheral atherosclerosis	0	+	+	++	0/+	0/+
Serum appearance	Creamy top layer	Clear	Clear	Turbid	Turbid	Creamy top layer and turbid bottom

6

Diseases of Immunity

1a. T-lymphocytes (2007)

- These are thymus-derived cells, which are mediators of cell-mediated immunity (CMI).
- They constitute 60–70% of circulating lymphocytes.
- They are present in paracortical region of lymph node and periarteriolar sheath of spleen.
- They are genetically programmed to recognize a specific cell-bound antigen by means of an antigen-specific T cell receptor (TCR).
- In 95% T cells, 'TCR' consists of a disulfide linkage made up of α and β polypeptide chains. In 5% T cells, the disulfide linkage is made up of γ and δ polypeptide chains.

- Each TCR is non-covalently linked to five polypeptide chains which form the CD3 complex and 'τ'-protein (TCR-complex). These are both identical in all T cells.
- In addition to CD3 proteins, T cells express a variety of other molecules, i.e. CD4, CD8, CD2, CD11a, CD28 and CD40.
- CD4 is expressed in 60% of mature CD3 + T cells and CD8 is expressed in 30% mature CD3+ T cells.

1b. B-lymphocytes

- These are mediators of humoral immunity.
- They are derived from progenitor B cells produced in the bone marrow.

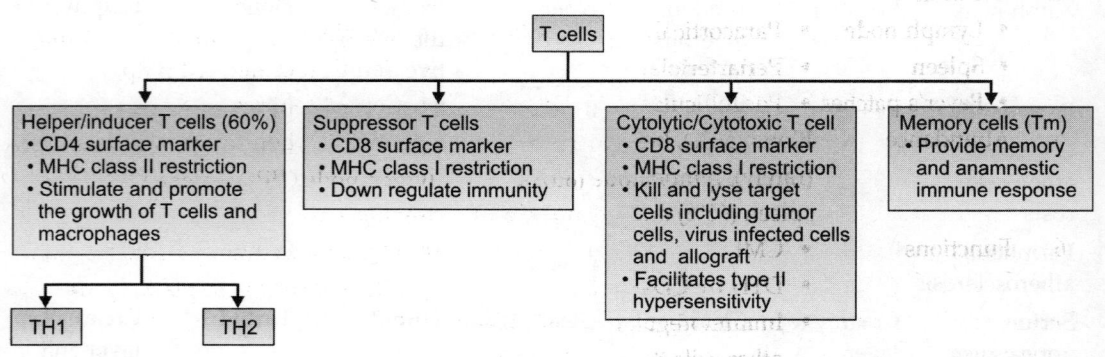

Fig. 6.1

- They constitute 10–20% of circulating lymphocytes.
- The principal function of B cells is to make antibodies against soluble antigens.
- They are present in lymph nodes (superficial cortex), spleen (white pulp), tonsils, bone marrow, and extralymphatic tissues, i.e. GIT.
- They are differentiated into two types: Plasma B cells (synthesize immunoglobulins) and memory B cells (remain in secondary lymphoid organs as memory cells are already activated by antigen and they produce quicker responses on later exposure of the same antigens).
- B cells recognize antigen BCR complex.

- Each BCR has a unique antigen specificity derived from rearrangement of Ig genes.
- Components of BCR complex:
  - Surface IgM (antigen binding component)
  - Igα and Igβ (required for signal transduction)
  - Complement receptor CD21 (EBV receptor)
  - Fc receptor
  - CD40 (member of TNF family)
- In contrast to TCR, BCR can be activated by Ag without MHC involvement, so Ag processing and presentation by APC do not occur for B cells.

2. Difference between T cell and B cell (1997, 90, 2000)

S. No.	Traits	T cell	B cell
1.	Origin	Originates from bone marrow, maturation in thymus	Origin and maturation both in bone marrow
2.	Life span	• T cell blasts—several days • Small T cell—month to years	• B cell blasts—several days • Small B cell—less than a month
3.	Surface markers		
	• Ag receptors	• Present	• Absent
	• Surface Ig	• Absent	• Present
	• Fc receptor	• Absent	• Present
	• Complement receptor	• Absent	• Present
	• CD marker	• Th: CD3, 4, 7, 2 • T suppressor: CD8, 3, 7, 2	• CD19, 21
4.	Location		
	• Lymph node	• Paracortical/Perifollicular	• Germinal center, medullary cords
	• Spleen	• Periarteriolar	• Germinal center, red pulp
	• Peyer's patches	• Perifollicular	• Central follicles
5.	Abundance	Blood (80%), bone marrow (rarely), lymph node (85%), spleen (65%) and thymus (90%)	Blood (20%), bone marrow (numerous). lymph node (15%), spleen (35%) and thymus (10%)
6.	Functions	• CMI • DTH by CD4+ cells • Immunoregulation of T, B and other cells through Th or T suppressor cells	• Humoral immunity—Ab secretion after converting to plasma cells.

3. Natural killer cells (NK cells)

- They make up 10–15% of peripheral blood lymphocytes.
- They are larger than small lymphocytes and contain abundant azurophilic granules (*Larger granular lymphocytes*).
- They don't have T cell receptor (TCR) like CD3, but they have CD16; it is Fc receptor for IgG responsible for antibody dependent cell-mediated cytotoxicity (ADCC).
- They are CD2, CD16 and CD56 positive.
- They take part in natural/innate immunity; no need for prior sensitization with antigens.
- *NK cells express receptors:* One that recognizes ill-defined molecules on the target cells and causing lysis (augmented by IL-2, IL-15); other receptor inhibits cell lysis by recognition of self-class I MHC. As all nucleated normal cells express MHC I on their surface, they are spared. In case of viral infected cells or tumor cells there is reduced MHC I expression and negative feedback to NK cells are interrupted resulting in lysis of such abnormal cells.
- It secretes TNF-α and granulocyte macrophage colony stimulating factor (GM-CSF), INF (differentiation of Th1 cells).
- Their activities are regulated by stimulatory (NKG2D) and inhibitory (killer cell Ig-like receptors and CD94 family of lectin receptor) influences.

4. Type I hypersensitivity/anaphylactic type (1990)

- It may be defined as "a rapidly developing immunologic reaction occurring within minutes after combination of an Ag with Ab bound to mast cells or basophils previously sensitized to the Ag".
- Reaction may be:
  - Systemic, if Ag is introduced directly into the circulation in a sensitized person like penicillin anaphylactic shock.

- It may be local reaction like skin allergy, allergic rhinitis, conjunctivitis, hay fever, bronchial asthma, etc.

Pathogenesis
- When an Ag comes in contact for the first time, Ab (IgE) against the Ag is formed. These IgE antibodies coat basophils/mast cells.
- Next time when same Ag comes in contact, it is presented by APC (Antigen presenting cells) in association with MHC II to T helper (Th) cells. Th cells get differentiated into Th-2 cells secreting IL-4 and 5 (act on B cells to convert it into plasma cells to produce Abs).
- Also Th2 secretes IL-3, 5, and GM-CSF to recruit eosinophils.
- Activated by TNF-α, mucosal lining produces eotaxin and RANTES (recruit eosinophils).
- Ab (IgE), thus formed acts on mast cells releasing IL-3 and 5 (recruit eosinophils).
- Cross-linking of IgE bound to mast cells/basophils causes degranulation and release of primary, and later on secondary mediators (Fig. 6.2).

Mediators
- *Primary mediators*
  - Histamine
  - Adenosine
  - Proteases
  - Proteoglycans like heparin and chondroitin sulfate
  - Eosinophil chemotactic factors
  - Neutrophil chemotactic factors
  - Other chemotactic factors
- *Secondary mediators*
  - Cytokines
  - Leukotrienes B4, C4 and D4
  - Prostaglandin D2
  - Platelet activating factors
- Eosinophils release major basic protein and cationic protein which aid to inflammation.

These mediators result in *two-phase response*:

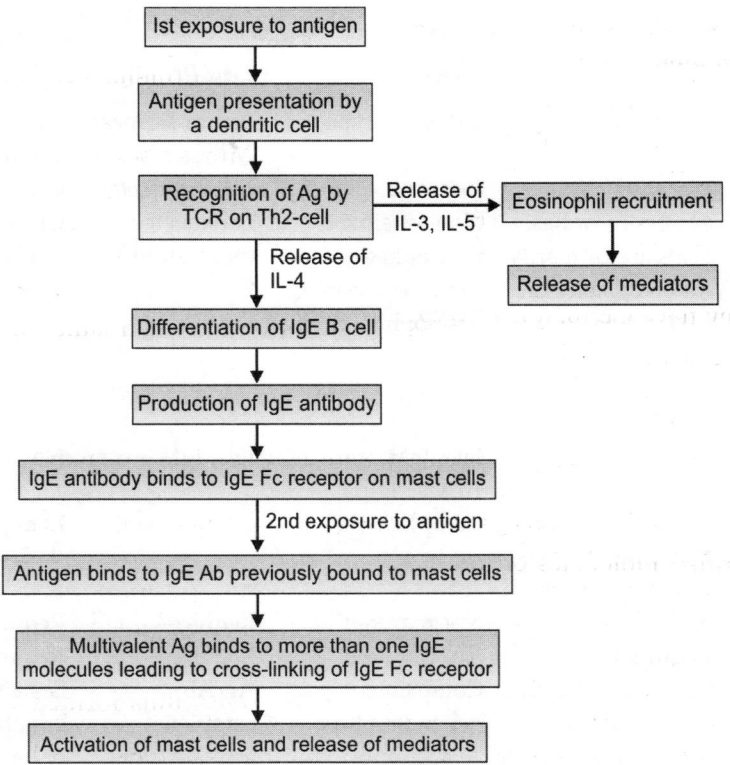

Fig. 6.2: Pathogenesis of type I hypersensitivity

- *Initial response*
  - Within 5–30 minutes
  - Subsides in 60 minutes
  - Vasodilatation
  - Vascular leakage
  - Smooth muscle spasm/glandular secretion
- *Late phase response*
  - After 8 hr for several days
  - Intense tissue infiltration by eosinophils, neutrophils, monocytes, basophils and CD4+ cells
  - Tissue destruction in form of mucosal damage

5. Difference between type I and type II hypersensitivities (1993, 98, 99, 2001, 07)

6. Difference between type II and type III hypersensitivities (1998, 94, 2004)

7. Difference between type I and type III hypersensitivities (1997)

8. Difference between type II and type IV hypersensitivities (2002)

9. Mechanism of type II hypersensitivity with examples (1994, 2000, 10)

10. Antibody dependent cell-mediated cytotoxicity (ADCC) (1989)

Type II hypersensitivity

Type II hypersensitivity is mediated by antibodies directed towards Ag present on the surface of cell or other tissue components. These Ag may be intrinsic to cell membrane or exogenous Ag absorbed on the cell surface (e.g. a drug metabolite). Reaction occurs when Ab binds to normal or altered cell surface Ag. The different antibody dependent mechanisms involved in this type of reaction are:

Types of hypersensitivity reactions: Summary

Traits	Type I	Type II	Type III	Type IV
Type	Anaphylactic type	Cytotoxic type	Serum sickness, Arthus reaction	Delayed type hyper-sensitivity
Definition	(*See short note*)	(*See short note*)	(*See short note*)	Cell-mediated
Cells involved	Mast cells or baso-phils are primarily involved, later on eosinophils, neu-trophils, monocy-tes, CD4+ cells, B cells	Non-sensitized macrophages, NK cells, neutrophils, eosinophils, B cells	Leukocytes (neutrophils), B cells	CD4+ T cells, APC (macrophages), CD8+ cells
Antibodies type	IgE	IgG, IgM, (rare in ADCC: IgE)	IgG, IgM	No
Chemical mediators	IL-3, 4, 5, histamine and other pharma-cological agents	Complements	Complements	Lymphokines, IL-12, IL–2, INF-γ, TGF-β and TNF-α
Ag presentation	By APC is required	Not required	Required	Required
Pre-sensitization	Required	Not required	Required	Required
Pathogenesis	Formation of IgE and immediate release of mediators to recruit inflamma-tory cells and in-flammatory changes	Complement dependent type, ADCC, anti-receptor antibodies type	Ag-Ab complexes → activate com-plements → attract neutro-phils → release of lysosomal en-zyme and other toxic agents	Sensitized T lymphocytes → release of lymphokines and T cell-mediated cytoto-xicity
Time of mani-festation	Minutes	Variable; hours to days	Variable; hours to days	Hours to days
Examples	Allergic bronchial asthma	Transfusion hemolytic reaction	Glomeruloneph-ritis, rheumatoid arthritis	Transplant rejection

i. Opsonization and complement and Fc receptor mediated phagocytosis.
  - Seen in cases of transfusion reaction, erythroblastosis foetalis, autoimmune hemolytic anemia/thrombocytopenia/agranulocytosis.
  - Most commonly involved in type II reaction (Fig. 6.3).
ii. Complement and Fc receptor mediated inflammation.

- In this, injury is due to inflammation and not because of phagocytosis (Fig. 6.4).
- Seen in glomerulonephritis, vascular rejection in organ graft.
iii. Antibody-mediated cellular dysfunction.
  - Antibodies against the cell surface receptor deregulate function without causing cell injury or inflammation, e.g. myasthenia gravis.
Another process called ADCC (Antibody dependent cellular cytotoxicity) (Fig. 6.5).

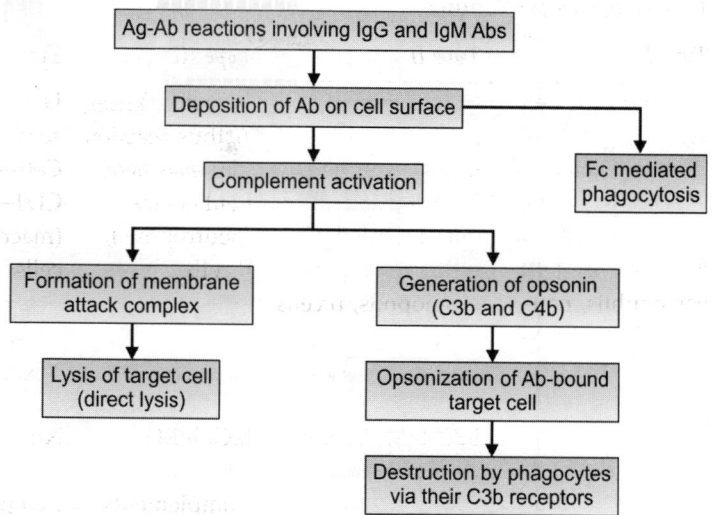

Fig. 6.3

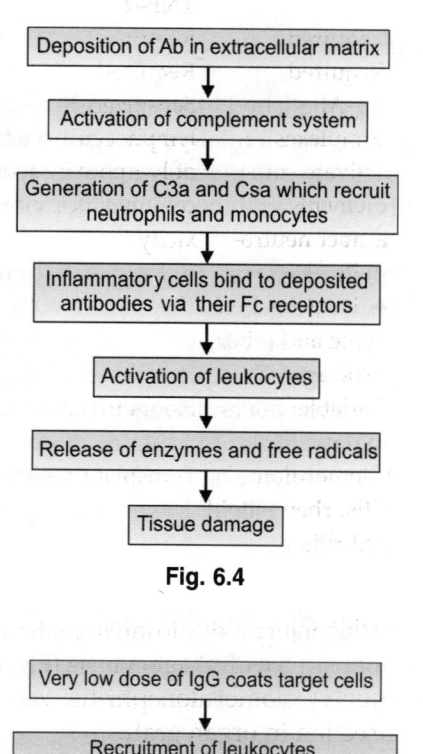

Fig. 6.4

Very low dose of IgG coats target cells

Recruitment of leukocytes
(Minimal/No activation of complement)

Activation of monocytes, neutrophils and NK cells which
bind to target cells via receptors for the Fc fragment of IgG

Cell lysis (by perforin) without phagocytosis

Fig. 6.5

This form of Ab-mediated injury does not involve complement fixation and it is not a type II hypersensitivity.

11. Difference between Arthrus reaction (1986, 87) and serum sickness

12. Type III hypersensitivity mechanism with examples (1998, 2008, 11)

- This is a type of hypersensitivity reaction in which Ag-Ab complexes produce tissue damage as a result of activation of complement system.
- The antigen may be exogenous like bacteria (poststreptococcal glomerulonephritis), viruses, parasites, etc. or drugs; or it may be endogenous like nuclear Ag in SLE.
- Immune complex may be generalized or it may be localized to a particular organ like kidney (glomerulonephritis), joints (arthritis), skin (local Arthus reaction), etc.

Systemic immune complex disease

Prototype disease: Acute serum sickness (large amount of foreign serum into the circulation directly) (Fig. 6.6).

Three Phases

i. *Formation of Ag-Ab complex* in the circulation: After exposure to Ag, Ab is formed against it. Ag-Ab complex is formed after combination of two.

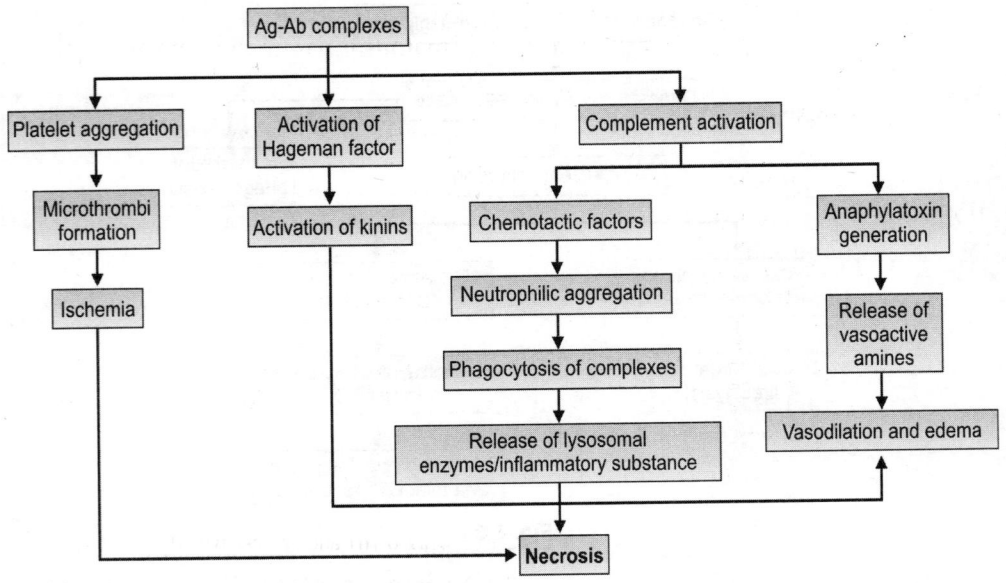

Fig. 6.6: Pathogenesis of systemic immune complex disease

ii. *Deposition of Ag-Ab complex* in various tissues and organs: When Ab is in excess, large complexes are formed and they are removed by mononuclear phagocytic system.

If intermediate or small-sized complexes are formed due to excess Ag and phagocytic system is impaired, they are deposited in their favored sites like joints, skin, heart, serosal surface and small blood vessels.

   Change in vascular permeability is must for complexes to be deposited outside vessels.

iii. *Generalized inflammatory reaction*
   – Clinical features: Fever, urticaria, arthralgia, lymph node enlargement, proteinuria, etc.
   – Activation of complement cascade
   – Activation of neutrophils and macrophages through Fc receptors
- Local immune complex disease or Arthus reaction
   – "It may be defined as a localized area of tissue necrosis resulting from acute immune complex vasculitis (inflammation of vessel wall)".

   – It can be elicited in an experimental subject having circulatory Ab against a particular Ag (due to prior exposure to it) by giving intracutaneous injection of same Ag.
   – Antibodies are in excess, when Ag diffuses through the vessel wall—Ag and Ab react to form large immune complexes. These complexes precipitate locally in wall and trigger inflammatory reaction similar to systemic type.
   – There is edema, severe hemorrhage and ulceration. Fibrinoid necrosis of vessels takes place.

13. DTH (Delayed type hypersensitivity) (1998)

- A type* of type IV hypersensitivity (cell mediated) reaction

   *Other type is direct cell cytotoxicity mediated by CD8+ T cells

- *Prototype:* Tuberculin reaction
- *Antigen:* Protein lipopolysaccharide component (purified protein derivatives, PPD)
- There is reddening and induration at the intradermal injection site and it is read at 72 hr after injection.

- *Microscopically*: There is accumulation of mononuclear cells around small blood vessels producing perivascular 'cuff'. Increased vascular permeability, escape of plasma protein (dermal edema), deposition of fibrin in interstitium (induration) and endothelium hypertrophy are seen.
- CD4+ T cells predominance.

- If Ag is persistent/non-degradable, granulomatous inflammation may take place.
- *Pathogenesis*: (Fig. 6.7)
  - On 1st exposure of Ag, APC presents these Ags in association with MHC II to CD4+ cells.
  - Naive CD4+ cells differentiate to Th1 cells, which is central to DTH.

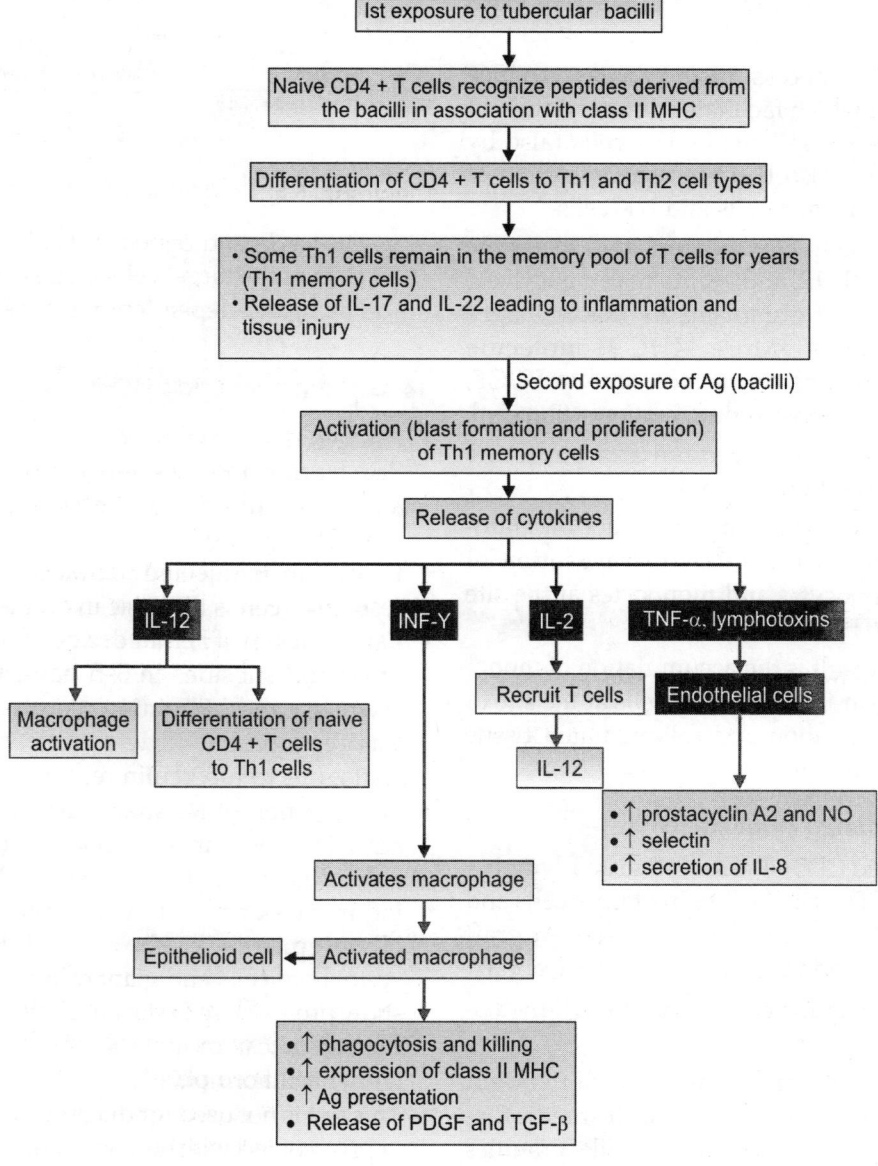

Fig. 6.7: Pathogenesis of DTH

– Some of Th1 cells remain as memory cells in circulation for years.

– On 2nd/subsequent exposure of the Ag, memory Th1 cells interact with Ag in association with MHC II of APC. Memory cells undergo blast transformation and proliferation to produce Th1 type cytokines (cell-mediated immunity).

– Resting macrophages (APC) during interaction with Ag try to phagocyte and kill the organism, but are unable to do so.

– In this process, macrophages produce IL-12 which facilitates differentiation of naive CD4+ cells to Th1 cells (also by INF-γ). Also IL-12 induces secretion of INF-γ from T cells and NK cells.

– INF-γ activates macrophages to secrete more IL-12, and ability to phagocytose; killing of organisms by macrophages increases. [More MHC II molecule expressions on surface; secrete PDGF, TGF-(fibroblasts proliferation—fibrosis)].

– IL-2 causes autocrine and paracrine proliferation of T cells.

– TNF-α and lymphotoxin act on endothelium to facilitate extravasation of lymphocytes and monocytes at the site of DTH.

– Net result is the accumulation of mononuclear inflammatory cells at the site of inflammation and cell-mediated tissue destruction.

T cell-mediated cytotoxicity

• Sensitized CD8+ T cells (cytotoxic T lymphocytes/CTL) kill Ag bearing target cells and seem to have an important role in graft rejection and resistance to viral infection.

• Two principal mechanisms of T cell-mediated damage are:
  – Perforins and granzyme dependent killing: These are soluble mediators contained in the lysosome-like granules of CTLs (Fig. 6.8).

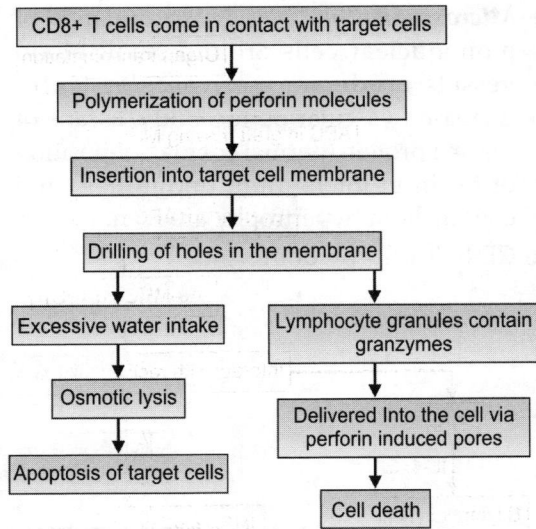

Fig. 6.8: T cell mediated cytotoxicity

– Fas-Fas ligand-dependent killing: Apoptosis of the target cells is caused by Fas-Fas ligand-dependent mechanism.

14. Lepromin reaction (1998)

• Antigen (lepromin) used is boiled, emulsified, lepromatous tissue-rich in lepra bacilli and standardized according to lepra bacilli contents.

• Lepromin is injected intradermally and response seen is biphasic in nature.

• Early reaction of Fernandez develops in 24–48 hr and subsides in 3–5 days. It shows erythema and induration. Poorly defined, this reaction has little significance. It is analogous to tuberculin reaction.

• Late reaction of Mitsuda starts in 1–2 wk, reaches its peak in 4th week and gradually subsides in next few weeks. There is indurated skin nodule, which may ulcerate. Histologically, it shows lymphocytes, epithelioid cells and giant cells. It does not show pre-existing DTH, but shows whether the person can mount the CMI against the lepra bacilli or not.

• This test is not used for diagnosis of leprosy or prior contact with the bacilli, it may be used to check CMI status against lepra bacilli.

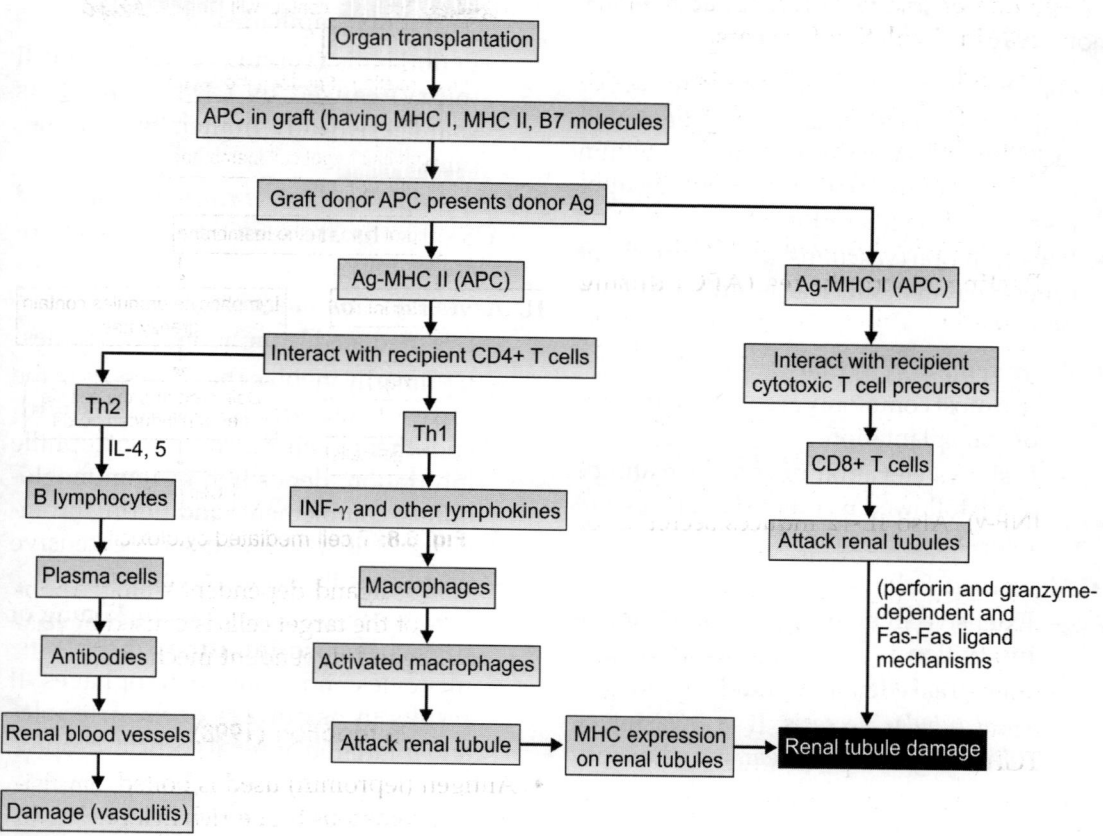

Fig. 6.9: Mechanism of transplant rejection

15. Acute transplant rejection (2008)

or

Transplant rejection—mechanism (2001, 04)

"Graft rejection depends upon the recognition by the host of the grafted tissue as foreign".

"Rejection is a complex process in which both cell-mediated and humoral immunity play a role; though T cell-mediated immunity is center to the transplant rejection".

- **T cell-mediated reaction**
  - *Direct pathway*
    - Certain cells in the graft express HLA Ag, like dendritic cells (APC).
    - T cells of recipient recognize Ag (HLA protein) on APC of donor tissue (Fig. 6.9).

  - *Indirect pathway:* APC of recipient processes the MHC molecules shed by the graft and it is presented as an antigen (as it happens in normal immune response to foreign antigens).

- **B cell-mediated**
  - *Hyperacute rejection*
    a. When preformed antibodies are present in the circulation of the recipient
    b. Arthus type reaction
  - *Acute rejection*
    a. Vasculitis is the outcome.
    b. Type II (all subtypes) and type III hypersensitivity reactions involved.

16. Renal pathology in acute graft rejection (1996)

- *Onset*: Acute graft rejection may occur within days of transplantation in untreated recipient or may appear suddenly within months or years later, after immunosuppression has been terminated.
- It has humoral (vasculitis) as well as cellular (interstitial mononuclear infiltration) components.

I. *Acute cellular rejection*
   - It is most commonly seen within months of transplantation.
   - It shows elevation of serum creatinine level; followed by other sign and symptoms of renal failure.

- *Microscopic features*
   - Extensive interstitial mononuclear cell infiltration
   - Interstitial edema and mild hemorrhage
   - *Focal tubular necrosis:* It is invasion of tubules by mononuclear inflammatory cells present in the glomerular and peritubular capillaries.
   - Endothelitis (vascular endothelial cell injury) caused by CD8+ cells. It is characteristically limited to endothelium.

- *Immunoperoxidase staining*: CD4+ and CD8+ T cells are seen on immunoperoxidase staining.

II. *Acute rejection vasculitis*
   - It is mediated by antidonor antibodies.
   - It primarily involves blood vessels in the form of necrotizing vasculitis with endothelial cell necrosis; neutrophilic infiltration; deposition of immunoglobulins, complements and fibrin; thrombosis. It is associated with extensive necrosis of the renal parenchyma.
   - Less acute vasculitis has thickening of intima by proliferating fibroblasts, myocytes and foamy macrophages. It results in narrowing of the arterioles and infarction or renal cortical atrophy.

17. Difference between acute and chronic transplant rejection (1994)

S. No.	Traits	Acute rejection	Chronic rejection
1.	Stage	2nd stage of rejection	3rd stage of rejection
2.	Onset	Occurs within days of transplant or suddenly after cessation of immunosuppressive therapy	Occurs over months to years after transplant
3.	Components	Two parts: Acute cellular (CD4+, CD8+ T cells) and acute rejection vasculitis (antibodies)	No division. Characterized by progressive organ dysfunction
4.	Mechanism	Interstitial mononuclear infiltration by CD4+ and CD8+ T cells , and antibody-mediated	Frequently mononuclear infiltrate with numerous plasma cells and eosinophils
5.	Morphology	Acute cellular: Damage tubular epithelium and vascular endothelial cells Acute rejection vasculitis: Necrotizing vasculitis, thrombosis or intimal thickening	Arterioles show dense intimal fibrosis leading to parenchymal ischemic injury

18. Graft versus host reaction (GVH) (1995, 97, 2002)

"This occurs in situations when immunologically competent cells like bone marrow grafting or their precursors are transplanted into immunologically suppressed recipient".

- There are three requirements for the GVH reaction to occur:
  - The graft must contain immunocompetent T cells.
  - The recipient must be immunocompromized.
  - The recipient must express antigens (e.g. MHC proteins) foreign to the donor, i.e. the donor T cells recognize the recipient cells as foreign. Even when donor and recipient have identical class I and class II MHC proteins, i.e. identical haplotypes, a GVH can occur because it can be elicited by differences in minor antigens.
- Acute GVH:
  - It develops within days to weeks of transplantation.
  - Organs affected are immune system, epithelium of skin, liver and intestines.
  - There is either infection by new organisms or activation of silent infection like CMV causing pneumonia (Immunosuppressed state).
  - *Skin:* Generalized rash; desquamation in severe cases
  - *Liver:* Destruction of small bile ducts (jaundice)
  - *GIT:* Mucosal ulceration (bloody diarrhea)
  - No heavy infiltration of affected organs by lymphocytes is seen.
- Chronic GVH:
  - It follows acute syndrome or may have insidious onset.
  - *Skin:* Extensive lesion, destruction of skin appendages, and fibrosis of dermis similar to systemic sclerosis.
  - *Liver:* Chronic parenchymal and bile duct damge (cholestatic jaundice)
  - *GIT:* Mucosal damage, esophageal stricture
  - *Involution of thymus:* Recurrent and serious infections
  - Autoimmune diseases

19. Immunological tolerance (2003)

20. Difference between clonal deletion and clonal anergy (2003, 07)

21. Difference between central and peripheral tolerance

S. No.	Traits	Central tolerance	Peripheral tolerance
1.	Site	Thymus/Bone marrow	Peripheral tissue
2.	Mechanism	Clonal deletion of self T/B cells	Clonal deletion, clonal energy, peripheral suppression by T cells
3.	Failure	Don't occur	May occur, autoimmune diseases

- Immunologic tolerance is characterized by a state in which the individual is incapable of developing an immune response to a specific antigen.
- Self-tolerance refers to tolerance against self-antigens. It is protective.
- *Mechanisms:*
  Central tolerance (Central clonal deletion): This refers to the clonal deletion of self-reactive T and B cells during their maturation in central lymphoid organs (thymus for T cells and bone marrow for B cells). Self-antigens or autologous self-Ag are processed and presented with self-MHC molecules. T cells having high affinity receptors for such self-Ag undergo Fas-mediated apoptosis and are negatively selected. Similarly, B cells coming in contact with membrane-

bound self-Ag undergo apoptosis. Cell clones of non-self reactive are transferred to periphery and participate in immunologic reactions.

Peripheral tolerance: Some of self-reactive T/B cells escape central clonal deletion, they reach circulation and are taken care by following mechanisms:

– *Clonal deletion* by activation-induced cell death: Self-peptide antigens are in abundance in body, it is presented by APC in association with self-MHC (to TCR of T cells). Also such APCs have B7 ligand, which bind to CD28 of T cells. This results in upregulation of Fas (CD95) receptor, and also expression of FasL on activated T cells. Repeated stimulus of T cells by Ag causes T cells to undergo apoptotic cell death by Fas/FasL system.

– *Clonal anergy:* "Prolonged or irreversible functional inactivation of lymphocytes, induced by encounter with antigens under certain conditions". In contrast to clonal deletion, Ag is presented by cells that do not bear the CD28 ligand (like B7), it results in a negative signal to T cells which become anergic—they fail to be activated even if competent Ag presenting cells present relevant Ag. As most of the normal tissue cells either don't express or weakly express B7 ligand like co-stimulatory molecules, encounter between autoreactive T cells and their specific self-Ag leads to clonal anergy. If B cells encounter Ag in the absence of specific helper T cells, the Ag receptor complex is down regulated and these cells never re-express their Ig receptors.

– *Peripheral suppression* by T cells: Down regulation of autoreactive T cells by secreting certain cytokines like IL-4, IL-10, TGF β, etc. by Th2 type cells.

– Antigen sequestration: Ags are hidden from immune system (testes, eye).

22. Mechanism of autoimmune disease (1999, 98, 2001, 07, 11)

• Breakage of central tolerance: No evidence, so no role

• Breakdown of peripheral tolerance:
  – Breakdown of T cell anergy: If APCs express B7 ligands and secrete IL-2 that stimulate Th1 cells like in case of CNS—multiple sclerosis.
  – Failure of *activation induced* cell death: It allows persistence and proliferation of autoreactive T cells in peripheral tissues.
  – Failure of T cell *mediated suppression.*
  – *Molecular mimicry:* Some exogenous Ag like viral/bacterial cell components share epitopes with self-Ag (cross-reacting Ag), e.g. RHD (Ab to streptococcal M protein cross reacts with cardiac glycoproteins).
  – *Polyclonal lymphocytes activation:* Super antigens (like TSST, Staphylococcus) activate a large pool of CD4+ cells in an antigen independent manner (stimulates very large number of T cells, without relation to their epitope specificity).
  – Release of *sequestered antigens:* Spermatozoa and ocular Ag that are completely sequestered during development act as foreign bodies and, if they come in contact with systemic circulation they cause an immune response.
  – Exposure of *cryptic self and epitope spreading:* Cryptic self means hidden epitopes or proteins that have not been exposed during embryonic life. Generally, each self-protein in the body expresses few epitopes to T cells during the embryogenic life and, thus these cells are either deleted in the thymus or undergo anergy in periphery. But sometimes during the adult life, the protein may present some uncommon epitopes which may lead to immunologic reactions.

23. Pathogenesis of SLE (systemic lupus erythematous) (2004, 10)

- SLE is a chronic disease characterized by acute/insidious in onset, remitting, relapsing, often febrile illness causing injury to skin, joints, kidney serosal membranes, etc.

- The exact cause of SLE remains unknown, but it is thought that there is failure of the regulatory mechanism that maintains self-tolerance. Antibodies against a number of self-antigens are formed (Fig. 6.10).
- It is a classical prototype of a multisystem disease of autoimmune origin.

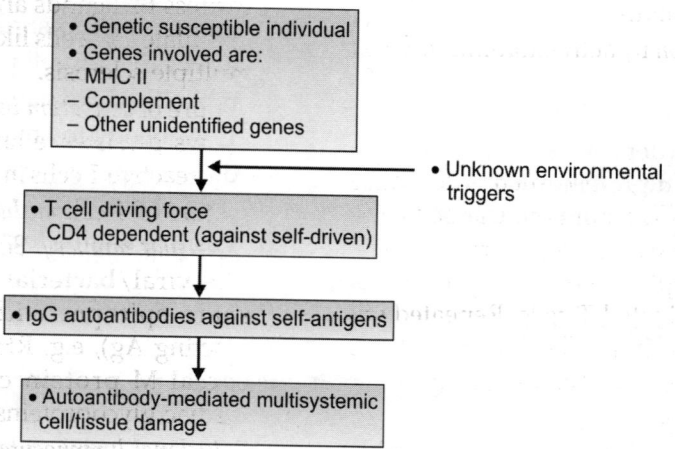

Fig. 6.10: Pathogenesis of SLE

24. Laboratory diagnosis of SLE (1999, 2010)

Blood	Immunological tests	Urine

• Hemolytic anemia (Increased reticulocyte counts and other features)
• Leukopenia
• Lymphopenia ($< 1500/mm^3$)
• Thrombocytopenia ($< 1,00,000/mm^3$)—↑ BT
• Uremia
• Ketoacidosis
• Electrolyte imbalances
	• Immunofluorescence: Self-antinuclear antibodies against:
	  – DNA
	  – Histone proteins
	  – Non-histone proteins bound to RNA
	  – Nucleolar antigen
	• Anti **Smith** (Anti-Sm) antigen anti-bodies against dsDNA—pathognomic of SLE
	• Antiphospholipids (present in 40–50% patients):
	  – Increase in IgG/IgM anticardiolipin Ab
	  – Lupus anticogulant anti-bodies interfering with clothing—↑ CT
	  – False positive serological test for syphilis for at least 6 months, but not positive for *T. pallidum* by immobilization test
		• Persistent proteinuria (> 0.5 g/day)
		• Cellular casts—RBC, tubular, granular or mixed casts
		• Hematuria
		
		Microscopic:
		• LE bodies
		• LE cells (1999)

- "For clinical diagnosis, person is said to have SLE, if any 4 or more of the following 11 features are present serially or simultaneously, during any intervals".

SLE Criteria

i. Malar rash
ii. Discoid rash
iii. Photosensitivity
iv. Oral ulcer
v. Arthritis
vi. Serositis
vii. Renal disorder
   a. > 0.5 g/d proteinuria or
   b. ≥ 3 + dipstick proteinuria or
   c. Cellular casts
viii. Neurologic disorder
   a. Seizure or
   b. Psychosis (without other cause)
ix. Hematological disorder
   a. Hemolytic anemia or
   b. Leukopenia (< 4000/cc) or
   c. Thrombocytopenia (< 1,00,000/cc)
x. Immunologic disorder
   a. Positive LE cell preparation or
   b. Antibody to native DNA or
   c. Antibody to Sm or
   d. False positive serological test for syphilis
xi. Positive antinuclear antibodies

Clinical manifestations of SLE

Systemic (in 95% patient)	Musculoskeletal (95%)	Cutaneous	Renal
• Fever • Malaise • Weight loss • Anorexia • Fatigue	• Arthralgia/myalgia • Non-erosive polyarthritis • Hand deformity • AVN of bone	• Malar rash • Photosensitivity • Oral ulcers • Alopecia • Discoid rash	• Proteinuria • Nephrotic syndrome • End stage renal disease • Hematuria
Hematological	Neurological	Cardiopulmonary	Others
• Anemia • Lymphopenia • Leukopenia • Thrombocytopenia • Hemolytic anemia • Splenomegaly • Lymphadenopathy	• Cognitive disorder • Mood disorder • Headache • Seizure • Mono- or polyneuropathy • Stroke, TIA • Aseptic meningitis	• Pleurisy, pericarditis • Myocarditis, endocarditis • Pneumonitis • Coronary artery disease • Interstitial fibrosis • Shrinking lung syndrome • Pulmonary hypertension	• Thrombosis (arterial/venous) • Sicca syndrome • Conjunctivitis • Episcleritis • GI involvement

25. HIV: Structure and antigenic factors, mechanism of pathogenesis, major abnormalities of immune functions (2001), phases/CDC classification (2003), opportunistic infections (1995, 1996, 2008) and Lab (2001) of AIDS. Modes of transmission of HIV infection (2009) and role of macrophages in HIV infection (1997, 2000)

- Causative organism: HIV I and II (Retro virus).
- Any HIV infected person with fewer than 200 CD4+ T cells/μl is considered to have AIDS.

Structure of HIV virus

- Spherical and contains an electron dense cone-shaped core. Virus core contains:
  - Major capsid protein p24

- Nucleocapsid protein p7/p9
- Two copies of genomic RNA
- Three viral enzymes (protease, reverse transcriptase and integrase)

- Viral core is surrounded by a matrix protein called p17.
- Viral envelop is studded with two glycoproteins, gp120 and gp41 which are critical for infection.
- HIV proviral genome contains non-structural and regulatory genes like LTR, vif, vpr, vpu, nef, rev, etc. which are codes for different viral proteins.

Gag gene	Capsid protein p24, matrix protein p17, nucleocapsid protein p7/9
Pol gene	Reverse transcriptase, protease, integrase, ribonuclease
Env gene	Envelope glycoprotein—gp160. Cleaved in ER to gp120 (mediates CD4 and chemokine receptor binding) and gp41 (mediates fusion)

Modes of HIV transmission

- Unprotected sexual intercourse
- Through blood/blood products (infected) other body fluids
- Needle stick injury
- From an infected mother to a newborn

Pathogenesis

- **Target**: 1. Immune system: CD4+ cells like CD4+ T cells, macrophages/monocytes, and dendritic cells/Langerhans cells and 2. CNS
- Viral particles enter into the host body and are taken to local lymph node/lymphoid organs.

  Viremia and widespread seeding of lymphoid tissue (*acute HIV infection*).

- *Entry of viral particles* into target cells.
  - "CD4+ molecule is a high affinity receptor for HIV".
  - HIV gp120 binds with CD4 molecules leading to a conformational change in gp120 and formation of a new recognition site on it.

- This new site binds to CCR5/CXCR4*—resulting in a conformational change in gp41 with the insertion of a fusion peptide present at the tip of gp41 into target cell membrane.
- Viral core containing genome enters cytoplasm of cell.

  *HIV may be M (macrophage) tropic—CCR5 (β-chemokine) receptors are present on monocytes/macrophages and freshly isolated peripheral blood T cells (not *in vitro* propagated T cell line).

  T cell tropic—CXCR4 (α-chemokine) receptors are present on T cells, both freshly isolated and retained in culture. M tropic viruses are more efficient in transmitting AIDS (90% cases) and are predominant in early phase than T cell tropic, but T tropic HIV gradually accumulates and cause the final rapid phase of disease (being more virulent).

- On internalization, viral genome undergoes reverse transcription to form cDNA. cDNA may remain in episomal form in quiescent T cells, but may be integrated into the host genome in dividing cells. After integration provirus may remain silent or it may transcribe and form viral particles in activated T cell (exposure to Ag/cytokines) (*Clinical latency/chronic infection*).
- Release of viral particles results in CD4+ cell lysis. There are also qualitative defects in T cells even in asymptomatic patients (*Clinical symptoms*).

- *Macrophages*
  - It acts as a factory and reservoir for virus.
  - It is a safe vehicle for HIV to be transported to other organs.
  - It provides a site for viral replication in the late phase of disease, when CD4+ cell count is greatly decreased.

- *Dendritic cell*
  - Mucosal Langerhans cells capture the virus and transport it to regional lymph nodes.

– Follicular dendritic cells in germinal center of lymph nodes are reservoirs of HIV.

- **CNS**
  – Viruses are brought by infected monocytes in circulation.
  – Exclusively by M tropic viruses

– Viruses infect macrophages and microgila; HIV does not infect neurons.
– Neurological deficit is due to direct effect of gp120 or indirectly by viral products and soluble factors (IL-1, TNF-α, IL-6) produced by macrophages/microglia. Nitric oxide produced is also held responsible.

- **Abnormalities of *immune functions***

Lymphopenia	Decreased T cell functions in vivo	Polyclonal B cell activation
• Selective loss of CD4+ Th-inducer cells	• Loss of memory T cells	• Hypergammaglobulinemia and circulating immune complexes
• Reversal of CD4+:CD8+ ratio	• ↑ Opportunistic infection	• ↓ Ab response to a new Ag
	• ↑ Neoplasm	• Loss of control/signal for B cell
Altered T cell function in vitro	• ↓ DTH reaction	function *in vitro*
	Altered monocytes/macrophages functions	
• ↓ lymphocyte proliferative response to mitogens and antigens	• ↓ Chemotaxis and phagocytosis	
	• ↓ HLA II expression	
• ↓ specific cytotoxicity	• ↓ Ag presentation	
• ↓ Th function aid to B cells	• ↑ IL-1, TNF-α, IL-6	
• ↓ IL-2 and INF-γ		

- **CDC classification categories of HIV infection**

Clinical categories	CD4+ T cell categories		
	1 > 500 cells/μl	2 499 to 200 cells/μl	3 < 200 cells/μl
A. • Asymptomatic cases • PGL (Persistent generalized lymphadenopathy)	A$_1$	A$_2$	A$_3$
B. Symptomatic cases other than those in A and C	B$_1$	B$_2$	B$_3$
C. AIDS indicator conditions (include many constitutional, neurological and neoplastic conditions)			

AIDS defining opportunistic infections

Protozoal and helminthic

- Cryptosporidiosis or isosporidiosis (enteritis)

- Toxoplasmosis (pneumonia or CNS infection)

Fungal

- Pneumocystosis (pneumonia or disseminated infection)

- Candidiasis (esophageal, tracheal and pulmonary infections)
- Cryptococcosis (CNS infection)
- Coccidioidomycosis (disseminated infection)
- Histoplasmosis (disseminated infection)

Bacterial infections

- Mycobacteriosis (atypical and mycobacterium tuberculosis, pulmonary and extrapulmonary)
- Nocardiosis (pneumonia, meningitis, and disseminated infection)
- Salmonella infection

Viral

- Cytomegalovirus (pulmonary, interstitial, retinal or CNS infection)
- Herpes simplex virus (localized or disseminated infection)
- Varicella zoster virus (localized or disseminated infection)
- Progressive multifocal leukoencephalopathy

AIDS defining neoplasms

- Kaposi sarcoma
- B cell non-Hodgkin's lymphoma
- Primary lymphoma of brain
- Invasive cancer of uterine cervix

Laboratory diagnosis

Non-specific tests

↓↓ TLC	T4:T8 ratio reversal	↓↓ CMI
↓↓ lymphocyte count (< 2000/cu mm)	Thrombocytopenia	LN, abnormality on biopsy
< 200 CD4+ T cells/μl	↓↓ IgG and IgA levels	↑ β_2 microglobulin level

Lymph node biopsy

Specific tests

- *Antigen detection*
  - Acute illness/seroconversion stage: p24 antigenemia and veremia, also appearance of IgM thereafter.
  - Asymptomatic phase: Decreased or absence of free p24, but Ab-bound p24 Ag may be demonstrated.
  - Stage of clinical disease: Highly increased free p24 Ag
  - Method: Antigen capture ELISA
  - In the first few weeks after infection and in terminal phase, the test is uniformly positive.
- *Antibody detection*
  - Simplest and most widely used method.

  - It is negative in *window period* that follows infection; time taken to appear antibodies (first IgM followed by IgG).

a. *ELISA*
  - More sensitive, but not so specific.
  - Types used: Direct solid phase antiglobulin ELISA, capture ELISA specific for IgM Ab, rapid tests like dipstick test, immunoperoxidase, cassette ELISA, etc.

b. *Western blot test*: "Gold standard test". More specific than ELISA.
  - *PCR*: Now "new gold standard" test for diagnosis in all stages of HIV.
  - *Viral isolation* and culture in neoplastic T cell line.

26. Difference between primary and secondary amyloidoses (1998, 2000)

S. No.	Traits	Primary (systemic) amyloidosis	Secondary amyloidosis
1.	Cause	30% associated with plasma cell dyscrasias, multiple myeloma, monoclonal gammapathies; rest is idiopathic	Associated with chronic inflammation, chronic non-infectious inflammatory condition of tumors

(Contd.)

Difference between primary and secondary amyloidoses (Contd.)

S. No.	Traits	Primary (systemic) amyloidosis	Secondary amyloidosis
2.	Chemical nature	AL	AA
3.	Chemically related precursor protein	Immunoglobulin light chain, chiefly lambda and kappa chains	SAA (serum associated amyloid from liver)
4.	Congo red	After prior treatment with permanganate on section, congo red stain is repeated— congo red positivity persists (*Congophilia*)	Turns negative for congo red
5.	Parts more severely affected	Affects skin, bowel, heart, skeletal muscles and less in solid abdominal visceral organs	More in solid abdominal visceral organs like liver, spleen, kidney, adrenals, etc.
6.	Condition associated	↑ed bone marrow plasma cells	In cases like RCC, HD, TB, chronic osteomyelitis, RA and bronchiectasis
7.	Distribution	Worldwide	More in developing and under-developed countries
8.	Frequency	Most common form of amyloidosis	Less common
9.	Pathogenesis	Stimulus → monoclonal B cell proliferation → excess light chains → partial degradation → insoluble AL fibrils	Stimulus → chronic inflammation → activation of macrophages → cytokines → partial degradation → insoluble AA

27. Etiopathogenesis of amyloidosis (2002, 09)

28. Chemical nature of amyloid. Its classification. Or physicochemical properties of amyloids (1999)

- Amyloid is a pathologic proteinaceous substance, deposited between cells in various tissues and organs of the body in variety of diseases.
- They are made of fibril material (95%) and remaining are P component and other proteins.
  - AL (amyloid light chain)—produced by plasma cells. It may be complete Ig chain or amino terminal fragment of light chain or mixed. Mostly λ type. Deposition associated with monoclonal B cell proliferation.
  - AA (amyloid associated) chain: Produced by liver.
  - Aβ amyloid found in cerebral lesion of Alzheimer's disease.
  - Transthyretin (TTR)
  - β_2 *microglobulin*

Two categories of amyloid proteins

i. Misfolded proteins (production of abnormal amount of normal proteins) are unstable and self-associate and form oligomers and fibrils.

ii. Mutant proteins (production of normal amount of mutant proteins) are structurally unstable, prone to misfolding and subsequently aggregates.

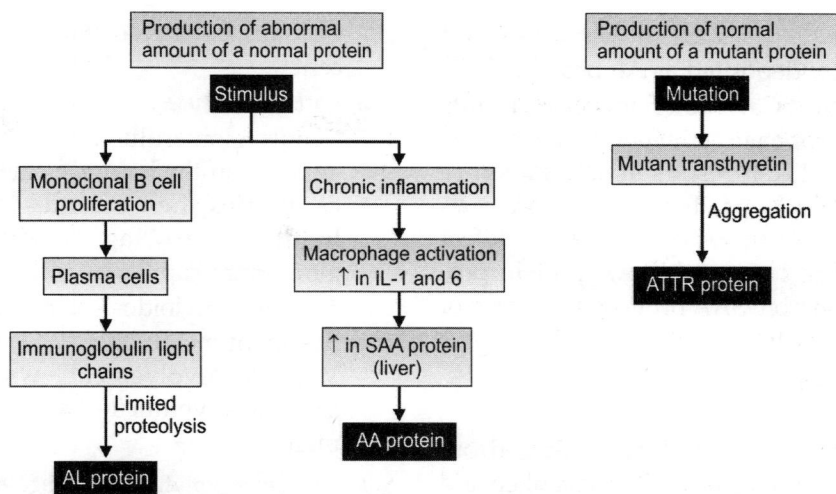

Fig. 6.11: Types of amyloid proteins

- **Classification:** (*see textbook*)

29. Stains of amyloids (1997, 98, 2001, 03, 08, 11)

Staining characteristics of amyloid

	Stain used	*Appearance*
Stain on gross	Lugol's iodine	Imparts purple color, on addition of dilute sulfuric acid turns blue
Hematoxylin and eosin	H and E	In light microscopy appears as extracellular homogeneous structureless eosinophilic hyaline material
Metachromatic stain (Rosamine dyes)	Methyl violet and crystal violet	Rose pink coloration of amyloid deposits
Congo red	Congo red	Ordinary light: Pink Polarized light: Apple green birefringence
Fluorescent stains	Thioflavin-T	Yellow under UV light
Immunohistochemistry	Various Ab stains against specific Ag protein type— anti-AA, anti-AL, anti-kappa	
Non-specific stains	von Giesen Immunoperoxidase Toluidine blue Alcian blue Periodic acid schiff (PAS)	Blue green color or orthochromatic blue

30. Changes and pathogenesis in kidney in amyloidosis

- Most common and potentially most serious form of organ involvement.

- **Pathogenesis**
  - *Primary*: Unknown agent results in monoclonal B cell proliferation—plasma cells producing Ig light chains that are

somewhat resistant to proteolysis and they are deposited as AL protein.

– *Secondary:* Chronic inflammation results in macrophage activation and release of IL-1 and 6. It results in stimulation of liver cells to produce SAA. There is an enzymatic (monocyte derived) defect resulting in insoluble AA protein production from SAA proteolysis instead of normal soluble protein.

• *Morphology*

  Gross

  – Size may appear normal or enlarged, but in the advanced case it is shrunken and contracted.

– Cut surface is pale, waxy and translucent.

Microscopic features:

– Mainly glomerulus involvement—first appears on the basement membrane of capillaries then extends to produce luminal narrowing and distortion of glomerular capillaries tuft.

– Tubule—amyloidosis starts from tubular basement membrane.

– Vascular involvement—wall of small arterioles, venules—narrowing of lumen.

Note: Spleen in amyloidosis—*sago* spleen and *lardaceous* spleen (*for viva*) (2000).

31. Difference between immunoglobulin allotype and idiotype (1995)

Idiotype	Isotype	Allotypes
Antibodies have antigen-binding sites called paratope. Specific antigenic determinant on the paratope is called idiotope. Sum of the total of idiotopes on an Ig molecule constitute its idiotype. It is of greatest biological importance.	Antigenic specificities, which distinguish the different classes and subclasses of Ig present in all normal individuals of a given species.	Differentiated between immunoglobulin type of individual. Antigenic specificities which distinguish Ig of the same class, betweem different groups of individuals in the same species.

32. Difference between helper T cell and cytotoxic T cell (1995, 2002)

33. Difference between helper T cell and suppressor T cell* (1989, 94)

S. No.	Traits	Helper T cells (T-DTH)	Cytotoxic T lymphocytes (T-CTL)
1.	CD type	CD 4 +ve; CD8 –ve	CD8 +ve; CD4 –ve
2.	% of peripheral T cells	60%	30%
3.	Ag recognition in association with	HLA class II	HLA class I
4.	Functions	Act by releasing lymphokines and activate macrophages, B cells and T-CTL. Central to immune response.	Act as cytotoxic cells by pore formation and release of granzymes/protease. Also Fas-Fas ligand dependent killing.
5.	Condition in AIDS	Impaired, CD4+ cell count ↓↓	Remains activated, plays important role in initial HIV containment. Count—normal

(*Contd.*)

Difference between helper T cell and suppressor T cell* (Contd.)

S. No.	Traits	Helper T cells (T-DTH)	Cytotoxic T lymphocytes (T-CTL)
6.	Function	Regulation of immune T, B cells, macrophages and NK cell functions. Mediate delayed type hypersensitivity like granulomatous inflammation	Specific cell-mediated cytotoxicity like graft rejection, virus infected cells, tumor cells death, etc.

*Suppressor T cell is type of CD8+, CD4– (as T-CTL) cells that act to inhibits B cell antibody synthesis and has other inhibitory functions.

34. Difference between Th1 cells and Th2 cells

S. No.	Traits	Th1 cells	Th2 cells
1.	IL-2 and interferon-γ	Secreted by it	Not secreted by it
2.	IL-4 and IL-5	Not secreted by it	Secreted by it
3.	Functions	Facilitating DTH, macrophage activation, synthesis of IgG2b Ab	Synthesis of other class Ig including IgE

35. Difference between hyaline and amyloid materials (1994) (rarely asked, see Textbook)

36. Difference between type I and type II major histocompatibility antigens (1998)

S. No.	Traits	MHC I	MHC II
1.	Location	Present on all nucleated cells of body and platelets. It may function as components of hormone receptors.	Found on antigen presenting cells—macrophages, dendritic cells, activated T cells and B cells.
2.	Structure	Alpha chains (α_1, α_2, α_3) and beta chain (β_2-microglobulin)	Alpha chain (α_1, α_2) and beta chains (β_1, β_2)
3.	Genes coding region	HLA-A, HLA-B, HLA-C	HLA-D (HLA-DP, HLA-DQ, HLA-DR)
4.	Ag presentation in its association to	CD8+ cells	CD4+ cells
5.	Functions	Graft rejection, cell-mediated cytolysis—virus infected, tumor cells, intracellular infected cell	Graft versus host response, immunologic reaction of CD4+ T cells—mixed leukocyte reaction (MLR)

37. Significance of HLA complex (1988)

38. Role of HLA in disease (2004)

- Association of diseases with HLA has been broadly classified into three groups:
  - Inflammatory disease like ankylosing spondylitis and postinfectious arthropathies
  - Inherited errors of metabolism like 21-hydroxylase deficiency
  - Autoimmune disease like endocrinopathies

- Summary of diseases and HLA:

Diseases	HLA allele	Diseases	HLA allele
Ankylosing spondylitis	B27	Chronic active hepatitis	DR3
Postgonococcal arthritis	B27	Primary Sjögren's syndrome	DR3
Acute anterior uveitis	B27	Insulin dependent DM	DR3, DR4, DR3/DR4
Rheumatoid arthritis	DR4	21-hydroxylase deficiency	BW47

39. Mechanism of action of CD4+ T cells (2004)

(How Ag is presented to T cells and how T cells response to Ag presentation, its action on T and B cells, other cells; see Microbiology: Immune Response–diagram of immune response against T cell dependent Ag).

40. Cell-mediated hypersensitivity (2007)

(*Refer to textbook*)

7

Neoplasia

Definitions

1. **Neoplasia:** Neoplasia (new growth) is excessive and unregulated proliferation that eventually becomes autonomous (independent of physiologic growth stimuli).

2. **Neoplasm:** A neoplasm is an abnormal mass of tissue, the growth of which it exceeds and is uncoordinated with that of normal tissue and persists in same excessive manner even after cessation of the stimuli which evoked the change.

3. **Tumor:** It means a swelling, which could be due to any cause, but this term is most commonly used for neoplasm.

4. **Benign tumor and malignant tumor:** Benign tumor is a type of localized neoplasm without potential to migrate to distant organ, while malignant tumor has the potential to spread to the distant organ.

5. **Cancer:** It is a common term for malignant tumor (derived from latin word crab—adherent to any part it seizes upon obstinately like a crab).

6. **Clonality:** A tumor is said to be clonal, if the entire population of cells within a tumor arises from a single cell that has incurred genetic changes.

7. **Desmoplasia:** Hyperplasia of fibroblasts and formation of abundant collagenous stroma as a reaction to infiltration by cancer is labelled as desmoplasia.

8. **Teratoma:** Tumors derived from a variety of cell types representing more than one germ cell layer, usually all three.

9. **Choriostoma:** An ectopic nest of a normal tissue, e.g. a nest of adrenal cells under the kidney capsule.

10. **Hamartoma:** An aberrant differentiation may produce a mass of disorganized, but mature, specialized cells/ tissue indigenous to the particular site (thought to an anomalous development or a neoplasm in origin), e.g. hamartoma of a lung.

11. **Aplasia:** Aplasia is defined as lack of differentiation. It is a hallmark of malignant transformation.

    Morphological features indicative of ana- plasia are:

    - Pleomorphism (variation in size and shape of cells)
    - Anisonucleosis (variation in size of nuclei)
    - Abnormal nuclear morphology includ- ing abundant and darkly stained (hyperchromatic) DNA, coarsely clum- ped chromatin, increased nucleocyto- plastic ratio (normal 1:4 to 1:6, may approach to 1:1).

- Numerous mitoses with abnormal, atypical, bizarre, tri-, quadri- and multipolar spindles.
- Loss of polarity (orientation of cell)

12. **Dysplasia:** Dysplasia is defined as loss of architectural orientation of cells with respect to one another and presence of pleomorphism, nuclear atypia, hyperchromatism and mitoses.

13. **Metaplasia:** It is a reversible change in which one adult cell type is replaced by another adult cell type.

1. Difference between hamartoma and neoplasia (1991)

S. No.	Traits	Hamartoma	Neoplasia
1.	Definition	Disorganized and excessive focal overgrowth of mature normal cells of tissues localized to particular site	Abnormal, excessive, uncoordinated, autonomous and purposeless proliferation of cells
2.	Malignancy	Totally benign	Benign or malignant
3.	Cell differentiation	Cells are completely differentiated and totally resemble normal counterparts.	Vary from completely differentiated to anaplastic
4.	Cell origin	Polyclonal	Monoclonal
5.	Examples	Hemangioma	Squamous cell carcinoma

2. Difference between dysplasia and anaplasia

S. No.	Traits	Dysplasia	Anaplasia
1.	Definition	Loss in the uniformity of individual cells (mainly epithelium) as well as loss in their architecture orientation. Cell character changes.	Anaplasia denotes lack of differentiation of cells. They deviate morphologically and functionally from original cells.
2.	Malignancy	A precancerous condition, which may or may not progress to neoplasm	Characteristics of most malignant tumors
3.	Pleomorphism	Present, but low grade	High degree of variation in size and shape of cell and nuclei
4.	Hyperchromatism	Present, but lesser degree	Highly pyknotic nuclei
5.	N:C ratio	Increased ($\uparrow$ed)	$\uparrow\uparrow\uparrow$ ed
6.	Nucleoli	Not so prominent	Very prominent, > 1
7.	Mitotic figures	Present, may be at abnormal places, but not atypical	Abnormal and atypical, having tripolar, quadripolar and multipolar spindles
8.	Tumor giant cells	Absent	Present
9.	Cytoplasmic organelles	Not lost	Cellular constituents may be lost with the loss of normal cellular functions
10.	Reversibility	Becomes irreversible, if involves whole thickness of epithelium; otherwise reversible	Irreversible
11.	Necrosis	Absent	Present
12.	Hemorrhage	Absent	Present

3. Metaplasia (1995, 2007)

4. Difference between metaplasia and dysplasia (1995, 99, 2008, 11)

S. No.	Traits	Metaplasia	Dysplasia
1.	Definition	Reversible change in which one adult cell type (epithelial or mesenchymal) is replaced by another adult cell type.	Loss in the uniformity of individual cells (mainly epithelium) as well as loss in their architectural orientation. Cell character changes.
2.	Pleomorphism	Absent	Regarding cell/nuclei size and shape present considerably
3.	Nuclei	Normal (like the type to which it has changed)	Hyperchromatic and abnormally large in comparison to cell size
4.	Mitotic figures	Very less and limited to normal places	Present at normal and also at abnormal place/sites
5.	Architecture of cells in tissues	Not lost	Anarchy, like loss of ordered maturation as in stratified squamous epithelium
6.	Reversibility	Reversible, if triggering factors are removed.	Becomes irreversible, if involves whole thickness of epithelium; otherwise reversible.
7.	Role	Adaptive change	Not adaptive
8.	Conversion to tumor	In chronic condition it may give rise to tumor.	Have more propensities
9.	Examples	Columnar to squamous epithelium in respiratory tract in chronic smokers Barrett's esophagus	Cervical intraepithelial neoplasia (CIN), dysplasia of squamous cells

5. Difference between benign and malignant tumors (1997, 2001)

S. No.	Traits	Benign tumor	Malignant tumor
1.	Gross		
	Boundaries	Encapsulated or well circumscribed/demarcated	Poorly circumscribed
	Size	Usually small	Often large
	Necrosis	Rare	Frequent
	Hemorrhage	Rare	Frequent
	Surrounding tissues	Often compressed	Infiltrated, invaded
2.	Microscopic		
	Pattern	Closely resemble the tissue of origin	Poorly resemble original tissue
	Basal polarity	Retained	Lost
	Pleomorphism	Usually absent	Often present
	N:C ratio	Normal (1:4–1:6)	Increases, approach 1:1
	Cytoplasm	Normal constituent usually present	Reduced or lost

(Contd.)

Difference between benign and malignant tumors (Contd.)

S. No.	Traits	Benign tumor	Malignant tumor
	Hyperchromatism	Absent	Present
	Nuclear chromatin	Fine	Condensed
	Nuclear shape	Regular	Irregular
	Nucleoli	May be present	Always present, prominent
	Mitotic figures	Present but typical/normal	Increased, atypical and abnormal
	Tumor giant cells	If present without nuclear atypia	Present with nuclear atypia
3.	Growth rate	Usually slow	Rapid (usually)
4.	Local invasion	Compresses local structures without infiltrating or invading	Infiltrate and invade surrounding structures
5.	Metastasis	Absent	Characteristics*
6.	Clinical function of organ	Usually retained	May be retained, lost or abnormal
	Prognosis	Better	Usually worse

*Gliomas and basal cell carcinoma are malignant, highly locally invasive, but do not metastasize (Viva).

6. Difference between epithelial and connective tissue tumors (2011)

7. Difference between carcinoma and sarcoma (1993, 95, 98, 99, 2001, 02)

S. No.	Traits	Carcinoma/Epithelial tumor	Sarcoma/Connective tissue tumor
1.	Definition	Malignant tumors of epithelial cell origin, derived from any of three germ layers.	Malignant tumors arising in mesenchymal tissue
2.	Age	> 40 yr	Earlier age of onset
3.	Growth	Slow	Rapid
4.	Microscopy	Groups of tumor cells forming structure or clusters are separated by connective tissues.	Each tumor cell is separated by mesenchymal tissues.
5.	Blood vessels	Less vasculature, confined to stroma	Highly vascularized, may invade beyond stroma
6.	Spread	Usually lymphatic	Usually hematogenous
7.	Immunocytochemistry	Shows presence of keratin	Shows presence of desmin
8.	Prognosis	Good	Poor
9.	Examples	Adenocarcinoma, squamous cell carcinoma	Fibrosarcoma, leiomyosarcoma

8. Difference between hyperplasia and neoplasia

S. No.	Traits	Hyperplasia	Neoplasia
1.	Definition	Increased number of cells due to cell division in tissues or organs in controlled manner	Uncontrolled cell division resulting in increased number of cells in tissue or organs.
2.	Cells status	Cells are differentiated	May be differentiated or undifferentiated
3.	Cell to cell contact	Present	Lost
4.	Cells type	Polyclonal	Usually monoclonal
5.	Effects of removal of stimulus	Stops, once stimulus removed	No effect. Continued cell proliferation
6.	Type	May be physiological or pathological	Always pathological
7.	Metastasis/ invasion	Always absent	Present in malignant cases, benign type shows pressure effects
8.	Organs involved	All cells except nerve cells, cardiac and skeleton muscles cells	No exception. All tissues are predisposed.
9.	Examples	Hyperplasia in uterus in pregnancy	Squamous cell carcinoma

9. Difference between hyperplasia and hypertrophy (1993, 96, 2002)

S. No.	Traits	Hyperplasia	Hypertrophy
1.	Definition	Increase in number of cells in an organ or tissue, which may lead to ↑ in its size	Increase in size of cells leading ↑ in the size of organ
2.	Process	Due to stimuli (physical/ hormonal), there is cell division in adaptation	Due to physical/hormonal stimuli, there is synthesis of cellular constituents resulting in increased size
3.	Cell features:		
	• Cell size	• Normal or slightly decreased	• Increased
	• Cytoplasm	• Reduced	• Increased
	• N:C ratio	• Normal/slightly increased	• Reduced
4.	Mitotic figures	Present	Absent
5.	Conversion to tumor	May occur	Never
6.	Examples	Hyperplasia (also hypertrophy) in uterus in pregnancy	In muscle after prolonged duration of exercise

10. Difference between hyperplasia and metaplasia

S. No.	Traits	Hyperplasia	Metaplasia
1.	Definition	Increased number of cells in an organ or tissue, which may lead to increase in its size	This is a reversible change in which one adult cell type (epithelial or mesenchymal) is replaced by another adult cell type
2.	Role	It may be pathological or physiological (adaptive).	Epithelial metaplasia is always reversible, while connective tissue metaplasia is irreversible
3.	Reversibility	Always reversible	
4.	Conversion to tumor	Present, but lesser	More
5.	Examples	Hyperplasia in uterus in pregnancy	Barrett's esophagus

11. Teratoma (1990, 96)
(*See male and female reproductive systems*)

12. Pathway of spread of tumors (1994, 97, 2001, 03, 07, 11)

Lymphatic spread
- Mainly carcinoma, but sarcoma may also take this path.
- The pattern of lymph node involvement follows the natural routes of drainage of that particular organ like cancer of upper outer quadrant of breast drain to axillary lymph node, while that of inner quadrant to internal mammary group.
- Tumor cells may grow in a continuous fashion (lymphatic permeation) or may form emboli in lymphatic channel. Such tumor emboli enter lymph node at its convex surface, first confined to subcapsular sinus, but later on involving entire node.
- In such cases there is lymph node enlargement, but this is not a characteristic of lymphatic spread of tumor as lymph node enlargement is also present in reactive hyperplasia (due to tumor cell debris or tumor Ag).
- Lymph node may act as a barrier to the spread of tumor though for only some time.
- Sometimes, lymph nodes may be bypassed (*skip metastasis*) due to venous-lymphatic anastomoses or obliteration of lymphatic channel.
- A "sentinel lymph node" is defined as the first node in the regional lymphatic chain to receive lymph flow from the primary tumor.

Hematogenous spread
- Mainly sarcoma, but carcinoma may also take this path.
- Cancer cells invade walls of capillaries, veins and venules readily than arteries (they have thick walls).
- *Favored sites*: Lung (all caval blood flow), liver (all portal blood), kidney, brain, bones; while spleen and skeleton muscles are rarely involved.
- Tumors like renal cell carcinoma invade branches of vein and grow in snake-like fashion even reaching to right side of heart. Likewise, hepatocellular carcinoma may penetrate portal and hepatic radicles to grow within them into main venous system. Such growth may occur without any widespread of tumor.

Seeding of body cavities and surface
- *Transcoelomic spread:* Such a tumor penetrates serosal layer to be carried to a distant place by coelomic fluids. Peritoneal cavity (most common), pleural and pericardial cavities are involved.

Examples: Ovarian tumor coats whole of peritoneal surface; are confined to surface only and may not penetrate into substance of organ.

- *Spread by CSF:* CNS tumors
- Spread along *epithelial lined surfaces:* Like tumor through bronchus to alveoli.
- Iatrogenic *implantation:* Surgical/any such clinical means

13. Enumerate cancer related genes

Genetic mutation of various genes results in loss of control of cellular proliferation/ differentiation or gain of cellular proliferation resulting in uncontrolled cellular growth.

- Excessive and autonomous growth: It involves growth promoting oncogenes.
- Refractoriness to growth inhibitors: It involves growth suppressing antioncogenes (Rb gene, p53, transforming growth factor-β, APC gene, WT-1 gene, NF gene, BRCA-1 and 2, VHL gene, PTEN, cadherins and KLF-6).
- *Evasion of cell death by apoptosis:* It involves genes regulating apoptosis and cancer.
- *Avoiding cellular ageing:* It involves telomers and telomerase.
- *Continued perfusion of cancer:* Angiogenesis
- Invasion and distant metastasis
- Damaged DNA repair system
- Cancer progression and tumor heterogenecity: Clonal aggressiveness

14. Oncogenes (2000)

- Oncogenes are cancer-causing genes, derivd from proto-oncogenes/cellular oncogenes (*c-oncs*).
- These proto-oncogenes are cellular genes that promote normal growth and differentiation of cells.
- Mechanism of activation of oncogenes from proto-oncogenes:

  – *Change in structure of genes:* Increased abnormal proteins (oncoproteins)
  – *Change in regulation of gene:* Increased normal growth promoting proteins
  Lesions resulting in above two conditions:
  1. *Point mutation: Ras* oncogene point mutation resulting in decreased GTPase activity.
  2. *Chromosomal rearrangement:* (translocation and inversion) Philadelphia chromosomes, Burkitt's lymphoma gene arrangement
  – Gene amplification
- Oncogenes are mutated and different from proto-oncogenes in following ways:
  – Presence of mutation in the structure of oncogenes is seen.
  – They have ability to promote cell growth in the absence of normal mitogenic signals and induces cancer.
  – They have ability to promote autonomous and excessive cellular proliferation, in the event of overexpression.

Oncoproteins

Oncoproteins are products of oncogenes, which resemble products of proto-oncogenes, but are devoid of important regulatory mechanisms.

- Growth factors (GFs) like PDGF, TGF-α, FGF
- Growth factor receptors like ErbB1 (EGF receptor) in squamous cell carcinoma, HER-2 (ErbB2) in carcinoma breast, lung, ovary and stomach.
- *Signal transduction proteins:* Mutated RAS gene
- Proteins involved in signal transduction
  – GTP-binding (K-RAS, H-RAS, N-RAS)
  – Non-receptor tyrosin kinase
- Nuclear regulatory proteins
  – Transcriptional activator (myc)
- Cell cycle regulators
  – Cyclins
  – Cyclins dependent kinase

15. Burkitt's Lymphoma genetic changes

- Example of translocation induced over expression of proto-oncogenes.
- *Genes involved*
  - *c-myc* gene located on the chromosome 8q24.
  - One of three immunoglobulin gene-carrying chromosomes.
- In normal position, the expression of *c-myc* gene is tightly controlled and it expresses only in certain stages of cell cycles.
- *Chromosomal abnormality*
  - There is translocation of *c-myc* containing segment (chromosome 8) to chromosome 14q band 32. This results in translocation of *c-myc* gene to chromosome 14 near immunoglobulin heavy chain gene.

- Regulatory element of Ig heavy chain allows high turnover of *c-myc* gene or there is mutation in the regulatory element of *c-myc* gene, producing increased quantity of *myc* protein; because in both cases the coding sequence remains intact.

16. Philadelphia chromosomes (1994, 95)
(*See disorders of white blood cells*)

17. Gene amplification

- (*see textbook for detail*)
- Activation of proto-oncogenes by reduplication and amplification of their DNA sequences.
- Examples of amplification are *N-myc* in neuroblastoma and *c-ErbB2* in breast cancers.

18. Difference between antioncogene and proto-oncogene (1995)

S. No.	Traits	Antioncogene	Proto-oncogene
1.	Synonyms	Cancer suppressor gene	Precursor genes for oncogene
2.	Normal functions	Its products apply brakes to cell. proliferation, and promotes differentiation and muturation of cells	Its products promote normal cell growth and differentiation
3.	Mutation	Homozygous inactivation, i.e. loss of both normal copies of gene is required for carcinogenesis	Mostly mutation in single copy leads to oncogenic conversion
4.	Mode of action	Acts passively, i.e. due to loss of its normal function, other cancer promoting factors dominate and lead to tumor.	Acts actively, i.e. gene products of oncogenes directly lead to tumor by some cellular alteration.
5.	Examples	p53, Rb gene, BRCA-1 and 2	myc, N-myc, ErbB/1/2/3, etc.

19. Tumor suppressor gene (2000, 04)

20. Rb Genes

- (*Also see retinoblastoma in chapter CNS and Eye*).
- *Location*: 13q14 (chromosome 13)
- First tumor suppressor gene to be discovered.

- *Mechanism of action:*
  - Its product *pRb protein* is a nucleoprotein, which is present in every type of cell and plays important role in regulation of cell cycle.
  - Quiescent cells (in G_0 and early G_1 phases) contain *active hypophosphorylated* form of *pRb*. In this form, it binds with

E2F transcription factor and prevents cell replication. When resting cells are activated by growth factors like increased D, E cyclins (activation of cyclin D/CDK4, CDK6, cyclin E/CDK2), pRb are phosphorylated (hyperphosphorylated form—inactive).

– The hyperphosphorylated form of *pRb* releases E2F transcription factors—promoting cell cycle into S and M phases.

– During the M phase, phosphate groups are removed from *pRb* by cellular phosphatase, thus regenerating dephosphorylated form of *pRb*—arrest of cell cycle.

21. p53 Genes

- *Location*: 17p13.1
- "A little over 50% of human tumors contain mutation in *p53 gene*".
- This gene acts as "gatekeeper gene"/"molecular policeman"/"guardian of the genome" that prevents the propagation of genetically damaged cells.
- Its product *p53* is a nucleoprotein localized to nucleus.
- In contrast to *pRb*, *p53* does not police normal cell cycle.
- Cell with *normal p53 gene*
  – Whenever there is DNA damage due to irradiation, UV light or chemicals or in case of hypoxia; there is activation of p53 gene.
  – p53 (protein) binds with DNA and stimulates transcription of several genes that mediate: Cells *cycle arrest* and *repair*.
  – p53 dependent transcription of CDK inhibitor p21 (it prevents phosphorylation of pRb necessary for cell to enter S phase): G_1 phase arrest—more time for cell repair.
  – Transcription of GADD45 (growth arrest and DNA damage) may repair cell by unknown mechanism.

– If repair fails to be achieved, injured cells undergo apoptosis with the help of GADD45 and bax gene.
- Cells with (homozygous loss of function) *mutated p53 gene*:
  – There is no activation of p53 dependent genes, no cell cycle arrest.
  – No repair of damaged DNA. Mutant cells undergo expansion.
  – In due course, there is additional mutation resulting in monoclonal malignant tumor.
- "Hypoxia selects for cells in which p53 gene is inactive and propagation of p53 deficient cells is favored" so, survival of tumor cells despite of initial hypoxic condition in and nearby lesion.

22. Telomeres

- Most cells have limited capacity to divide; and after a fixed number of divisions, cells are arrested in a non-dividing terminal stage (*cellular senescence*).
- Many postulations have been given to explain how these cells "count number of divisions"—most interesting and consistent finding have been *shortening of telomeres after each cell division*.
- Telomeres are present at the end of each chromosome. They consist of short and repeat TG-rich sequence. Human telomeres have variable number of repeat sequences 5'-TTAGGG-3'. They are important for integrity of chromosomes as they prevent end-to-end chromosomal fusion.
- When telomeres are reduced to a certain short length by a fixed number of cell divisions, telomeres loses its function. There is end-to-end chromosomal fusion and net result of cell death by apoptosis.
- *Telomerase (enzyme)* prevents shortening of telomeres in normal rapidly/continuously dividing cells like germ cells/bone marrow cells. They are absent from somatic cells and, hence no reparative elongation of telomeres after cell cycle in such cells.

- But as we know tumor cells undergo continuous and rapid cell division. These tumor cells must have some mechanism to prevent shortening of telomeres (i.e. telomerase or alike activity).
- This is the subject of interest as *"telomere shortening is a tumor suppressive mechanism"*.

23. Mechanism of invasion and metastasis of malignant tumor

Stages
- *Invasion of extracellular matrix*
  This is an active process having following steps from its primary growth:
  a. Detachment (loosening up) of tumor cells from each other—breaking of epithelial cadherin, a transmembrane glycoprotein adhering two adjacent cells.
  b. Adhesion to and invasion of basement membrane.
  c. Attachment to matrix components— tumor cell's integrins attaches to ECM like fibronectin.
  d. Degradation of extracellular matrix (proteolytic enzyme by tumor cells or induced normal cells like stromal/ macrophages—most important of being metalloproteinase and MMP including collagenase IV).
  e. Migration of tumor cells through extracellular matrix to reach blood vessel or lymphatic channel.
- *Vascular dissemination*
  - Intravagation by permeating through the vessel wall.
  - Formation of tumor emboli (homotype adhesion of tumor cells together and heterotype adhesion of tumor cells and blood components like platelet, RBC and WBC) resulting in averting immune phagocytosis.
- *Homing of tumor cells at secondary sites*
  - Exact mechanism remains unclear regarding selection of some preferred sites for homing.
  - Adhesion molecule CD44 on endothelium may be used for extravasation as do lymphocytes.
  - Metastatic deposits in secondary sites and proliferation of tumor cells.
  - Angiogenesis.
  - Secondary tumor results.

24. Chemical carcinogens and carcinogenesis (1994, 99, 2008, 11)

Chemical carcinogens

Direct acting carcinogens[1*]	
Alkylating agents:	*Acylating agents:*
• Dimethyl sulfate • Anticancer drugs like cyclophosphamide, nitrosoureas • β-propiolactone	• 1-acetyl-1-imidazole

[1*]: They are highly reactive electrophilic groups that can react with nucleophilic sites like nucleotides in the cells producing covalent adducts.

Indirect acting[2*]	
Polycyclic, heterocyclic aromatic hydrocarbons:	*Aromatic amines, amides, azo dyes:*
• Benzanthracene • Benzopyrene • Dibenzanthracene	• β-naphthylamine • Benzidine • Azo dyes like butter yellow

[2*]: Agents that require metabolic activation before they can act as carcinogens.

Natural plants and microbial products	*Others*
• Aflatoxin	• Nitrosamine and amides
• Griseofulvin	• Vinyl chloride
• Betel nuts	• Insecticides, fungicides
• Actinomycin D	• Metals like nickel, chromium

Chemical carcinogenesis

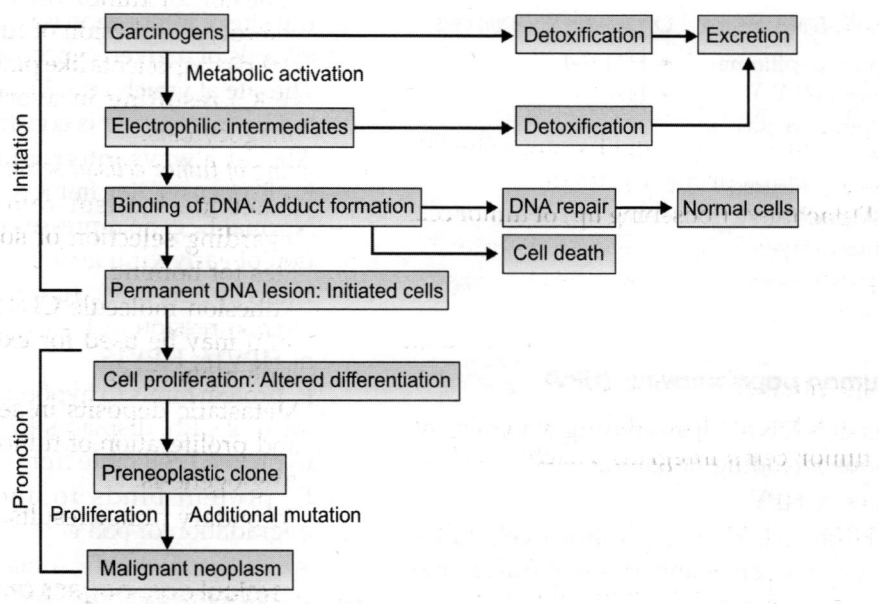

Fig. 7.1: Chemical carcinogenesis

25. Difference between initiators and promoters

S. No.	Traits	Initiators	Promoters
1.	Sequence of application	Applied first	Applied after initiator
2.	Mechanism	Induction of mutation	Not mutagenic; instead they are mitogenic. They induce cell cycling and reinforce the action of initiators.
3.	Dose	Single for a short time	Repeated over a long time
4.	Response	Sudden	Delayed
5.	Molecular change	Permanent/irreversible	Reversible
6.	Examples	Most chemical carcinogens	Hormones

26. Mechanism—how ionizing radiation causes cancer

(*See chapter 'Environmental and Nutritional Pathological'*)

27. Role of DNA viruses in neoplasia (1993, 95, 99, 2000, 02, 03, 04, 08, 11) or classify oncogenic viruses (1990, 99) or viral oncogenesis (1994)

Oncogenic DNA viruses	Oncogenic RNA viruses
• Human papilloma-viruses (HPVs)	• HTLV-1
• Epstein-Barr viruses (EBVs)	• HIV
• Hepatitis viruses (HBV and HCV)	
• Human herpes simplex viruses (HSV 8)	

28. Human papillomavirus (HPV)

- This is a DNA virus causing a variety of lesions including neoplasm.
- *Types* of HPV
  - High-risk HPV: Squamous cell carcinoma of cervix and anogenital area; oral and laryngeal cancer.
  - Low-risk HPV: Benign warts and pre-neoplastic lesions (HPV genome as episome non-integrated form)
- *Carcinoma cervix*
  Mechanism of action of virus:
  - HPV genome integrates with host genome.
  - Integration is must for malignant transformation.
  - Site of integration in the host genome cell differs in different persons.
  - But site of integration is identical within all cells of a given cancer in a person.
  - The site at which viral DNA is interrupted by integration is constant.
  - Almost always interruption is within E_1/E_2 open reading frame of viral genome.
  - Normal E_2 gene represses the transcription of early viral gene E_6/E_7.
  - Interruption of E_2 function results in overexpression of E_6/E_7 gene products of HPV16, HPV18.
  - E_7 protein binds to hypophosphorylated form of pRb, displaces E2F and frees it to proceed cell cycle from G_1 to S phase.
  - E_6 protein binds to and facilitates degradation of p53 gene product.
  - All these cause carcinoma of cervix.

Sequences producing neoplasms:

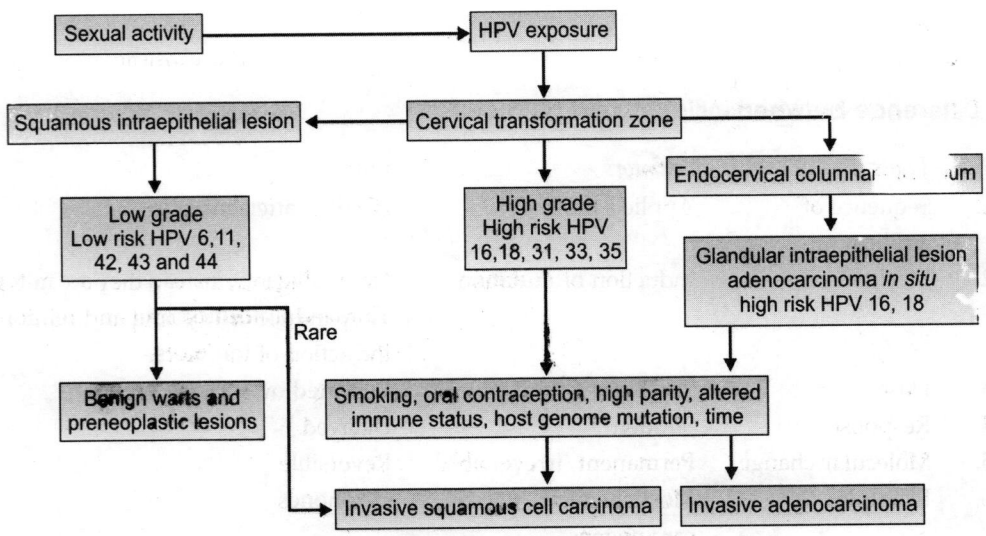

Fig. 7.2: HPV and carcinoma cervix

29. Epstein-Barr virus (EBV) (1998, 2002)

- DNA virus, a member of herpes family.
- Tumors associated with EBV:
  - African form of Burkitt's lymphoma
  - B cell lymphoma in immunosuppressed person like HIV or organ transplantation
  - Some Hodgkin's disease
  - Nasopharyngeal carcinoma
  - Gastric carcinoma
  - NK cell lymphoma
- *Pathogenesis*
  - EBV infects epithelial cells of oropharynx and B lymphocytes.
  - It enters B cells with the help of CD21 receptors present on every B cell.
  - Within B cells, the linear genome of EBV circularizes to form episome in host cell nuclei.

- There is no replication of virus or no host cell death (latent infection).
- Latent B cells are *immortalized* and acquire the *ability to propagate* indefinitely *in vitro*.
- *The mechanism of immortalization:* It is proposed that several viral genes dysregulate the normal proliferative and surviving signals in such host cells. For example, latent membrane protein (LMP-1) can induce cell growth and survival.

- EBV infection has been strongly associated with *Burkitt's lymphoma*, but this infection is *one of many* factors responsible for this lymphoma (Fig. 7.3).
  - EBV infection causes polyclonal B cell proliferation and failure of immunoregulation of proliferative cells.

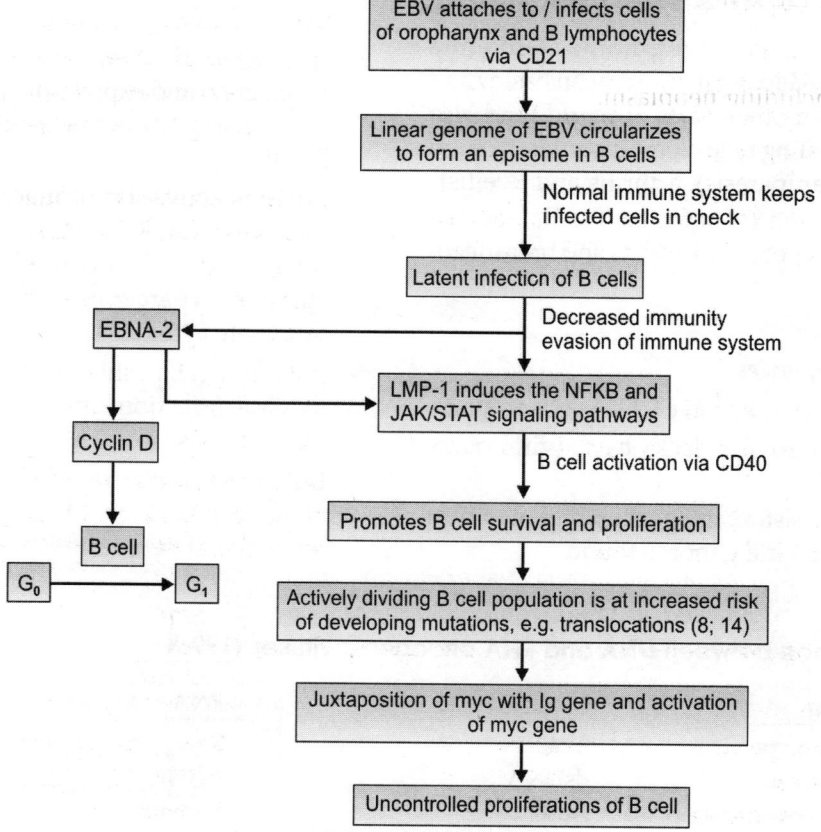

Fig. 7.3: Mechanism of EBV oncogenesis

- Any condition like chronic malaria that *further promotes* proliferation of B cells may result in mutation in rapidly dividing B cells and further propagation of such mutated cells, producing monoclonal proliferation.
- Now by chance/other means if *c-myc translocation* occurs in any of above monoclonal cells, it produces a subset of monoclonal cells with that mutation.
- Again if it is followed by *N-Ras* mutation in any of these subset of monoclonal cells, it results in monoclonal proliferation of B cells with accumulation of all mutations required for Burkitt's lymphoma.

30. Mechanism of RNA virus oncogenesis (1990, 2010)

31. Human T cell leukemia virus type I (HTLV-1)

- It causes T cell lymphoma/leukemia endemic in Japan and Caribbean basins and sporadic in other parts of world [and also demyelinating neurologic disorder (tropical spastic paraparesis), arthritis and uveitis].
- Transmission (of infected T cells): Sexual intercourse, blood products and breastfeeding

Pathogenesis
- *Virus properties*
  - These viruses have CD4+ cells tropism.
  - This retrovirus lacks *v-onc* (viral oncogenes).
  - No consistent integration region of host cells to viral genome found.

- But genomic integration shows clonal pattern in all tumor cells of one host.
- It has gag, pol, env, and LTR genes, but most important for pathogenesis is *tax* gene.

Tax gene
- Its product is essential for viral replication.
- Stimulates transcription of viral mRNA
- Stimulates transcription of several host cell genomes producing some bioactive substances like IL-2 and its receptors, GM-CSF.
- It prevents formation of complex between CDK4 and its inhibitor p16: Cell cycle becomes dysregulated.

- *Sequence*
  - HTLV-1 infection stimulated proliferation of T cells.
  - Increased IL-2 secretion, increased production and expression of IL-2 receptors causing 'autocrine' proliferation of T cell.
  - There is activation of macrophages by increased GM-CSF. Activated macrophages secrete IL-1 which in turn "extra stimulate" (paracrine activation) T cells to secrete cytokines.
  - Initially T cell proliferation is polyclonal as viral infection causes activation of many T cells.
  - But in due course, rapidly dividing cells acquire mutation to transform into monoclonal neoplasm.

32. Difference between DNA and RNA oncogenic viruses (1996)

S. No.	Traits	DNA oncogenic virus	RNA oncogenic virus
1.	Prototype virus	SV40	Rous sarcoma virus
2.	Genome	dsDNA	ssRNA
3.	Reverse transcriptase	Absent	Present

(Contd.)

Difference between DNA and RNA oncogenic viruses (Contd.)

S. No.	Traits	DNA oncogenic virus	RNA oncogenic virus
4.	Interaction with host genome	Linear DNA genome forms a double stranded circle within the infected cell and then covalently integrated into the host genome	First RNA is transcripted into dsDNA and then integrate into the host genome
5.	Name of gene	Early region A gene	src gene
6.	Name of protein	T antigen	src protein
7.	Function of protein	Protein kinase, ATPase activity, binding to DNA and stimulation of DNA synthesis	Protein kinase that phosphorylate tyrosine—disturbs the growth control process
8.	Location of protein	Primarily nuclear, but sometimes in plasma membrane	Plasma membrane
9.	Required for viral growth	Yes	No
10.	Genes have cellular homologue	No	Yes

Note: Protein products from both types of viruses are required for cell transformation.

33. Cancer cachexia

Characterized by
- Progressive loss of body fat and lean body mass
- Profound weakness
- *Anorexia*
  - No GIT obstruction generally
  - Abnormality in taste has been found
  - Central control of appetite is disturbed.
  - Increased BMR—increased calorie expense.
  - Equal loss of fat and muscle mass (protein)
  - This is due to TNF-α secreted by macrophages or tumor cells.
  - IL-1 or TNF-γ may synergy its action.
  - Other directly acting factors to mobilize fat and muscle masses are found.
  - Protein mobilizing factors have been found in some cases.
- *Anemia*
  - Due to action of soluble factors from tumor cells in response to tumors
  - Not due to nutritional demand of tumor

34. Paraneoplastic syndromes (2000, 04, 07)

- Paraneoplastic syndromes are group of conditions in cancer bearing patients that cannot be explained either by local or distant spread of the tumor or by the elaboration of hormones indigenous to the tissue from which the tumor has arose.
- *Importance*
  - Earliest manifestation of hidden cancer in some cases
  - May represent clinical problems due to excessive production of that hormone
  - May mimic metastatic disease
- The syndrome can be classified into: (see table on next page).
- *Endocrinopathies*
  - The most significant finding is the ectopic hormone/hormone-like substance production by cells of non-endocrine origin.
  - For example, in case of small cell carcinoma of lung, pancreatic or neural tumors; tumor cells produce ACTH or ACTH-like substance resulting in Cushing's syndrome.

Classification of paraneoplastic syndrome

Syndromes	Major forms of underlying cancer
Endocrinopathies	
Cushing's syndrome	Small cell ca of lung, pancreatic carcinoma
SIADH	Small cell ca of lung, intracranial neoplasm
Hyperkalcemia	Squamous cell ca of lung, breast ca, renal ca
Carcinoid syndrome	Bronchial adenoma, pancreatic adenoma, gastric ca
Neuromuscular	
Myasthenia	Bronchogenic ca of lung
Cerebellar degeneration	Small cell ca of lung
Lambert-Eaton syndrome	Small cell ca of lung
Peripheral neuropathy	Small cell ca of lung
Skin	
Acanthosis nigricans	Gastric carcinoma, bronchogenic carcinoma
Dermatomyositis	Bronchogenic carcinoma, breast ca
Osseous, articular	
Hypertrophic osteoarthropathy	Bronchogenic ca
Hematologic and vascular	
Venous thrombosis	Pancreatic ca, bronchogenic ca

Note: ca: carcinoma

– Similarly, in squamous cell carcinoma of lung, breast, renal, ovarian carcinoma; tumor cells produce excess of parathormone or related hormone, TNF-α, TGF-α, IL-1 causing hyperkalcemia (most common paraneoplastic syndrome).
– Gastric and bronchial carcinoid syndromes are subset of endocrinopathies related paraneoplastic syndromes.

35. Enumerate methods to diagnose cancer

1. Histological methods
2. Cytological methods: (FNAC, exfoliative cytology) (1987, 95)
3. Histochemistry and cytochemistry
4. Immunocytochemistry
5. Molecular diagnostic technique
6. Flow cytometry
7. Tumor markers
8. Radiological methods (for some aspects of tumor)

36. Histological method

• This method is the most often used and most valuable in arriving at the accurate diagnosis of tumor with support of clinical and other investigations.
• This method is based on the microscopic examination of properly fixed tissue.
• *Sample collection:* This is an important step because quality and type of sample will decide the result.
  – Methods are *excision or biopsy or needle aspiration:* Care has to be taken that the sample is taken from the appropriate site of lesion as central part of tumor would be necrotic and margins may show normal appearance.
  – Similarly, if lymph node biopsy is taken, cancer may be masked by reactive hyperplasia of LN.
• *Preservation of sample:* Formalin solution or special preservatives like glutaraldehyde for electron microscopy or quick frozen

section for quick staining and examination of sample to access that margins are devoid of cancer lesion after surgery is used.

- *Staining*: Special stains like PAS may be used, otherwise H and E staining is universally used.
- *Examination*: Usually examined in light microscope.
- *Histochemistry/Cytochemistry (special stains)*

These are diagnostic tools for identifying chemical composition of cells, for the purpose of tumor diagnosis and classification.

Substances	Stain
Basement membrane and collagen	PAS
	Reticulin
	van Gieson
	Masson's trichrome
Glycogen	PAS with diastase loss
Glycoproteins	PAS
Mucin of epithelial origin	Mucicarmine
Acid mucin of mesenchymal origin	Alcian blue
Argyrophillic/ Argentaffin granules/ Fungi	Silver stains
Fat	Oil red O, Sudan black B

37. Fine needle aspiration cytology (FNAC) (1998, 2000, 01)

Procedure

A syrine (10 ml) with a well-defined 23 gauge (or thicker) fine needle is used to aspirate the fluid/cells from the lesion that are palpated, if deep seated with the help of radiological images. Dry and wet (pap) smears are made and stained.

Applications

- *Routine uses:* For the diagnosis of palpable masses like lymph nodes, breast masses, enlarged thyroid, superficial soft tissue masses, salivary glands, palpable abdominal mass, testicular lesions.

Samples from prostate, pelvic organs, bones or joint spaces, lungs or retroperitoneum may also be obtained.

- *Special uses:* For non-palpable lesions, help of radiology may be taken.
  - Plain X-ray: Lesions of bones and some lesions of lung
  - CT scan: Chest and abdomen
  - Ultrasonography (USG): Extremely valuable for thyroid nodule, soft tissue masses, intraabdominal lesions and intrathoracic lesions about chest wall, but ineffective in deep-seated intrathoracic lesions and bony lesions

Advantages of FNAC

- It is an OPD procedure, no hospitalization or any special preparation.
- Quick, safe and little invasive—less pain.
- No anesthesia is required.
- Cost effective (low cost)
- Procedure can be repeated, not inconvenient.

Disadvantages

- Problem in deep-seated lesion, though radiology may reduce this problem.
- Reliablity of test varies much, as only small portion of cell representative of that particular place (not whole lesion) is aspirated. So sample from *"not exact place"* of lesion may give false negative result despite of clinical findings. In such cases, FNAC should be repeated or biopsy may be taken.

38. Pap smear/Exfoliative cytology (1990, 96, 99)

"Exfoliative cytology is a branch that deals with the study of cells, spontaneously shed off due to continuous growth of epithelial linings from epithelial surface into body cavity or body fluids; cells may also be obtained by scraping, brushing and washing mucosal structures."

Examples

- *Pap smear*
- Gastric lavage, scraping from oral cavity.

- Respiratory tract—sputum, aspiration/ brushing during bronchoscopic procedures
- Body fluids like effusion, CSF, seminal fluids
- Buccal smear for sex chromatin bodies

Cells shed in all these above specimens are looked for any specific abnormalities.

Papanicolaou smear

Method: The patient is placed in the dorsal position, the labia parted and the Cusco's self-retaining speculum gently introduced without the use of lubricants or jelly. The cervix is exposed; the squamocolumnar junction is now scrapped with the Ayre's spatula. The scraping are evenly spread onto a glass slide,

and immediately fixed by dipping the slide in the jar containing equal parts of 95% ethanol and ether.

Staining: Three stains—one nuclear stain (Harris' stain) and two cytoplasmic stains (orange G: orange color to cytoplasm; eosin alcohol: cyanophilic tint to cytoplasm) are used.

Observations
- *Cytohormonal evaluation*
  - Acidophilic index (relative proportion of acidophilic cells).
  - Pyknotic index (relative number of cells having small, dark nuclei).
  - Maturation index.

- *Non-neoplastic abnormal findings*

Non-specific inflammatory changes		Specific inflammation by	
Acute	*Chronic*	*Bacterial*	*Viral*
Squamous cells show:	Squamous cells show:	• N. gonorrhoea	• Herpes simplex
• Increased number of parabasal bodies	• Nuclear enlargement	• M. tuberculosis	• HPV
• Cytoplasmic acidophilia	• Hyperchromatism	*Fungal*	*Parasitic*
• Cytoplasmic vacuolization	• Nucleolar prominence	• Candida albicans	• Trichomonas vaginalis
• Leukocytic migration	• Multinucleation		• E. histolytica
• Nuclear pyknosis			
• Perinuclear halo			

- *Neoplastic abnormalities*
  - Squamous cell carcinoma or carcinoma *in situ* (CIN)
  - Squamous cells have decreased cohesiveness.
  - Cells show anaplasia.
  - Here *diagnosis* has to be made by seeing only one cell/a clump of few cells without the supporting evidence of architectural disarray, loss of orientation of one cell to another or evidence of invasion.
  - This method differentiates among normal, dysplastic, cancerous cells and cellular changes that are characteristics of carcinoma *in situ*.

- (*Also see CIN in female reproductive system*)
- Endocervical and endometrial adenocarcinoma may also be detected in pap smear.

39. Immunocytochemistry

In this method, monoclonal antibody is used to identify cell products or surface markers using fluorescence dyes or enzymes linked substrates.

- *Uses*
  - Categorization of undifferentiated malignant tumors: Highly anaplastic tumors of diverse origin tend to resemble

each other are difficult to be diagnosed in H and E stained smears. Some cell products like presence of keratin points to tumor of epithelial origin, whereas desmin is specific for tumor muscle cell origin.
- Categorization of leukemia and lymphomas.
- Determination of site of origin of metastatic tumors: When primary lesion is not obvious.

- Detection of molecules that have prognostic or therapeutic values: Estrogen receptor positive tumors of breast have better prognosis, while breast cancers with overexpression of *c-ErbB2* protein have poor prognosis.
• Intermediate filaments of cytoskeleton are formed by a family of related proteins which enhance structure integrity and stability of cells. They are five major antigens used in immunohistochemistry:

Cytokeratin	Carcinoma, mesothelioma, non-seminomatous GCT
Vimentin	Sarcoma (tumor of mesenchymal cells), melanoma, seminomas, lymphoma
Neurofilaments	Neural tumors
Glial fibrillary acid proteins (GFAP)	Non-neural brain tissue (astroglial origin → astrocytoma, ependymomas, medulloblastoma, oligodendroglioma)
Desmin	Leiomyoma and rhabdomyoma

40. Electron microscopy

This technique is used for confirming or substantiating tumor diagnosis based on:
• Presence and type of cell junctions
• Presence of microvilli
• Shape of nucleus, features of nuclear membrane and nucleoli
• Cytoplasmic organelles
• Presence of dense bodies in the cytoplasm

41. Molecular diagnosis

(*See textbook for details*)
• Diagnosis and differentiation of malignant tumor from each other and to know chromosomal abnormalities
• Prognosis of malignant neoplasm
• Detection of minimal residual disease after surgery or chemotherapy
• Diagnosis of hereditary predisposition to cancer

42. Flow cytometry

This is a newer technique to study the properties of cells suspended in a single moving stream.

Apparatus: (*Flow cytometer*)
• Laser light source (fluorescence)
• Cell transportation system in a single layer stream
• Monochromatic filters
• Lenses
• Mirrors
• Computer for analysis
Flow cytometer allows cell of a single layer to flow in a single direction, which can be viewed for individual cell characteristics like membrane antigen and DNA content of tumor cells.

Advantages
• Rapid
• Quantify results
• No subjective errors

Disadvantages
• Its use is limited to flow assay (as single cell suspensions are required) like WBC, RBC and their precursors, body fluids; sometimes solid tissues that can be made into cell suspension.

Uses
• Immunophenotyping of various hematopoietic cells and neoplasm.

- Diagnosis and prognosis of immunodeficiency like CD4+ T cells in AIDS.
- Diagnosis of autoantibodies.
- Measurement of nucleic acid contents and DNA ploidy.
- Diagnose the cause of allograft rejection by CD4+ T cell count as in renal transplant.

43. Tumor markers (1987, 88, 89, 91, 93, 97, 2000, 03, 04, 07, 10)

- Some tumors produce or elicit the production of markers that can be measured in blood or urine or other fluids.
- Tumor markers include surface antigen, cytoplasmic proteins, enzymes, and hormones.
- In practice, this refers to biochemical assay of these substance.

Uses of tumor markers

- These tumor markers may also be produced by normal cells or other non-neoplastic cells under certain circumstances. So, tumor markers cannot be used as a sole diagnostic tool for tumor. They may support the diagnosis.
- Their levels are used to monitor the response of therapy: Decreasing levels may suggest tumor is responding to therapy.
- Reappearance of tumor markers indicates relapse of tumor after therapy.
- To determine the prognosis preoperative— Higher levels suggest high tumor burden.
- To determine the growth of tumor—increasing levels suggest increase in growth.
- Examples of some tumor markers:

Tumor markers		Associated cancer
Hormones	Human chorionic gonadotropin	Trophoblastic tumors, non-seminomatous testicular tumor
	Calcitonin	Medullary carcinoma of thyroid
	Catecholamines and its metabolites	Pheochromocytoma
	Ectopic hormones	Paraneoplastic syndromes
Oncofetal protein (1990, 94)	α-fetoprotein	Liver cell carcinoma, non-seminomatous testicular tumor
	Carcinoembryonic antigens	Carcinoma of colon, pancreas, lung, stomach and breast
Isoenzymes	Prostatic acid phosphatase	Prostate cancer
	Neuron specific antigen	Small cell carcinoma of lung, neuroblastoma
Specific proteins	Prostate specific antigens	Prostate cancer
	Immunoglobulins	Multiple myeloma and other gammopathies
Mucin and other glycoproteins	CA-125	Ovarian cancer

44. Alpha-fetoprotein (1986, 90, 94, 95, 96)

- This is a glycoprotein synthesized normally early in fetal life by yolk sac, fetal liver and fetal GIT.

- Abnormal increase in plasma level are seen in cancers arising in:
  - Liver
  - Germ cells of testes

- Carcinoma of colon, lung, pancreas (less commonly)
- Non-neoplastic conditions related to increased level:
  - Cirrhosis
  - Toxic liver injury
  - Hepatitis
  - Pregnancy (fetal death or fetal stress)
- Though specificity is not high, but marked rise in its level is a strong indicator of hepatocellular or testicular tumors. Its serial level is useful in prognostic value after surgery or in response to therapy.

45. Carcinoembryonic antigen (CEA) (1995)

- This is a glycoprotein normally produced in embryonic tissues of gut, pancreas and liver during the first-two trimesters.
- Abnormal increase in plasma level are seen in cancers arising in:
  - Colorectal carcinoma
  - Gastric carcinoma
  - Pancreatic carcinoma
  - Breast carcinoma
- Non-neoplastic conditions related to increased level:
  - Alcoholic cirrhosis
  - Ulcerative colitis
  - Hepatitis
  - Crohn disease

- CEA assay lacks both specificity and sensitivity required for the detection of early cancers.
- Its level (high or low) may have prognosis/burden level of tumors.
- In patients of CEA positive colon cancers, presence of elevated level of CEA after 6 wk of surgery indicates residual disease.
- Serum CEA is also useful in monitoring the treatment of metastatic breast cancer.

46. Carcinoma *in situ* (1986, 91, 95)

This is a severe form of dysplasia where dysplasia involves all layers of epithelium, but there is not invasion of basement membrane. This is a preneoplastic lesion that has high risk to be converted into a cancer lesion, but all carcinoma *in situ* do not get converted into cancer.

(*For more details see from various chapters including female reproductive system—CIN*)

47. Difference between hyperplasia and dysplasia (1998)

48. Occupational cancer (2000)

49. Aflatoxin (1991)

(*See textbook or Chapter on Liver; not important*)

8

Infectious Diseases, Environmental and Nutritional Pathology

1. Difference between tubercular leprosy and lepromatous leprosy (1993, 94, 97, 2004, 08, 10)

S. No.	Traits	Tubercular leprosy	Lepromatous leprosy
1.	T-cell mediated immunity, lepromin test	Present — Strongly positive	Absent/very weak — Negative
2.	Skin lesion	Asymmetrical, single or few lesion, hypopigmented and erythematous macular lesion	Symmetrical, multiple, hypopigmented, erythematous, maculopapular or nodular lesion
3.	Granuloma formation	Present like TB	Absent
4.	Microscopic features of lesion	Hard tubercle similar to granuloma (epithelioid cells macrophages, giant cells) eroding the basal layer of epidermis, no clear zone. *Paucibacillary*	Foamy macrophages/lepra cells in the dermis separated from epidermis by a clear zone. *Multibacillary*
5.	CD4+ cells	Present at the periphery of granuloma	Almost absent
6.	CD8+ suppressor cells	Very few; at center of lesion	Present (more in number) in diffuse manner
7.	Infectivity	Low	High
8.	Involvement	Mostly nerve (severely affected, may be destroyed), skin	Skin, peripheral nerves, anterior eye, upper airways, testes, feet, hands
9.	Complications	Related to nerve damage like paralysis, distinct sensory disturbances	Ag-Ab complex mediated erythema nodosum leprosum, vasculitis, glomerulonephritis besides nerve related
10.	Prognosis	Milder disease; better prognosis	Extensive, progressive disease; bad prognosis

2. Primary complex (1997, 98, 2001)

3. Difference between primary TB and secondary TB (1990, 93, 98, 2002, 07)

(*See lung, but prepare these questions for paper I, as these have been asked many times as mentioned here in paper I*)

4. Biological effects and mechanism of action of ionizing radiations (1990, 96)

Ionizing radiations have short wavelength and high frequency. They have sufficient energy to remove tightly bound electrons from an atom. The collision of electrons with other molecules releases electrons in a reaction cascade, referred to as ionization. Sources of ionizing radiations are X-ray, gamma-rays, high-energy neutrons, alpha-particles and beta particles.

5. Hazards of radiations (1988, 92)

6. Pathogenesis of radiation damage and relative radiosensitivity of tissues (2002)

7. Acute radiation syndrome/radiation sickne (1998, 2004, 07, 08, 09, 11)

Acute radiation syndrome (ARS), also known as radiation poisoning, radiation sickness or radiation toxicity, is a constellation of health effects which present within 24 hr of exposure to high amounts of ionizing radiation. They may last for several months.

Major morphological consequences of radiation injury

Brain	Skin	Lungs
Adult-resistant	Erythema, edema (early)	Edema
Embryonic-destruction of neurons and glial cells	Dyspigmentation (weeks to months)	ARDS
	Atrophy, cancer (months to years)	Interstitial fibrosis (late)
Lymph nodes	**Gastrointestinal tract**	**Blood and bone marrow**
Acute tissue loss	Mucosal injury (early)	Thrombocytopenia
Atrophy and fibrosis (late)	Ulceration (early)	Granulocytopenia
	Fibrosis of wall (Late)	Anemia, lymphopenia

		Gonads	
	Testes		*Ovaries*
Early	Destruction of testes		Destruction of ovaries
	– Spermatogonia		– Germ cells
	– Spermatids		– Granulosa cells
	– Sperm		
Late	Atrophy and fibrosis of testes		Atrophy and fibrosis of ovaries

Effects of total- body ionizing radiation (Acute radiation syndrome)

	0–1 Sv	1–2 Sv	2–10 Sv	10–20 Sv	> 50 Sv
Main site of injury	None	Lymphocytes	Bone marrow	Small bowel	Brain
Sign and symptoms	None	Moderated granulocyto-penia, lymphopenia	Leukopenia, hemorrhage, hair loss, vomiting	Diarrhea, fever, electro-lyte imbalance, vomiting	Ataxia, coma, convulsions, vomiting
Time of development	–	1–1 wk	2–6 wk	5–14 days	1–4 hr
Lethality	None	None	Variable (0–80%)	100%	100%

- Main determinants of the biologic effects of ionizing radiations:
  - Rate of delivery and field size of exposure.
  - Cell proliferation: Highly proliferative cells are more prone to cell damage.
  - Oxygen contents of tissue: High oxygen contents of tissue have high chance of producing reactive oxygen, hence damage.
  - Vascular damage: Damage to moderately sensitive endothelial cells may cause narrowing or occlusion of blood vessel leading to impaired healing, fibrosis and chronic ischemic atrophy.

Mechanism of action of ionizing radiations:
- At very high dose (> 10 Gy) it produces cell/tissue necrosis.
- At intermediate dose (1–2 Gy) it kills the highly proliferating cells.
- At lower doses it causes subcellular damages like:
  - DNA-protein cross-linking
  - Cross-linking of DNA strands, single base-damage
  - Oxidation or degradation of bases
  - DNA strand breaks (most serious damage)

- Free radical like oxygen free radical
- Formations of lipid-derived free radicals
- Breaks the covalent bonds that hold the ribose phosphate chain together
- Alter the electrons in the bases and, thus changes their hydrogen bonding (wrong pairing of bases)
- Depending upon the dose of ionizing radiation, p53 gene and other cell cycle regulator's functional status; the cell may be repaired or may undergo apoptosis (if extensive DNA damage). It may not follow either of these two paths; it may show the delayed signs of injury like mutation, chromosomal aberrations, and genetic instability and may transform into tumor.
- Radiations have the ability to induce fibrosis and replace the normal parenchymal tissues by fibrosis resulting in scarring or loss of functions.

8. Kwashiorkor (1987, 92, 2008)

9. Marasmus

10. Difference between kwashiorkor and marasmus (1988, 91, 93, 98, 2004)

S. No.	Traits	Kwashiorkor	Marasmus
1.	Age	< 5 yr	0–2 yr
2.	Deficiency	Protein deprivation is greater than carbohydrate deprivation	Protein and carbohydrate both deficient
3.	Cause	Weaning of child in early age without proper food	Weaned children on only carbohydrate-rich food, chronic diarrhea—no protein absorption or chronic protein losing disease
4.	Skeleton muscles	Relatively spared	Catabolized, loss of muscles
5.	Visceral protein compartment/ liver protein stores	Markedly deprived/reduced, sometimes life threatening	Depleted only marginally; almost preserved for survival
6.	Serum protein levels	Markedly decreased	Normal/slightly decreased
7.	Subcutaneous fat	Spared	Mobilized for energy

(Contd.)

Difference between kwashiorkor and marasmus (Contd.)

S. No.	Traits	Kwashiorkor	Marasmus
8.	Hypoalbuminemia/ edema	Present; edema may be generalized or dependent.	Absent
9.	Extremities	Edematous	Looks emaciated; head appears too large as compared to body
10.	Growth/mental retardation	Present, but much lesser	Present; more severe
11.	Life threatening	More severe form as severe loss of visceral protein compartment	Less as visceral protein compartment is preserved for emergency
12.	Weight loss	60–80% of normal weight for the age and sex	Falls below the 60% of normal range
13.	Skin lesions	"Flaky paint" appearance—alternating zone of hyperpigmentation, desquamation and hypopigmentation	No such characteristics
14.	Hair changes	Loss of color, alternating bands of pale and darker hair (flag sign), hair easily fall, straightening, etc.	Dry and wrinkled skin; may be loose
15.	Hepatomegaly	Present with fatty changes	No such abnormality
16.	Appetite	Loses; patient is apathy, listlessness	Hungry and alert
17.	Small bowel	Decreased in mitotic index in crypt of glands, associated with mucosal atrophy and loss of villi	Rare
18.	Thymic and lymphoid atrophy	More marked	Less marked
19.	Immune deficiency/ recurrent infections	Present, lesser	Immune deficiency (mostly T cell) present, prone to recurrent infection

11. Eye changes in vitamin A deficiency

- Ocular changes due to vitamin A deficiency are collectively known as *xerophthalmia* (dry eye).
- First change is dryness of the conjunctivae (*xerosis*)—normal lacrimal and mucus secreting epithelium are replaced by keratinized epithelium.
- It is followed by accumulation of keratin debris as small opaque plaque called **Bitot spots**.
- There is erosion of roughened surface of cornea-*corneal ulcer*.
- Softening and destruction of cornea (*keratomalacia*) follow it.
- Blindness is the final outcome.
- First symptom of vitamin A deficiency is night vision (vision in deem light) becomes difficult.

12. Predisposing factors for rickets and osteomalacia

- Inadequate synthesis or dietary deficiency of vitamin D
  - Inadequate exposure to sunlight
  - Limited dietary intake of fortified foods
  - Poor maternal nutrition during pregnancy and breastfeeding
  - Dark skin pigmentation

- Decreased absorption of vitamin D (fat soluble)
  - Cholestatic liver disease
  - Biliary tract obstruction
  - Pancreatic insufficiency (fat digesting enzymes decreased)
  - Diseases of small intestine.
- Deranged vitamin D metabolism
  - Impaired synthesis of 25-(OH) vitamin D
  - Increased degradation of vitamin D and 25-(OH) vitamin D
  - Decreased synthesis of 1,25-$(OH)_2$ vitamin D
- Resistance to 1, 25-$(OH)_2$ vitamin D action
- Phosphate deficiency
  - Decreased absorption from GIT
  - Increased excretion from kidney.

13. Osteomalacia (1995)

(*See bones*)

14. Bone changes in rickets (1989, 98, 2010) or Rickets (1993, 2004)

- Overgrowth of epiphyseal cartilage
- Irregular and distorted masses of cartilage persist which may project into marrow cavity
- Osteoid matrix are deposited on inadequate mineralized cartilaginous remnants
- Disruption of the orderly replacement of cartilage by osteoid matrix
- Abnormal overgrowth of capillaries and fibroblasts in the disorganized zone
- Deformity of skeleton like craniotabes, frontal bossing, squared appearance of frontal head, rachitic rosary, pigeon chest deformity, Harrison groove, lumbar lordosis, bowing of the legs, etc.

15. Diet and cancer (1991)

- *Exogenous carcinogens in the diet:*
  - *Aflatoxins:* Present in *Aspergillus flavus*; food contaminated with it has high incidence of hepatocellular carcinoma.
  - Other substances like food additives, pesticides in food or artificial sweeteners increase the chances of developing cancer.
  - Pickled or salty foods contain nitrates, which have been implicated in gastric cancer.
  - Burnt or barbecued foods contain a group of carcinogenic substances called polycyclic aromatic hydrocarbons, which are produced, if food is overheated.
- *Cancer preventing diets*
  - *Retinoic acid* promotes differentiation of mucus secreting epithelial cells. So diet containing β-carotene and retinoic acid reverse the metaplasia and precancerous lesions of respiratory tract.
  - Low *fiber* contents with high animal fat contents in the diet predispose to colon carcinoma.
  - *High fat content* means high level of bile salts and acids in the intestine; thus altering the intestinal flora and favoring aerobic conditions—free radicals and carcinogenic by-products of bile acid metabolism by bacteria.
  - *Fibers* bind with carcinogens and also bile products to decrease its effect on GIT mucosa. It also increased stool bulk and decreases the transit time (decreasing the contact time of carcinogens with GIT mucosa).
  - Some antioxidants like β-carotene, vitamins C and E prevent free radical damage to cell and its DNA: Preventing from 'cancer initiation'.
  - Vitamin A enhances immunity and other related retinoids; may control free radical production by modulating inflammatory reactions.
- Fruits and vegetables in the diets are thought to *lower* the risk of cancer.
- *Despite of the proclamations* by many 'health-food' industries, it has not been possible to ascertain the exact role and mechanism of 'diet in the prevention of cancer'. In some cases, 'diet therapy' was found to be harmful.

9

Diseases of Infancy and Childhood

1. Neonatal respiratory distress syndrome (RDS)/hyaline membrane disease

Formation of pulmonary hyaline membrane resulting in acute respiratory distress syndrome. It is associated with conditions:
- Pre-term infants.
- Infants born to diabetic mothers.
- Cesarean section delivery.
- Excessive sedation of mother during labor resulting in infant respiratory depression.
- Other birth related asphyxia.
- Male predominance than female (unknown cause).

Clinical features
- Dyspnea just after birth or after some time in apparently normal infants accompanied with tachypnea, hypoxia, and cyanosis.
- It may be fatal in severe cases.

Sequence of development
- Premature birth (much before 35 wk of gestation period).
- Reduced surfactant synthesis, storage and release resulting in decreased alveolar surfactant.
- Causes increased alveolar surface tension and atelectasis.
- Uneven perfusion and hypoventilation causes hypoxemia and CO_2 retention.
- Acidosis and further reduced surfactant synthesis.

- Pulmonary vasoconstriction and hypoperfusion.
- Endothelial and epithelial damage.
- Leakage of plasma into alveoli.
- Fibrin and necrotic cells.
- Resulting in hyaline membrane formation.

Morphology
- *Gross:* Lung or its part(s)
  - Normal size
  - Reddish purple in color
  - Solid
  - Sinks in water
  - Airless

- *Microscopic features*
  - Collapsed alveoli
  - Neutrophilic infiltration
  - Eosinophilic hyaline membrane in the terminal bronchiole ducts and alveolar ducts/alveoli.

2. Define fetal hydrops. Enumerate and describe the two types of hydrops

Fetal hydrops refer to accumulation of edema fluid in the fetus during intrauterine growth. Fluid accumulation may vary from progressive generalized edema of the fetus (hydrops) to a more localized isolated pleural/peritoneal collection.

It may be immune or nonimmune in origin.

Nonimmune hydrops
- Major cause include cardiovascular defects, chromosomal abnormalities (Turner syndrome, trisomies 18 and 21), and fetal anemia (α-thalassemia resulting in intrauterine cardiac failure.
- Transplacental infection with parvovirus B19 is emerging as an important cause of fetal hydrops.

Immune hydrops is also known as erythroblastosis fetalis (described below).

3. Erythroblastosis fetalis (1997, 2000)

or

Hemolytic disease of newborn (1987, 93, 08)

- Hemolytic disease in the newborn is caused by blood group incompatibility between mother and child.
- *"Immunization* of the mother by blood group antigens on fetal red cells and the free passage of antibodies from the mother through the placenta to the fetus" is basis of the disease.
- Antigen (RBC) may reach maternal circulation in the last trimester (weak placental barrier) or during childbirth (injury).
- Red cell antigens derived from father act as foreign antigen to fetus-bearing mother, if these cross placenta.
- Most common incompatibility is Rh (D); followed by ABO blood group, if any.

Rh incompatibility (*pathogenesis:* 1987, 93):
- *Conditions* when disease develops:
  - When an Rh⁻ mother is sensitized by Rh⁺ blood by prior transfusion: even *first* Rh⁺ child may be affected.
- When mother is Rh⁻ and first child/fetus is Rh⁺ then first child is almost unaffected, but all pregnancies in future with Rh⁺ fetus will be affected *except* administration of Rhesus immune globulin (RhIg) containing anti-D antibodies are administered within 72 hr of delivery and (or) at 28th week of pregnancy to Rh⁻ mothers.

- Such sensitized mother forms antibodies against Rh antigens.
- Antibodies (Ab) cross placenta during the first Rh⁺ pregnancy, but it happens in late 3rd trimester, IgM isotype is the first antibody to be formed which does not cross placenta—so first child is mostly unaffected; but if there is heavy and early sensitization of mother, then hemolytic symptoms are also visible in the first child due to IgG formation (which is capable of crossing placenta).
- Second Rh⁺ fetus causes large amount of IgG antibodies formation. These antibodies cross placenta and attach to Rh⁺ fetal RBCs. Destruction of such RBCs leads fetal anemia and hemolytic jaundice. In severe cases, jaundice may lead to kernicterus and mental retardation; anemia may cause extramedullary hematopoiesis and (or) cardiac decompensation leading to *hydrops fetalis*.

ABO incompatibility
Very less due to:
- Anti-A and anti-B antibodies are IgM type that do not cross placenta.
- Neonatal RBCs express blood group antigens A and B poorly: less sensitization of mother.
- Many cells other than RBCs express A and B antigen, so they cross-react with antibodies that cross placenta.
- ABO hemolytic disease occurs exclusively in infants born to O blood group mothers (IgG type anti-A and anti-B antibodies).

4. Neuroblastoma (1990, 2008, 10)

- One of the most common solid tumors of childhood.
- *Age:* Childhood, most common in infants (<1 year age).
- Mostly sporadic, rarely familial with autosomal dominant transmission.
- *Sites*
  - *Most common*—adrenal medulla.

- Other sites—anywhere along sympathetic chain (paravertebral region of posterior mediastinum and lower abdomen).
- *Morphology*
  Gross
  - Size: Varies from *in situ* lesion (small nodules) to large mass.
  - *In situ* lesion may regress to present only small foci of fibrosis and calcification (spontaneous regression or therapy induced maturation): otherwise may form benign ganglioneuroma.
  - Some tumors may appear encapsulated and sharply demarcated, others are highly infiltrative.
  - Cut section: Soft gray, brain-like tissues. Areas of necrosis and hemorrhage are present in large tumor masses.

  Microscopic features
  - Tumor cells are present in sheets.
  - Tumor cell is small; primitive-looking cells having dark nuclei, scant cytoplasm and poorly defined cell margins.
  - Eosinophilic fibrillary background (neutrophil or neurotic processes of primitive neuroblasts) is indicative of a neural origin.
  - Homer-Wright pseudorosettes (tumor cells are arranged around a central space filled with fibrillar extension of tumor cells).
  - Differentiation of tumor cells varies from well differentiated to poorly differentiated.

  Electron microscopy: Neurosecretory granules in the cells are found.
- *Clinical features*
  - Large abdominal mass
  - Fever
  - Weight loss
  - Elevation of urinary catecholamines as 90% of tumors produce catecholamines
  - Metastases may cause hepatomegaly, ascites and bone pain.

  In neonates, disseminated neuroblastoma may present with multiple cutaneous metastasis and deep blue discoloration of the skin (blueberry muffin baby).

Prognostic factors is neuroblastoma

Variable	Favorable	Unfavorable
Stage	Stage 1, 2A, 2B, 4S	Stage 3.4
Age	≤ 1 yr	> 1 yr
Histology		
• Evidence of schwannian stroma and gangliocytic differentiation	Present	Absent
• Mitotic rate	Low	High
• Mitosis-karyorrhexis index	≤ 200/500 cells	> 200/500 cells
• Intramural calcification	Present	Absent
DNA ploidy	Hyperploid or near triploid	Diploid, near diploid or near tetraploid
N-myc	Not amplified	Amplified
Chromosome 17q gain	Absent	Present
Chromosome 1p loss	Absent	Present
Trk-A expression	Present	Absent
Telomerase expression	Low/absent	High expressed
MRP expression	Absent	Present
CD-44 expression	Present	Absent
Serum biochemical marker		
Ferritin	Normal	Elevated
Lactate dehydrogenase	≤ 1500 U/ml	≥ 1500 U/ml

10

Disorders of Red Blood Cells

1. Normal cell sequence: Hematopoiesis (2002)

See Fig. 10.1.

2. Normal values (Harrison's internal medicine)

Hb:

Adult male: 13.3–16.2 g/dl

Adult female: 12.0–15.8 g/dl

RBC count: Adult male: 4.30–5.60 × 10^{12}/l, adult female: 4.00–5.20 × 10^{12}/l

Hematocrit: Adult males: 38.8–46.4, adult females: 35.4–44.4

Hemoglobin electrophoresis:

Hemoglobin A: 95–98%, hemoglobin A_2: 1.5–3.1%,

Hemoglobin F: 0–2.0%, hemoglobins other than A, A_2, or F: Absent

Mean corpuscular volume (MCV): 79–93.3 μm^3

Mean corpuscular hemoglobin (MCH): 26.7–31.9 pg/cell

Mean corpuscular hemoglobin concentration (MCHC): 32.3–35.9 g/dl

RBC diameter: 6.7–7.7 μm

Red cell distribution width: 11.5–14.5

RBC life span: 120 days

Reticulocye count: Adult males: 0.8–2.3% red cells, adult females: 0.8–2.0% red cells

WBC count: 3.54–9.06 × 10^3/mm^3

DLC: (Adult): Neutrophil: 2.0–7.5 × 10^9/l (40–75%)

Lymphocytes: 1.5–4.0 × 10^9/l (20–45%)

Monocytes: 0.2–0.8 × 10^9/l (2–10%)

Eosinophils: 0.04–0.4 × 10^9/l (1–6%)

Basophils: 0.02–0.1 × 10^9/l (1%)

Platelet count: 165–415 × 10^3/mm^3

ESR: Westergren (1 hour at 20 ± 3°C)

Adult male: 0–15 mm/h, adult female: 0–20 mm/h , children:0–10 mm/h

Prothrombin time (PT): 12.7–15.4 s

Partial thromboplastin time with kaolin (PTTk): 26.3–39.4 s

Plasma fibrinogen: 1.5–4 g/l

3. Classify anemia according to morphology/Wintrobe classification

	Hypochromic	*Normochromic*
Normocytic	Chronic hemorrhage	Acute hemorrhage, all hemolytic anemia except thalassemia, aplastic anemia
Macrocytic	Secondary to (2°) liver diseases	Megaloblastic anemia
Microcytic	IDA, thalassemia	Chronic infections

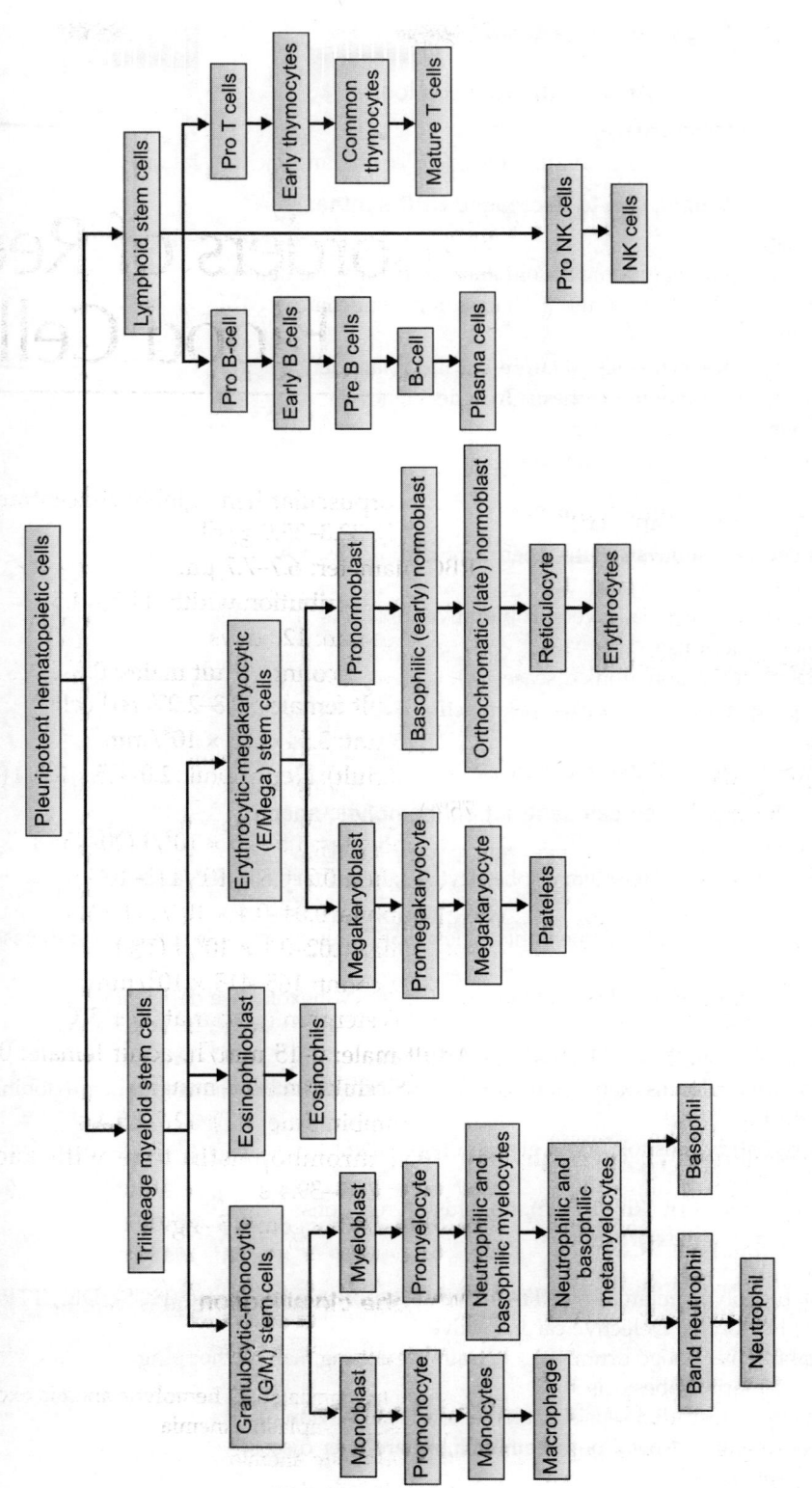

Fig. 10.1: Hematopoiesis

4. Classify anemia according to etiology (2002)

Anemia due to blood loss

- Acute blood loss: Trauma (hemorrhage)
- Chronic blood loss: GIT bleeding, menstruation blood loss or helminthic infestation

Anemia due to decreased RBC synthesis

- Inherited genetic defect
  Defect leading to stem cell depletion: Fanconi anemia, telomerase defects
  Defect leading to erythroblast maturation: Thalassemia syndrome
- Nutritional deficiency
  Deficiencies affecting DNA synthesis: Vitamin B_{12} and folate deficiency
  Deficiencies affecting hemoglobin synthesis: Iron deficiency
- Erythropoietin deficiency:
  Anemia of chronic disease, renal failure
- Immune mediated injury of progenitors
  Aplastic anemia, pure red cell aplasia
- Inflammation-mediated iron sequestration: Anemia of chronic disease
- Primary hemopoietic neoplasms
  Acute leukemias, myelodysplasia, myeloproliferative disorders
- Space occupying marrow lesions
  Metastatic neoplasms, granulomatous disease
- Infection of red cell progenitors: Parvovirus B19 infection
- Unknown mechanism
  Endocrine disorders, hepatocellular liver diseases

Increased red cell destruction/ hemolytic anemia

- Inherited genetic defect
  Red cell membrane disorders: Hereditary spherocytosis, hereditary elliptocytosis
  Enzyme deficiencies
    Hexose monophosphate shunt enzyme deficiencies: G6PD deficiency, glutathione synthetase
    deficiency
    Glycolytic enzyme deficiencies: Pyruvate kinase deficiency, hexokinase deficiency
  Hemoglobin abnormalities
    Deficient hemoglobin synthesis: Thalassemia syndromes
    Structurally abnormal globins (hemoglobinopathies): Sickle cell anemia, unstable hemoglobins
- Acquired genetic defects
  Deficiency of phosphatidylinositol-linked glycoproteins: PNH
- Antibody mediated destruction
  Hemolytic disease of newborn (Rh disease), transfusion reactions
  Drug induced, autoimmune disorders
- Mechanical trauma
  Microangiopathic hemolytic anemias (MAHA): Hemolytic uremic syndrome (HUS), DIC, TTP
  Cardiac traumatic hemolysis: Defective cardiac valves
  Repetitive physical trauma: Bongo drumming, marathon running, karate chopping
- Infection of red cells: Malaria, babesiosis
- Toxic or chemical injury: Clostridial sepsis, snake venom, lead poisoning
- Membrane lipid abnormalities: Abetalipoproteinemia, severe liver disease
- Sequestration: Hypersplenism

5. Classify hemolytic anemia according to extrinsic and intrinsic causes (2001, 02, 04, 11)

Intrinsic/intracorpuscular abnormalities

Hereditary
- Red cell membrane disorders
  - Membrane cytoskeleton disorder: Spherocytosis, elliptocytosis
  - Lipid synthesis disorder: Increase in membrane lecithin
- Red cell enzyme deficiency: Pyruvate kinase, hexokinase G6PD, glutathione synthetase
- Disorders of hemoglobin synthesis
  - Deficient globin synthesis: Thalassemia syndrome
  - Structural abnormality of globin chain (hemoglobinopathies): Sickle cell anemia

Acquired
Membrane defect: PNH

Extrinsic/extracorpuscular abnormalities

- Antibodies mediated
  - Isohemagglutinins
    - Transfusion reaction
    - Erythroblastosis fetalis
  - Autoantibodies
    - Idiopathic, SLE, drug associated
    - Malignant neoplasm
- Mechanical trauma to red cells
  - Microangiopathic hemolytic anemia (MAHA)
    - Thrombotic thrombocytopenic purpura (TTP)
    - DIC
  - Cardiac traumatic hemolytic anemia
- Infection
  Malarial, bacterial infection (sepsis)
- Chemical injury
  Lead poisoning
- Sequestration in mononuclear phagocyte system
  Hypersplenism

6. Clinical signs and symptoms of anemia

Acute anemia: Shortness of breath, respiratory distress, congestive heart failure, shock.

Chronic anemia
- Fatigue, lassitude, dyspnea, palpitation, dizziness, headache, syncope, tinnitus, vertigo, irritability, sleep disturbances, lack of concentration and paresthesia
- Anorexia, nausea, bowel disturbances
- Symptoms of cardiac failure
- With hemolysis: Jaundice, gallstones, skeletal abnormalities due to expansion of marrow, growth retardation
- With defective erythropoiesis: Iron overload, heart and endocrine failure

Signs of anemia
- Pallor of skin and mucus membranes, nail beds, palmar creases
- Tachycardia with wide pulse pressure
- Ejection systolic murmur
- Cardiomegaly and other signs of cardiac failure
- Edema
- Koilonychia (in iron deficiency)

7. Morphological abnormalities of red cells in different types of anemias

Common cell	Morphology	Disorders
Burr cell (echinocyte)	Speculated erythrocyte with short equally-spaced projection	Uremia, MAHA, pyruvate kinase deficiency, liver disease

(Contd.)

Morphological abnormalities of red cells in different types of anemias (Contd.)

Common cell	Morphology	Disorders
Spur cell (acanthocyte)	Blunted spicules of varying length, irregularly distributed over cell surface	Liver disease, lipid disorders, hemangiosarcoma, DIC
Elliptocyte (ovalocyte, pencil cell, cigar cell)	Oval to elongated ellipsoid erythrocyte with central area of pallor and hemoglobin at both ends of cell	Herediary elliptocytosis, iron deficiency
Sickle cell (drepanocyte)	Crescent shaped with pointed ends	Sickle cell anemia
Fragmented cell (schistocyte)	Fragmented erythrocyte	DIC, microangiopathic hemolytic anemia (MAHA), severe burn, uremia
Target cell (codocyte)	Flat red cells with a central mass of hemoglobin (dense area) surrounded by a ring of pallor (pale area), and an outer ring of hemoglobin (dense area)	Liver disease, iron deficiency, post-splenectomy, thalassemia
Stomatocyte	Red cell with central area slit like or mouth like appearance	Alcoholism
Bite cell	Red cell appearing to have a bite of cytoplasm removed	G6PD deficiency
Teardrop cell	Red cells in the shape of tear drop	Infiltrative disorders of marrow
Punctate basophilia or basophilic stippling	Presence of fine or coarse purple-blue granules in cytoplasm of red cells, representing ribosomal aggregates	Severe anemia, β-thalassemia, chronic lead poisoning
Howell-Jolly body	These are remnants of nuclear material left in erythrocytes, after the nucleus is extruded. Normally removed by spleen and not seen in circulation	Absent spleen (asplenia/post-splenectomy), megablastic anemia
Heinz body	These are formed in red cells from denatured aggregated hemoglobin	Thalassemia, asplenia, chronic liver disease
Spherocytes	Dark appearing (dense hemo-globin) with no central pallor	Immune hemolytic anemia, hemolytic disease of newborn, burns, hereditary spherocytosis
Polychromatophils or polychromasia	Red cells staining bluish-gray. They represent young reticulo-cytes	Accelerated eryhtropoiesis

8. Causes of intravascular hemolysis (2001)

- Mechanical trauma to red cells (defective cardiac valves, thrombus in microcirculation)
- Thermal injury
- PNH
- March hemoglobinuria (vigorous exercise)
- Microangiopathic hemolytic anemia (sickle cell anemia, DIC, TTP)
- G6PD deficiency
- Pregnancy induced hypertension (PIH, HELLP syndrome)
- Infection—*P. falciparum* malaria, *Clostridium perfringens*
- Autoimmune hemolytic anemia (AIHA; Ab and complement mediated)
- Disseminated carcinomatosis
- Hemolytic uremic syndrome
- Clostridial toxin

9. Causes of extravascular hemolysis (2000)

- All red cell membrane defects like HS
- Splenomegaly (hypersplenism)
- Sickle cell anemia
- Premature destruction of RBC—thalassemia, or other Hb synthesis disorders
- Drug induced immune hemolytic anemia

- Autoimmune hemolytic anemia
- G6PD deficiency

10. Lab diagnosis of hemolytic anemia (2001)

Characterized by
- Premature destruction of red cells ($\downarrow t\frac{1}{2}$)
- Accumulation of hemoglobin catabolic products
- Increased erythropoiesis in bone marrow.

Test for increased RBC breakdown
- Serum bilirubin: Increased (mainly unconjugated)
- Fecal stercobilinogen: Increased
- Urine urobilinogen: Increased (no bilirubinuria)
- Plasma LDH: Increased ($LDH_2 > LDH_1$)
- Characteristics of intravascular hemolysis:
  - Serum haptoglobin and hemopexin (hemoglobin binding proteins): Decreased or absent
  - Hemoglobinemia
  - Jaundice
  - Hemoglobinuria
  - Hemosiderinuria
  - Methemoglobinemia

(*See* Fig. 10.2)

Extravascular hemolysis versus intravascular hemolysis

S. No.	Traits	Extravascular hemolysis	Intravascular hemolysis
1.	Site of hemolysis	RE cell organs like spleen and bone marrow	In circulating blood vessels
2.	S. methemalbumin	–ve	+ve
3.	Plasma haemoglobin	–ve	+ve
4.	S. ferritin	N or ↑	↓
5.	S. haptoglobin	↓	↓
6.	S. bilirubin (unconjugated)	↑↑	↑
7.	S. LDH	↑	↑↑
8.	Urine hemoglobin	–ve	+ve
9.	Urine hemosiderin	–ve	+ve
10.	Tissue iron (spleen, liver)	↑ed	↓ed
11.	Diseases	Thalassemia	G6PD deficiency

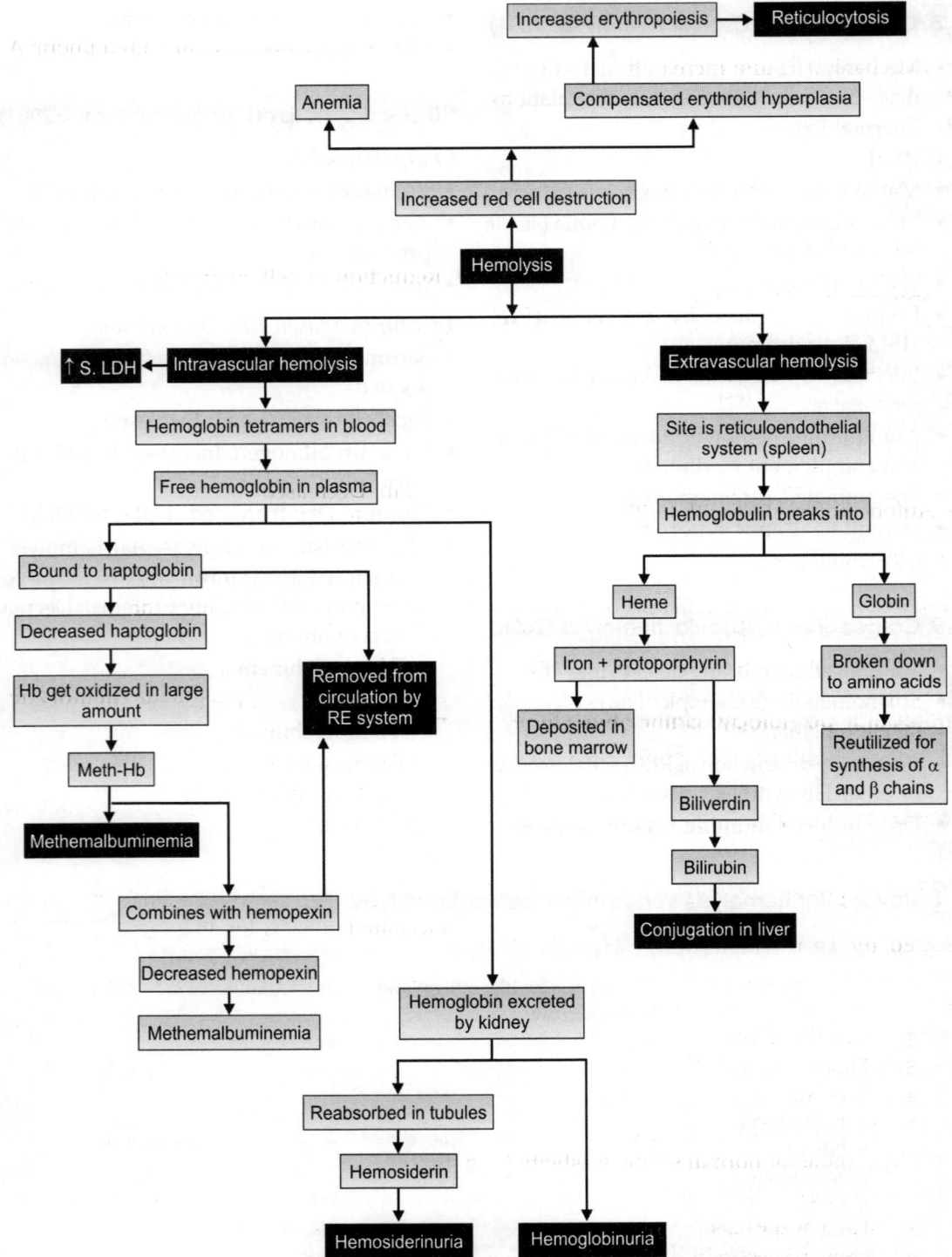

Fig. 10.2: Pathophysiology of hemolysis

Test for increased red cell production
- Reticulocyte count: Increased.
- BM: Erythroid hyperplasia.
- PBS: Macrocytosis, polychromasia, aniso-poikilocytosis (spherocyte, acanthocyte, echmyocyte, sickle cell, autoagglutinated cells) and normoblasts. Increased erythroid creatinine.
- X-ray: Expansion of bone marrow (crew cut appearance of facial bones).

Test for damage to red cells: (Shows underlying causes)
- Osmotic fragility test
- Coombs' test
- Electrophoresis and estimation of abnormal Hb like HbA$_2$, HbF
- Autohemolysis test with/without glucose
- Sickling test
- Test for G6PD deficiency

Test for shortened red cell life: Decreased t½ to 30–40 days in mild case (normal 120 days).

11. Hereditary spherocytosis: Definition, molecular pathology, pathophysiology, laboratory diagnosis and clinical features

or

Laboratory diagnosis of hereditary spherocytosis (2010)

Definition: This is autosomal dominant (75%, remaining recessive) inherited disease characterized by an intrinsic defect in red cell membrane that renders RBC spheroidal, less deformable, and vulnerable to splenic sequestration and destruction.

Structural defects in HS
- Membrane cytoskeleton that lies closely opposed to the internal surface of plasma membrane is responsible for normal shape, elasticity/flexibility and strength of red cell membrane.
- Membrane skeleton consists of:
  - Spectrin: The chief protein component
  - Ankyrin and band 4.2: Binds spectrin to band 3
  - Band 3: A transmembrane ion transport protein

  - Band 4.1: Binds spectrin to glycophorin A, a transmembrane protein
- Any defect in these cytoskeleton proteins (Ankyrin defect is the most common finding followed by band 3) is associated with reduced membrane stability and loss of membrane fragments as the cells are exposed to shear stress in the circulation.
- Reduction in cell surface to volume ratio forces cells to assume shape of least surface area for given volume, i.e. sphere.

Pathophysiology
(*See* Fig 10.3)

Laboratory diagnosis
- *Complete blood count (CBC)*
  - Hb: Decreased
  - MCHC: Increased
  - MCV: Normal or slightly decreased
  - Reticulocyte count: Increased
- *PBS:* Anisocytosis microspherocytosis—dark appearing spherocytes with no central pallor.
- *BM:* Erythroid hyperplasia (hemolytic picture).
- *Osmotic fragility test:* Highly increased osmotic fragility of RBC due to spheroidal shape, and thus decreased margin for expansion of RBC volume without rupture.
- *Autohemolysis test:* Highly increased spontaneous autohemolysis when blood is incubated at 37 °C for 48 hours (10–15% of RBC) as compared to normal (<4%).
- *Direct Coombs' test:* Negative; differentiate it from acquired spherocytosis of AIHA in which Coombs' test is positive.
- Measurement of spectrin and other cytoskeleton.
- Other: Serum bilirubin: Increased.
- Features of extravascular hemolysis.

Clinical features
- Crisis (aplasia, hemolytic anemia)
- Splenomegaly
- Jaundice: Intermittent jaundice
- Gallstones
- *Treatment:* Splenectomy (after splenectomy, spherocytes persist but anemia is corrected).

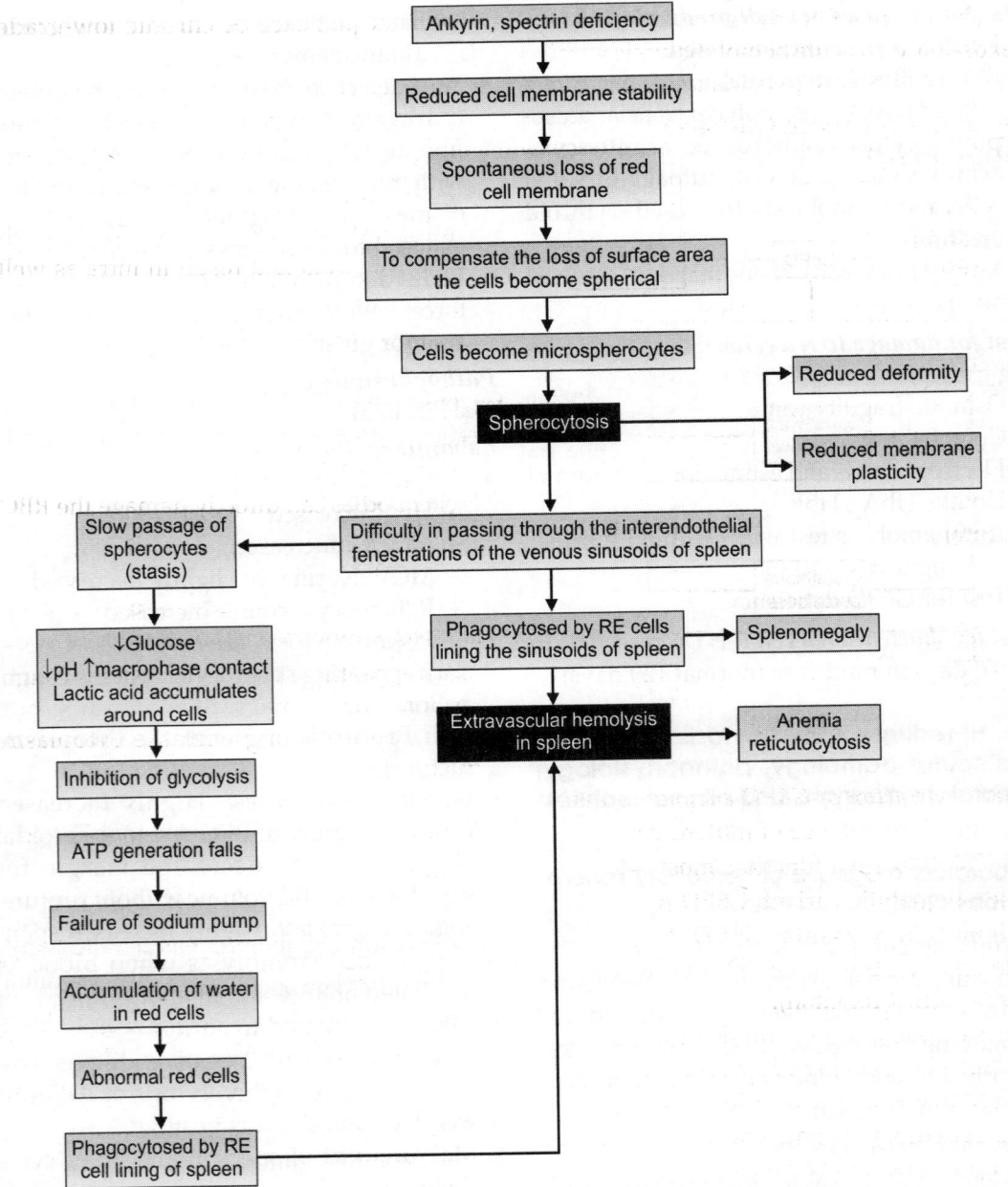

Fig. 10.3: Pathophysiology of HS

12. G6PD (Glucose-6-phosphate dehydrogenase) deficiency anemia (1990, 93, 94, 2003, 07)

13. Mechanism of anemia in G6PD deficiency (2000)

- Erythrocytes are vulnerable to oxidative injuries by a variety of endogenous and exogenous oxidants.
- G6PD prevents such oxidative damage by maintaining the supply of reduced glutathione which inactivates such oxidants.

In absence of G6PD therefore, patient may experience an acute hemolytic crisis within hours of exposure to oxidative stress.

Role of G6PD enzyme (glucose-6-phosphate dehydrogenase)

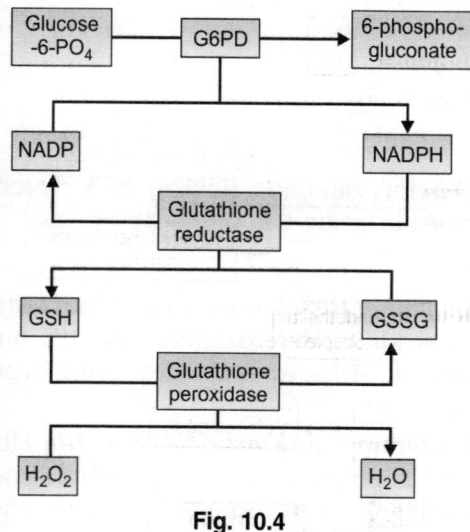

Fig. 10.4

Genetic variation of G6PD enzymes

- X-linked inheritance of mutant gene.
- *G6PD B:* Normal function, most common.
- Non-hemolytic variant: G6PD A$^+$.
- Hemolytic variants: G6PD A$^-$ (10–60% deficit functions), G6PD Mediterranean (90% deficit function).
- In all these cases synthesis of enzymes is normal but stability (decreased t½) of these abnormal enzymes affected.
- So reticulocytes and younger cells have normal functioning enzymes but older cells lose enzymes as no new enzymes can be synthesized in non-nucleated RBC.

Induction of hemolysis

- *Drug induced*: Antimalarial drugs like primaquine and chloroquine, sulfonamides, nitrofurans, acetyl salicylic acid, etc.
- *Infection*: Viral hepatitis, pneumonia, typhoid fever.
- *Food*: Fava beans.

- Neonatal jaundice or chronic low-grade hemolytic anemia.

Mechanism

- RBC having normal enzymes can easily withstand oxidative stress due to any conditions including above.
- Abnormal enzymes cannot deal with oxidative stress and result in intra as well as extravascular hemolysis.
- Infection or oxidant results in oxidation of sulfhydryl group of globin chain.
- Denaturation of Hb chain and its precipitation into *Heinz bodies* (appear as dark inclusion within cells).
- Heinz bodies can directly damage the RBC membrane sufficiently to cause intravascular hemolysis.
- Attachment of Heinz bodies to membrane aids to deformity of the RBC.
- Otherwise, these cells when pass through splenic cords, macrophages pluck out Heinz bodies along with the cytoplasm giving appearance of *'bite cells'*.
- Loss of membrane results in formation of spherocytes, further causing extravascular hemolysis.

14. Laboratory diagnosis of G6PD deficiency anemia (2002)

During normal phage: No anemia is evident but red cell survival is decreased. Defective variant enzymes can be detected by molecular technique.

During hemolytic phage

- *CBC*
  - Features of *intravascular hemolysis.*
  - Rapid fall of hematocrit.
  - During recovery phage—reticulocytosis.
  - MCV, MCH, MCHC—are normal as it is mostly acute condition which subsides once oxidative stresses are removed; so no morphologic changes are seen as seen in chronic hemolytic anemia.

- *PBS*
  - Heinz bodies (by supravital stains like crystal violet).
  - Bite cells (red cells with a 'bite' of membrane).
  - Blister cells (red cells with surface blistering of membrane).
  - Irregular shaped small cells.
- *G6PD assay*
  - Indirect method: Based on decreased ability to reduce dye. Methods used are: Methemoglobin Reduction Test (MRT), fluorescent screening test and ascorbate cyanide screening test.
  - Direct enzymes assay of RBC: In conditions where enzyme level is very low.
- *Electrophoresis of serum:* Based on altered mobility of different isoenzyme types.

Methemoglobin (MetHb) reduction test

- In this test Hb is converted into MetHb by addition of sodium nitrite. If the enzyme levels are normal, MetHb is reduced to normal Hb in the presence of a reducing dye (methylene blue); otherwise MetHb remains which is of brown color. Positive and negative controls are also set up.
- In males: Brown color of solution: Deficiency of enzymes.
- In homozygous female: Brown color solution: Deficiency of enzyme.
- In heterozygous female: Intermediate color between red and brown is seen.

---

15. Clinicopathological features of sickle-cell anemia (2008)

or

Molecular changes and pathophysiology in sickle cell disease

Molecular change

- A type of hereditary hemoglobinopathy (structurally abnormal hemoglobin production).
- Point mutation—substitution of normal glutamic acid (CTG) by valine (CAG) at 6th position in β-globin chain.

- If an individual is homozygous for sickle cell mutation almost all the hemoglobin in red cell is HbS, there is no normal β chain, so no HbA type of Hb in this condition.
- In heterozygous individual only 40% of hemoglobin is HbS, remainder being normal HbA.

Pathophysiology

(See Fig 10.5)

---

16. Factors affecting sickling and clinical features in sickle cell anemia

Factors

- *Amount of HbS:* The most important factor for sickling. Heterozygote has little tendency to sickle except under severe hypoxia.
- *Interaction with other type of Hb:* HbF inhibits polymerization of HbS and hence sickling (so, newborn shows disease after 5–6 months of life). HbC and HbD promote sickling. HbSC is more severe form of disease. HbA also has an inhibitory effect on polymerisation and sickling. Deoxy HbS molecule copolymerizes most effectively with other HbS molecules and in decreasing order, with HbC, D, O, Arab, A, J and F.
- *Hb concentration of cell/MCHC:* The rate of HbS polymerisation is strongly dependent upon the Hb concentration per cell, i.e. MCHC. Any condition (like dehydration) that increases MCHC increases sickling. Any condition (α-thalassemia) that decrease MCHC decrease sickling.
- The length of time red cells are exposed to low oxygen tension.
- pH: Fall in pH increases sickling.
- Oxygen concentration: The most important physiological determinant of HbS sickling. Polymerisation occurs only with deoxygenation. Any condition that decreases oxygen affinity of Hb (like acidosis or increased 2, 3 DPG) increases sickling.

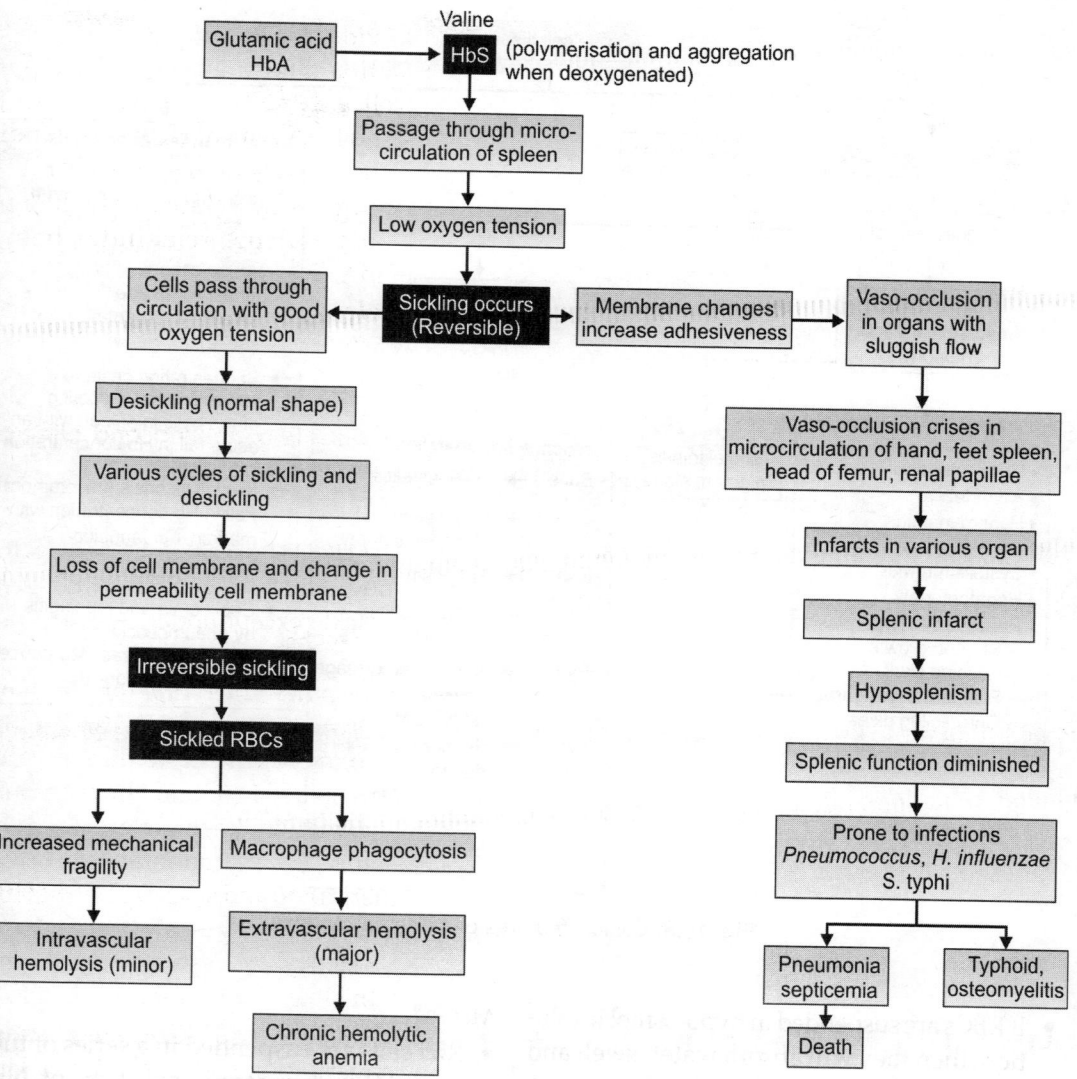

Fig. 10.5: Pathophysiology of sickle cell anemia

Clinical features

(See Fig 10.6)

Susceptibility to infection is due to:

1. Impaired splenic function due to erythrophagocytosis.

2. Autosplenectomy: Removes organ of bacterial filtration of blood.

3. Defect in alternate complement pathway (opsonisation defect of bacteria).

17. Osmotic fragility test (2007)

or

Lab diagnosis of sickle cell anemia (2001, 02, 11)

The osmotic fragility test is a measure of resistance of erythrocytes to hemolysis by osmotic stress.

Principle

• 0.9% NaCl is almost (slightly hyperosmolar) iso-osmolar to blood. RBCs suspended in 0.9 NaCl do not hemolyse.

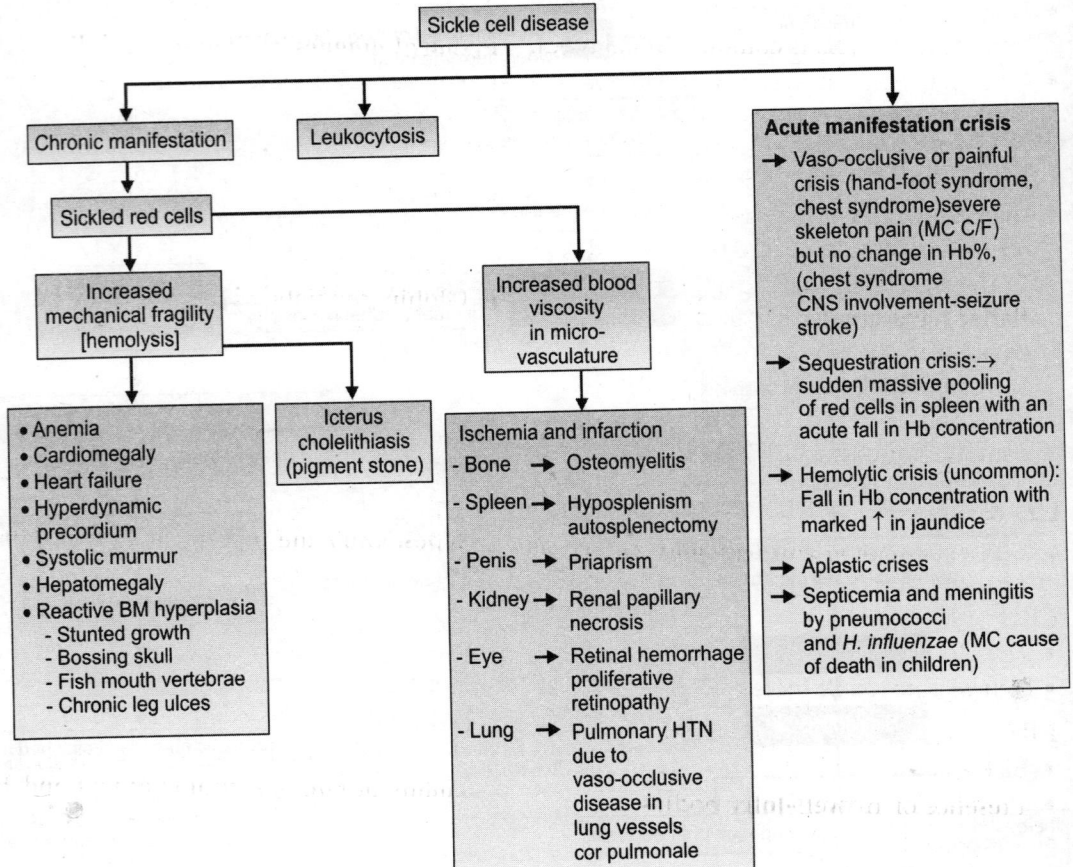

Fig. 10.6: Clinical features of sickle cell anemia

- If RBCs are suspended in hypo-osmolar solution, then they will absorb water, swell and after certain limit will burst and get hemolysed.
- Similarly, if they are kept in hyperosmolar fluid, they will shrink due to outflow of water from RBCs.

Method
- Red cells are suspended in a series of tubes containing hypotonic solution of NaCl varying from 0.9 to 0%. The degree of hemolysis is then measured for each NaCl concentration.

Increased osmotic fragility	Decreased osmotic fragility
Hereditary spherocytosis	Iron deficiency anemia
Hemolytic anemia (acquired immune)	Sickle cell anemia
Hemolytic disease of newborn	Thalassemia
Malaria	Asplenia
Severe pyruvate kinase deficiency	Liver disease
	Reticulocytosis
	Hemoglobinopathies, HbC, HbS

Interference

- Normally RBCs begin to hemolyse at 0.5 NaCl and the hemolysis is complete at 0.3 NaCl.
- Cells that are more spherical with a decreased surface/volume ratio have a limited capacity to expand in hypotonic solution and so lyse at higher concentration of NaCl than normal biconcave cells do. These cells are said to have increased osmotic fragility.
- Conversely, cells that are hypochromic and flatter have greater capacity to expand in hypotonic solution and so they lyse at a lower concentration than do the normal cells. These cells are said to have decreased osmotic fragility.

Lab diagnosis of sickle cell anemia

(*General features of intravascular as well as extravascular hemolysis*)

CBC
- *Hb:* Moderate to severe decrease (6–8 g/dl)
- *Reticulocyte count:* Increased

PBS
- Sickle cells
- Presence of **Howell-Jolly bodies**
- Target cells
- Nucleated RBC

Sickling test: Using reducing substance like sodium metabisulfite: Increased sickling tendency.

Hb electrophoresis
- Highly decreased or absent HbA (normal adult Hb)
- Highly increased HbS (abnormal Hb)
- Increased HbF (2–20%, compensatory ↑)

Solubility test: In reducing substance like sodium dithionite, HbA gives clear solution, whereas HbS polymerizes to produce turbid solution.

Osmotic fragility test: Highly decreased osmotic fragility due to sickle shape (as has large reserve for expansion of volume without rupture of cell).

X-ray: Crew cut appearance of facial bones.

Molecular method: To demonstrate mutation in gene or separation of HbS.

Prenatal diagnosis: Diagnosis of disease by molecular study of fetal DNA.

18. Hemoglobin: Summary

- Hemoglobin is a conjugated protein which consists of heme as prosthetic part and globin as the protein part.
- Globin consists of two pairs of similar polypeptide chain. Each of the polypeptide is attached with heme. Thus one hemoglobin molecule contains four heme units.
- Heme consists of iron plus porphyrin.
- Normal human hemoglobin is of several types. The heme group is identical in all types. Only the protein or globin part of these hemoglobin vary.

Adult hemoglobin (HbA)
- HbA is the major adult hemoglobin. It normally constitutes approximately 96% of the total adult hemoglobin.
- The globin part consists of four polypeptide chains of two identical α chains and two identical β chains.

Fetal hemoglobin (HbF) **(1988)**
- It is the major hemoglobin of fetus and newborn infants.
- The globin part consists of four polypeptide chains having two identical α chains similar to HbA and two identical γ chains in place of β chains of HbA.
- During fetal life, production of γ chains are high, so fetal hemoglobin is the predominant Hb in fetal life. As gestational age increases γ chain production decreases and β chain production increases. By 6–9 months after birth its value is significantly lower.
- Fetal hemoglobin resists alkali denaturation (adult hemoglobin does not)
- It has less ability to bind with 2, 3 DPG, and thus HbF has high affinity for oxygen.
- Quantitative estimation by Betke's method (adult N< 2 g%) and Singer's method (N< 4 g%)

- Increased HbF is seen in thalassemia major and minor, persistence of fetal hemoglobin (hereditary disease), hyperthyroidism, sickle cell disease, HbH disease, juvenile myeloid leukemia with absence of Philadelphia chromosome, anemia as a compensatory mechanism (pernicious anemia, PNH, sideroblastic anemia), aplastic anemia, myeloproliferative disorders, multiple myeloma, lymphoma.

Minor hemoglobin (HbA$_2$) **(2003)**

- It normally constitutes less than 3.5% of total adult hemoglobin.
- Globin part consists of two α (alpha) and δ (delta) chains.
- The level HbA$_2$ increases during the first year of life at which time the adult value is reached.
- Increased HbA$_2$ is seen in β-thalassemia major, minor and intermedia, HbA/S (sickle cell trait) (15–45%), HbS/S (sickle cell disease) (2–6%), megaloblastic anemia, hyperthyroidism, vitamin B$_{12}$ or folate deficiency.
- Decreased HbA$_2$ is seen in untreated iron deficiency anemia, sideroblastic anemia, HbH disease, erythroleukemia.

19. Common types of thalassemia

i. α-thalassemia
   - α-thalassemia trait
   - Hemoglobin H disease
   - Hemoglobin Bart's (hydrops fetalis)
ii. β-thalassemia
   - β-thalassemia minor (trait)

β-thalassemia-molecular pathology

- β-thalassemia intermedia
- β-thalassemia major.

20. β-thalassemia: Molecular changes

"There is a total lack or a reduction in the synthesis of structurally normal β-globin chains with normal synthesis of α-chain."

- Normal Hb found in adults is HbA (two α chains and two β-chains).
- β-chains are coded by two globin genes each located on one of the two chromosomes 11, whereas α-chains are coded by two pairs of genes located on each chromosomes 16.
- Thalassemias are autosomal recessive disorder. β-thalassemia is caused by point mutation while α-thalassemia is caused by gene deletion.

Molecular pathology

- β^0 thalassemia: Total absence of β-chain in homozygous state.
- β$^+$ thalassemia: Reduced β-chain in homozygous state.
- β-thalassemia is mainly due to point mutation (in contrast to gene deletion in α-thalassemia).
- Promotor region mutation lead to β$^+$ thalassemia.
- Chain terminator mutation leads to β^0 thalassemia. Either of two mechanisms:
  1. Frame shift mutation (introduction of stop codon).
  2. Splicing mutation (most common cause of thalassemia).
  At junction of exon and intron—β^0 thalassemia. In intron—β$^+$ thalassemia.
- Translation defect of exon leads to β^0 thalassemia.

	β-globin genes	HbA	HbA$_2$	HbF
Normal	Homozygous β	97–99%	1–3%	<1%
Thalassemia major	Homozygous β^0	0%	4–10%	90–96%
	Heterozygous β$^+$ (mild)	0–30%	0–10%	60–100%
Thalassemia intermedia	Homozygous β$^+$ (mild)	0–30%	0–10%	60–100%
Thalassemia minor	Heterozygous β^0	80–95%	4–8%	1–5%
	Heterozygous β$^+$	80–95%	4–8%	1–5%

21. β-thalassemia major: Pathogenesis and clinical features

Pathogenesis: (*See* Fig. 10.7)

Clinical features of thalassemia major

- Age of manifestation: 6–9 months after birth (as HbF ↓↓ es).

- Severe anemia, requires regular transfusion.
- *Untransfused patients*
  - Fails to thrive
  - Growth retardation
  - Die at early age
  - Bone marrow expansion (crew cut appearance of face on X-ray)

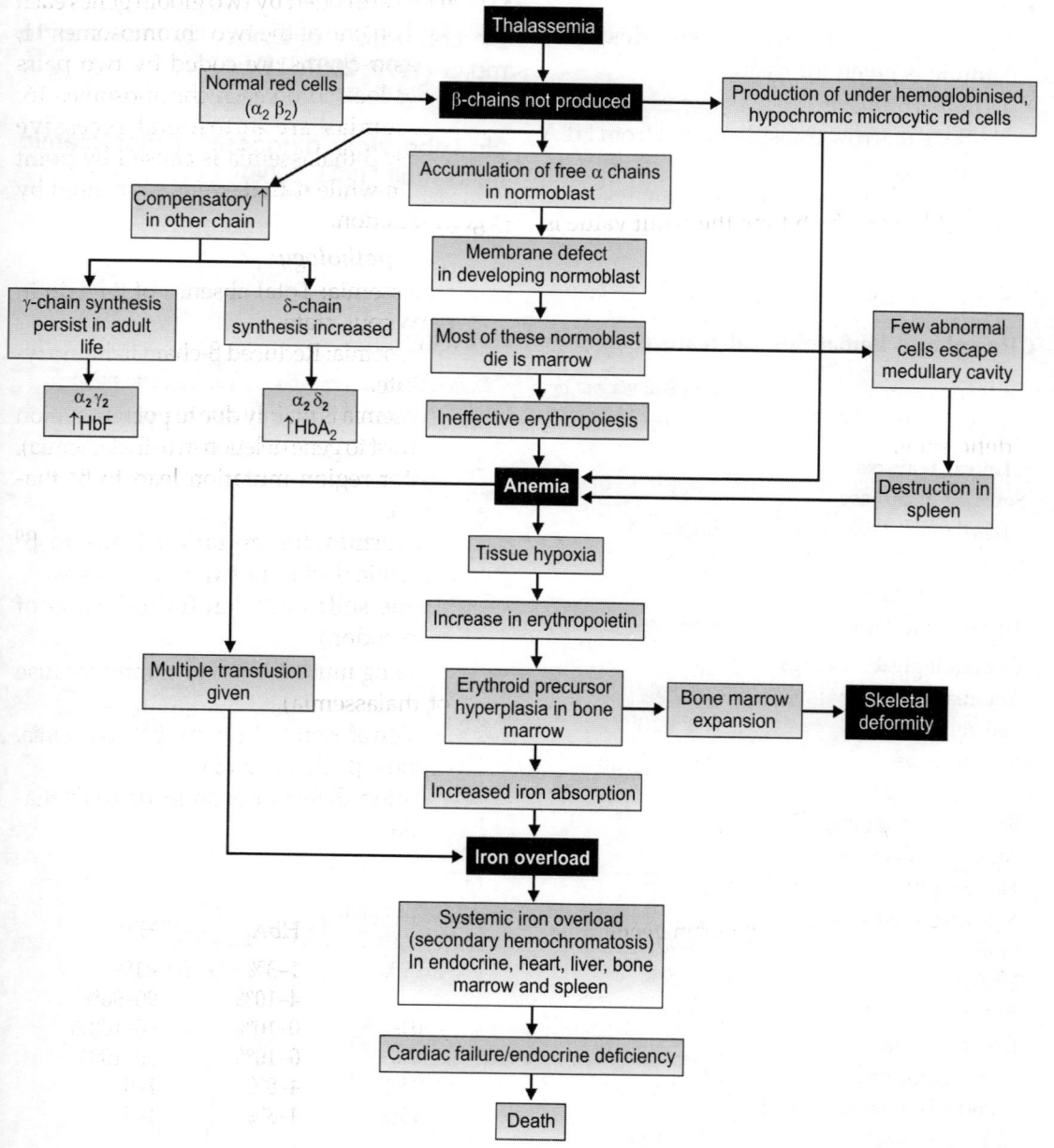

Fig. 10.7: Pathophysiology of thalassemia

- Hepatosplenomegaly (erythrophago-cytosis, extramedullary erythropoiesis)
- Recurrent infections, spontaneous frac-tures, leg ulcers.
- Mongoloid or thalassemia facies (due to marrow expansion, patients have skull bossing, hypertrophied maxillae and hair on end appearance on X-ray).
- *Transfused patients*
Secondary hemochromatosis (desferro-xamine is given for treatment)
- *Definite treatment*
  - Bone marrow transplantation from HLA identical sibling.
  - Prenatal diagnosis by DNA analysis and abortion.

22. β-thalassemia minor: Clinical features

- Asymptomatic, mild or no anemia
- Are diagnosed accidentally looking for some other disease in blood smears.

23. Lab diagnosis of thalassemia (2003)

24. Laboratory diagnosis of thalassemia major (1993, 2001, 11)

25. Laboratory diagnosis of thalassemia minor/trait (1993, 2008)

(*See* Table below)

Clinical and hematological features of β-thalassemia

	Thalassemia major	*Thalassemia intermedia*	*Thalassemia minor*
Genetics	Homozygous	Double heterozygous	Heterozygous
Clinical features			
Severity of disease	++++	++	±
Growth and development	Impaired	Normal	Normal
Splenomegaly	++++	++	–nt
Skeletal changes	+++	±	–nt
Thalassemia facies	+++	+	–nt
Hematological findings			
Anemia (Hb)	< 7 g%	7–10 g%	> 10 g%
Red cell count	$< 4 \times 10^{12}/l$	$< 5 \times 10^{12}/l$	$> 5.5 \times 10^{12}/l$
Microcytosis	+++	++	+
Hypochromia	+++	++	+
Basophilic stippling	++	+	+
Anisopoikilocytosis	+++	++	±
Target cells	+++	++	+
Nucleated red cells	++	–nt/occasional	–nt
HbF	30–90%	20–100%	0–5%
HbA_2	< 3.5%	< 3.5%	3.6–8%
BM iron	++++	++	±
Iron overload			
– myocardium	+	–nt	–nt
– endocrine involvement	+	–nt	–nt
Life expectancy	20–28 yrs	Normal	Normal
Blood transfusion	Repeated BT	No regular BT	No BT

β-*thalassemia major*
- *CBC*
  - Hb: 3–6 g/dl
  - MCV: ↓↓ed
  - MCH: ↓↓ed
  - MCHC: ↓↓ed
  - RCB: count ↓↓ed
  - Hematocrit: ↓↓ed (severely)
  - WBC: ↑ed (often), shift to left of neutrophil series, with presence of myelocytes and metamyelocytes.
  - Platelet count: normal/↓ed (if massive splenomegaly).
- *PBS*
  - Severe microcytic hypochromic anemic picture
  - Marked anisopoikilocytosis
  - Basophilic stippling
  - Fragmented red cells
  - Normoblasts
  - Target cells
  - Pencil cells
  - Nucleated RBCs
  - Tear-drop cells
  - Cells with Cabot's ring
- *BM*
  - Normoblastic erythroid hyperplasia
  - Myeloid/erythroid ratio (3:1) reversal
  - Ineffective erythropoiesis
  - Predominance of intermediate and late normoblast (smaller in size than normal)
  - ↑↑ed reticuloendothelial iron
  - Sideroblast: Uncommon
  - Siderotic granules in cytoplasm of normoblasts
  - Increase in bone marrow iron because of hemolysis and repeated transfusion.
- *Hb electrophoresis*
  - HbA: absent/↓↓ed, (0–30% of total Hb)
  - HbA$_2$: Normal/↓ed/↑ed, (0–10% of total Hb)
  - HbF: ↑↑ed (60–100% of total Hb)
- *Biochemical findings*
  - S. bilirubin (unconjugated): ↑ed

- S. iron: marked ↑ed
- Urine urobilinogen: ↑ed
- Percentage transferrin saturation: > 70%
- S. ferritin: 300–3000 mg/dl (↑↑ed)
- *Osmotic fragility*: ↓ed osmotic fragility of red cells

β-thalassemia trait
- *CBC*
  - Hb: mild ↓ed
  - Hematocrit: ↓ed
  - Reticulocyte count: ↑↑ed
  - MCV, MCH, MCHC: ↓↓es out of proportion to degree of anemia
  - RBC: ↑ed count (it is differentiating features from IDA, despite ↓ in Hb, RBC ↑es here)
- *PBS*
  - Minor abnormality as compared to thalassemia major
  - Hypochromic, microcytic RBC
  - Tear-drop cells
  - Cells with Cabot's ring
  - Target cells
  - Pencil cells
  - Nucleated RBC
  - Basophilic stippling
  - Irregularly contracted cells
  - Anisopoikilocytosis may be present
- *BM*: Mild erythroid hyperplasia
- *Hb electrophoresis:* HbA$_2$: Highly increased (3.6 – 9%) (Normal 1–3.5%)
- *Osmotic fragility test*: Decreased fragility
- Molecular technique: Prenatal diagnosis, mutation detection (point mutation)
- Iron profile: (See comparative table of microcytic hypochromic anemia).

26. Paroxysmal nocturnal hemoglobinuria (PNH): Pathology and lab diagnosis (2002)

"Only example of acquired defect in red cell membrane".

Pathology
- Mutation in phosphatidylinositol glycan A (PIGA) gene that codes for GPI protein.

- Glycosylphosphatidylinositol (GPI) protein acts as an anchor of GPI linked proteins to the cell membrane.
- GPI linked proteins that regulate complement factors are absent in PNH (complement regulatory proteins) and their effect:
  - CD55 or decay-accelerating factor (increased hemolysis)
  - CD59-membrane inhibitor of reactive lysis inactivation of C3 convertase of alternative complement pathway (increased hemolysis).
  - C8 binding protein
  - Urokinase plasminogen activator receptor (promotes thrombosis).
  - Neutrophil alkaline phosphatase (decrease in neutrophil alkaline phosphatase score).

  The somatic mutation occurs in pleuripotent stem cells, hence all clonal progeny, i.e. RBCs, platelets, granulocytes are more sensitive to complement lysis when these proteins are absent.

Laboratory diagnosis
- General picture of intravascular anemia
- Hb: ↓ed
- RBC count: ↓ed
- WBC count: ↓ed
- Platelet count: ↓ed (pancytopenia)
- Reticulocyte count: ↑ed

- HbF: occasionally raised
- Serum bilirubin: ↑ed
- *PBS*
  - Anemic picture
  - Moderate macrocytosis
  - Polychromasia
- *BM*
  - Hypercellular marrow
  - Some dyserythropoiesis
  - Normoblastic erythroid hyperplasia
  - Iron store: ↓ed
  - Bone marrow is sometimes aplastic
- *Hams test:* Screening test for PNH.
  Principle: The patient's cell undergo hemolysis in compatible acidified serum at 37°C. The serum may be the patient's own or from another normal subject. 10–50% lysis is usually observed in a positive test. Hemolysis is by alternative complement pathway.
- *Sucrose hemolysis test:* Screening test for PNH. More sensitive than Hams test, though lacks specificity. PNH red cells are lysed when suspended in isotonic solutions of low ionic strength if serum is also present. If whole blood screening test (the sugar water test) is positive then confirmatory sucrose lysis test is done to find out degree of hemolysis (>10% hemolysis: Diagnostic of PNH, 5–10: borderline). Hemolysis is by classic pathway of complement.

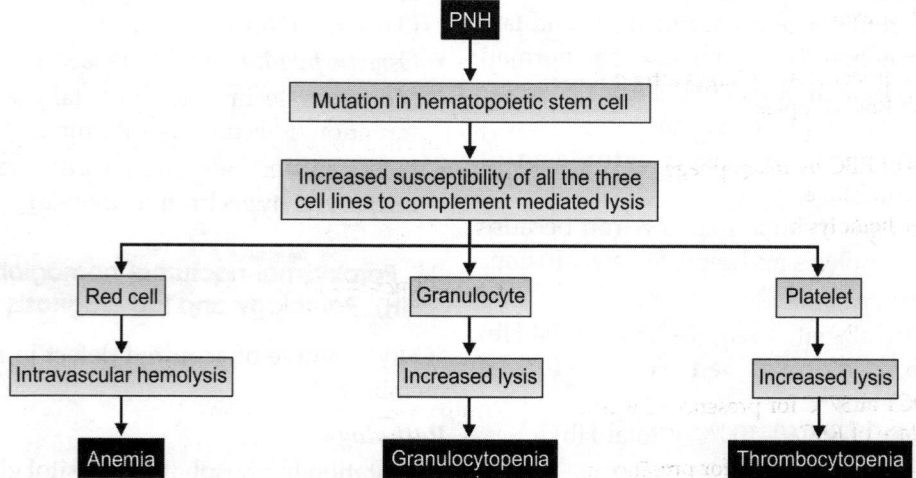

Fig. 10.8: Pathology of PNH

- Now the diagnosis of PNH depends upon analysing the expression of GPI-AP on the hematopoietic stem cells using monoclonal antibodies and flow cytometry. The simplest method is to analyse the expression of CD59 on erythrocytes.
- Leukocyte alkaline phosphatase: ↑ed LAP
- Coombs' test: In some cases direct antiglobulin test is positive.
- Hemoglobinuria and hemosiderinuria is common.

Clinical features

- Intravascular hemolysis: It is paroxysmal and usually occurs at night.
- Intermittent clinical hemoglobinuria, acute hemolytic episodes occur at night (mostly) identified by passage of brown colored urine in the morning. During sleep at night,

the pH of blood gets slightly reduced, low pH leads to activation of complement.
- Thrombosis: Despite the presence of thrombocytopenia, PNH is associated with venous thrombosis. The absence of CD59 on platelets results in externalization of phosphatidyl serine, a site for prothrombin complexes and thus increases the propensity for thrombosis. The thrombosis occurs most commonly in intra-abdominal vein (Budd-Chiari syndrome/hepatic vein thrombosis) followed by cerebral vein and intradermal vein.

27. Autoimmune hemolytic anemia (AIHA)

- AIHA are a group of diseases in which hemolysis occurs as a result of presence of autoantibodies, with specificity against

Idiopathic warm autoimmune hemolytic anemia	Idiopathic cold hemagglutinin disease
Binding of autoantibodies to red cells membrane occurs maximally at 37°C	Binding of autoantibodies to red cells membrane occurs maximally at 4°C
These autoantibodies are usually IgG type	These autoantibodies are usually IgM type
Disease associated:	**Disease associated:** Cold hemagglutinin disease,
Malignant lymphoma, CML, myeloma, SLE, PAN, RA	*Mycoplasma pneumonia*, malignant lymphoma, infectious mononucleosis
Mechanism of hemolysis	**Mechanism of hemolysis**
RBCs coated with IgG type antibody	RBCs coated with IgM antibody at low temperature
At higher temperature	↓
↓	Activation of complement
Pass through spleen	↓
↓	C3 binds to RBC membrane
Fc receptor of spleen macrophages attract Fc portion of Ab-RBC complex	↓
↓	While traveling through warm area, weakly bound IgM are released, but C3b remains attached to RBC
Phagocytosis of RBC by macrophage	↓
↓	Splenic macrophages have receptors for activated C3 (CR1 and CR3)
Extravascular hemolysis	↓
	Coated RBCs are phagocytosed
	↓
	Extravascular hemolysis
Diagnosis	**Diagnosis**
• Positive DCT at 37°C for presence of warm Ab on surface of RBC	Positive DCT for detection of C3 on the red cell surface, but IgM responsible for coating on red cells is not found.
• Positive indirect CT at 37°C for presence of large quantities of warm Ab in serum	

blood group antigen. These autoantibodies are detected by Coombs' test, therefore these are also called Coombs' positive hemolytic anemias.

- Based on the maximum binding of these autoantibodies to erythrocyte membrane at two specific temperature (37°C and 4°C), these are classified as idiopathic warm autoimmune hemolytic anemia and idiopathic cold hemagglutinin disease.

28. Coombs' test (1995, 96, 2002, 04, 09)

"This test is used to detect the incomplete antibodies present in serum. These antibodies coat antigens, but do not agglutinate them".

Principle: When human gammaglobin (antiglobin, Coombs' serum, complete antibodies) directed against such incomplete antibodies, are made to react with these incomplete antibodies and agglutination takes place.

Methods: Two types are:

1. *Direct Coombs' test (DCT)*
   - This method detects the incomplete antibodies coated on the surface of red cells (as in hemolytic disease of newborn, maternal antibodies have already coated the baby's RBCs).
   - RBCs are separated from the blood of such patients, and suspension is prepared in normal saline.
   - Now, antibodies against the incomplete antibodies coating RBCs are added,

which bind with these incomplete antibodies and lead to agglutination of RBCs. This is *positive* Coombs' test.

- In case incomplete antibodies coating RBCs are absent Coombs' test will be negative.

Indications
- Hemolytic disease of newborn
- Autoimmune hemolytic anemia

2. *Indirect Coombs' test*
   - Here we detect the incomplete antibodies present in a person's sera (as in case of a Rh negative mother whose 1st child is Rh positive, and wants second conception).
   - The serum from the patient is taken and added to suspension of O⁺ RBCs. If the serum contains incomplete antibodies against Rh antigen, it will coat the O⁺ RBCs. The suspension is washed many times to remove excess unbound antibodies in the serum.
   - Thereafter, Coombs' serum is added. If agglutination occurs, the test is said to be positive.

Indications
- In cross matching of blood to detect incomplete antibodies in donor's serum.
- In case of Rh negative mother whose 1st child is Rh positive, and wants second conception.

Interpretation

IgG	Anti-C3 antibodies	Conditions
Positive	Negative	1. Idiopathic 2. Secondary to lymphomas or autoimmune (like SLE) or drugs
Negative	Positive	1. Acute conditions like MI 2. Chronic conditions—idiopathic or may be associated with lymphoma
Positive	Positive	Viral infection, *Mycoplasma pneumoniae*, and paroxysmal cold hemoglobinuria

*IgG and anti-C3 antibodies are incomplete antibodies.

29. Megaloblastic anemia (1995): define and causes (1998)

1. **Macrocyte:** It is characterized by increased volume (MCV > 100 fl), diameter (>8.5 µl), and thickness of red cell (MCH > 31.5 pg; MCHC: Normal). Increased thickness is perceived as a loss of central pallor.

2. Megaloblastic anemia constitutes a group of diseases having impaired DNA synthesis and abnormally large erythrocyte and its precursor cells.
3. Megaloblast: An erythrocyte in which maturation of nucleus lags behind maturation of cytoplasm due to impaired DNA synthesis caused by deficiency of vitamin B_{12} and folate.

30. Causes of macrocytic anemia (1995)

Vitamin B_{12} deficiency	Folate deficiency
Decreased intake	Decreased intake
Inadequate diet, vegetarianism	Inadequate diet, alcohol, infancy
Impaired absorption	Impaired absorption
Intrinsic factor deficiency	Malabsorption state, intestinal disease
Pernicious anemia	Oral contraceptives, anticonvulsants
Gastrectomy	Increased loss: Hemodialysis
Malabsorption	Increased requirement
Diffuse intestinal disease like lymphoma, ileal resection, ingestion of corrosives	Pregnancy, infancy, disseminated cancer, markedly increased hematopoiesis
Parasites like fish tapeworm	Impaired use—antagonists (methotrexate)
Small bowel bacterial overgrowth	**Non-vit B_{12} non-folate**
Increased requirement	Metabolic inhibitors like
Pregnancy, hyperthyroidism, malignant disseminated cancer	Fluorouracil, mercaptourines
	Unexplained
	Acute erythroleukemia
	Pyridoxine and thiamine-responsive megaloblastic anemia
Liver diseases	**Hypothyroidism**
Disorders of red cell production	**Idiopathic**
Aplastic anemia	Pregnancy
Pure red cell aplasia	Chronic lung disease
Myelodysplastic syndromes	Cancer
Myeloproliferative disorders	Multiple myeloma
Sideroblastic anemia	
Drugs inhibiting DNA synthesis	**Others drugs**
Purine antagonist	Phenytoin
6-Mercaptopurine, azathioprine	Primidone
Pyrimidine antagonist	Phenobarbitone
5FU, cystosine arabinose	Nitrous oxide
Other	
Procarbazine, hydroxyurea, acyclovir, zidovudine	

31. Pathogenesis of megaloblastic transformation of red cells (2000)

- Vitamin B_{12} and folic acid are coenzymes for DNA synthesis. Its absence or decreased level impairs DNA synthesis and hence nuclear maturation.
- Delayed nuclear maturation results in delayed cell division.
- As such these vitamins have no role in RNA formation and protein synthesis, so cytoplasm are formed normally on time.
- Delayed cell division results in 'extra-accumulation' of cytoplasmic contents and its disproportionate enlargement with the net result of increased cell size, i.e. megaloblastic anemia.

32. Laboratory diagnosis of megaloblastic anemia (1993, 97, 98, 2000, 02, 04, 07)

33. Investigations in case of vitamin B_{12} deficiency (2004)

CBC
- RBC count: ↓ed
- Hb: ↓ed
- TLC: Normal/↓ed
- Platelet: Normal/↓ed
- MCV: >100 fentoliter (fl) is suggestive of megaloblastic anemia; if >110 fl, it indicates more of megaloblastic anemia than any liver disease, aplastic anemia, etc.
- MCH: ↑ed
- MCHC: Normal/↓ed
- Reticulocyte count: ↓ed/normal
- Severe megaloblastic anemia is associated with pancytopenia.

PBS
- Macrocytosis of red cells is a characteristic feature. Macrocytes are larger in diameter, thickness and volume. Hb content in cell is proportionately increased, therefore, MCHC remains normal.
- Moderate to marked degree of aniso-poikilocytosis seen.

- Red cells are variable in size with majority being macro-ovalocyte (diagnostic of megaloblastic anemia)
- Tear-drop cells
- Evidence of dyserythropoiesis like elongated red cells with inclusion like Howell-Jolly bodies, basophilic stippling, and cabot's ring.
- Few large hypersegmented neutrophils (characteristic feature, one of the first manifestations of megaloblastic anemia): They have 6–10 nuclear lobes.

BM
- Bone marrow: Hypercellular with megaloblastic predominence
- M:E ratio = ↓ed up to 1:1 (normal 3:1)
- Megaloblasts are abnormal, large, nucleated, have nuclear-cytoplasmic maturation asynchrony, nuclear chromatin failing to mature because of impaired DNA synthesis, while cytoplasm gets hemoglobinized, nuclear chromatin more dispersed than expected.
- Degenerated erythroid precursor cells (ineffective erythropoiesis)
- Abundant stainable iron found
- Megakaryocytes: Large, multilobulated nuclei
- Giant form of metamyelocytes and band cells may be present
- Increase in number and size of iron granules in erythroid precursor cells (Prussian blue staining)

Special tests
A. Biochemical test
   1. *Serum*
      a. *Microbiological assay*: Use of *Euglenia gracilis* or *lactobacillus*. Incubate serum with these organisms and look for turbidity. A value of less than 100 ng/l indicates megaloblastic anemia.
      b. *Radioassay*: Use serum with vitamin B_{12} and folic acid labelled with cobalt (radio labelled). We look for serum and red cell value of these enzymes.

c. *Measurement of serum cobalamin and folate:*
  • Normal S. cobalamin: 200–900 pg/ml (<100 pg/ml is significant for the disease).
  • Normal S. folate: 6–20 ng/ml (<4 ng/ml is significant).
  • Measurement of RBC folate level provides useful information, as it is not subjected to short-term fluctuation.
  • Red cells folate is decreased both in vitamin B_{12} and folate deficiency.
d. *Other serum tests:*
  • Serum iron: Normal/↑ed
  • Serum ferritin: Normal/↑ed
  • Bilirubin (unconjugated): ↑ed
  • LDH: ↑ed ($LDH_1 > LDH_2$)
  • Serum methylmalonate and homocysteine level are increased in cobalamin deficiency; only homocysteine is increased in folate deficiency.

2. Urine
a. Methyl malonyl urea (methylmalonate in urine): Vitamin B_{12} deficiency.
b. Increased exretion of FIGLU after administered dose of histidine: Folate deficiency.

B. Other special test
  • Schilling test
  • Deoxyuridine (DU) suppression test: Less suppression in case of megaloblastic anemia than normal.
  • Clinical: No neurologic deficit in folate deficiency as compared to vitamin B_{12} deficiency.

Clinical features of megaloblastic anemia (vit B_{12})
  • Pallor of gradual onset
  • Glossitis and angular cheilosis
  • CNS manifestation: Subacute combined demyelination of posterolateral column of spinal cord resulting in unsteadiness of gait and altered sensorium. There may be dementia (reversible).
  • Peripheral neuropathy: Numbness and tingling
  • Thrombosis

34. Schilling test (radioisotope absorption test)

Schilling test
  • This test is done in patients of megaloblastic (vitamin B_{12} deficiency) anemia to rule out pernicious anemia (intrinsic factor deficiency) or malabsorption of vitamin B_{12}.
  • This test is done in two parts:

Part 1: Oral versus intramuscular
  • 0.5–2.0 µg oral dose of radiolabelled vitamin B_{12} (Hot B_{12}) is given.
  • At the same time, intramuscular unlabelled vitamin B_{12} (Cold B_{12}), 4 gram (large dose) is given to saturate the tissue store with normal B_{12} so that orally given radiolabelled vit B_{12} cannot bind to body tissues, and if absorbed, it will pass into urine.
  • Normally, ingested radiolabelled B_{12} will be absorbed into the body. Since the body already has liver receptors for vitamin B_{12} saturated by injected unlabelled B_{12}, much of the labelled B_{12} is excreted through urine.

Part 2: Vitamin B_{12} versus IF
  • If the abnormality is found in part 1, the test is repeated, this time with additional oral intrinsic factor.
  • This step differentiate between pernicious anemia (IF deficiency) from malabsorption.
  • In some places an additional stage 3 test is done before labelling malabsorption of vitamin B_{12}. The whole test is repeated after a course of treatment with antibiotics or anti-inflammatory drugs, if the excretion becomes normal; it was malabsorption vitamin B_{12} (*see* Fig. 10.9).

35. Vitamin B_{12}: Its absorption, biochemical functions

  • Active absorption of vitamin B_{12} is a highly efficient mechanism responsible for the absorption of physiological amount of vitamin B_{12} (*see* Fig. 10.10).

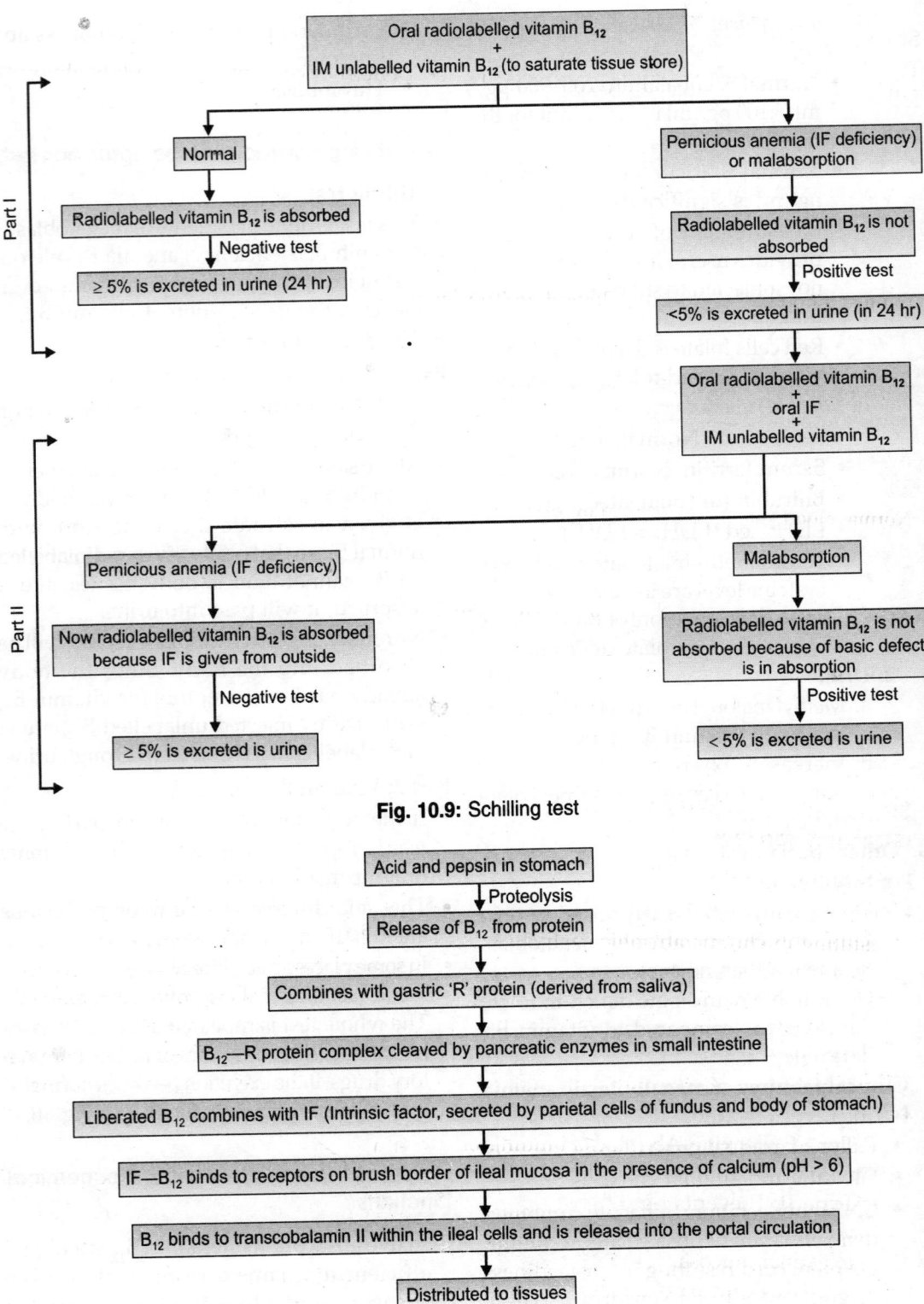

Fig. 10.9: Schilling test

Fig. 10.10: Vitamin B_{12}—absorption and transport

Storage of vitamin B_{12}

The liver stores large amount of vitamin B_{12}, followed by kidneys, heart and brain.

Functions of vitamin B_{12}

- As a co-factor in the formation of succinyl CoA from methylmalonyl CoA.
- DNA synthesis
- Deficiency of vitamin B_{12} leads to abnormal myelin lipids synthesis (myelin degeneration and neurological abnormalities), impaired DNA synthesis and trapping of folate as methyltetrahydrofolate.

Features	Vit B_{12}	Folate
Content in food	*Vegetables:* Poor source	*Vegetables:* Rich source
	Meat: Rich source	*Meat:* Moderate source
	Milk: Rich source	*Milk:* Poor source
Effect of cooking	10–30% loss	60–90% loss
Adult: Daily requirement	2–4 µg	200 µg
Adult: Daily intake	5–30 µg	100–500 µg
Site of absorption	Ileum	Duodenum and jejunum
Normal blood level	140–180 pg/ml	165–760 ng/ml
Body stores	2–5 mg	5–10 mg
	Adequate for three years	Adequate for 4 months
Function	Myelin synthesis	DNA synthesis
	DNA synthesis	
Deficiency	Megaloblastic anemia	Megaloblastic anemia
	Neurological symptoms	

36. Pernicious anemia: Pathogenesis and diagnostic features

Pathogenesis

- Antibody mediated autoimmune disease resulting in chronic atrophic gastritis, loss of parietal cells, and prominent infiltration of lymphocytes and plasma cells.
  - It leads to deficiency of intrinsic factor (IF)/its function.
  - Impairment of vitamin B_{12} absorption.
- Three types of autoantibodies:
  - Type I: Blocking Ab (blocks binding of vitamin B_{12} to IF).
  - Type II: Prevents binding of IF or IF-vitamin B_{12} complex to IF receptors of intestinal mucosa.
  - Type III: Parietal canalicular Ab (against alpha and beta subunit of gastric proton pump).

Diagnostic features

- Moderate to severe megaloblastic anemia
- Leucopoenia with hypersegmented neutrophils
- Mild to moderate thrombocytopenia
- Neurologic changes mainly involving posterolateral spinal tract
- Achlorhydria even after histamine stimulation
- Schilling test (inability to absorb oral vitamin B_{12})
- Striking improvement in anemic condition after parenteral administration of vitamin B_{12}
- Low level of serum vitamin B_{12}
- Excretion of methylmalonic acid in urine
- Presence of autoantibody against IF

37. Difference between megaloblast and normoblast (1988, 94, 98, 2004, 07, 09, 11)

S. No.	Traits	Megaloblast	Normoblast
1.	Produced in conditions	In deficiency of folic acid and vitamin B_{12}	Normal red cells
2.	Size (MCV)	Larger than normal (> 100 fl)	Normal (78–100 fl)
3.	*Nucleus*		
	Size	3/4th of cell volume	Very small
	Chromatin	"Opened"	Clumped, pyknotic
	Nucleoli	2–3 in number	Absent
4.	*Cytoplasm*		
	Amount	Less as compared to cell size	More
	Staining	Deep basophilic	Less basophilic

38. Causes of microcytosis (1990, 99)

39. Causes of microcytic hypochromic anemia (2002)

Disorders of iron metabolism	Disorders of globin synthesis	Disorders of porphyrin and heme synthesis
• Iron deficiency anemia	• Thalassemia	• Sideroblastic anemia
• Anemia of chronic disease	• HbE trait and disease	• Defective δ aminolevulinic acid
• Atransferrinemia	• HbC disease	• Defective ALA synthatase activity
• Shahidi-Nathan-Diamond syndrome	• Unstable Hb disease	• Deficiency of ferrochelatase
	Unknown mechanism:	• Vitamin B_6 deficiency
	Aluminum intoxication	• Lead poisoning

40. Iron deficiency anemia (IDA): Causes and lab diagnosis (1990, 94, 97, 99, 2002, 09)

Causes

Decreased iron intake	Increased blood loss
• Inadequate diet	• Gynecological and obstetrics
Impaired absorption	Excessive menstruation
• Achlorhydria	• GIT bleeding
• Gastric surgery	Hemorrhoids, parasitic infestation
• Celiac disease	ulcers, ulcerative colitis
• Anorexia	Malignancies, esophageal varices
Increased requirement	• Renal tract bleeding
• Growth phase of infancy, childhood, and adolescence	Hematuria, hemoglobinuria
• Pregnancy	• Hemoptysis
• Lactation	• Repeated epistaxis
	• Frequent blood donation

Laboratory diagnosis

CBC

- Hb: ↓ed
- Hematocrit: ↓ed
- RBC count: ↓ed
- WBC count: Usually normal
- Platelet count: Normal
- MCV: ↓ed
- MCH: ↓ed
- MCHC: ↓ed
- RDW (RBC distribution width): ↑ed
- Reticulocyte count: Normal/↑ed or ↑ed after hemorrhage
- Platelet count: Normal/↑ed in patients who had bleeding
- ESR: Normal/slightly ↑ed

PBS

- Microcytic, hypochromic red cells
- Poikilocytosis (variation in shape)
- Anisocytosis or variation in cell size (indicated by increased RDW)
- Elliptical form RBC
- Target cells, pencil cells
- Polychromatic cells

BM

- Erythroid hyperplasia (increased cellularity)
- M: E ratio decreased
- Normoblastic erythropoiesis with predominance of small polychromatic normoblasts: Micronormoblasts (cytoplasmic maturation lags behind: pyknotic nucleus but persistent of polychromatic cytoplasm)
- Dyserythropoiesis: Seen (mild)
- Sideroblast: Reduced
- Cytoplasmic basophilia: Present

Serum iron studies:

(See comparative table of microcytic hypochromic anemia)

Bone marrow iron (Prussian blue/Pearl reaction): ↓ed

Others

- Serum bilirubin: Normal/slightly ↓ed

- Plasma in hematocrit tube is paler or even colorless
- Transferrin receptors (thought to be most accurate): ↑ed

41. Iron metabolism (1999)

(See Fig. 10.11)

Serum iron and transferrin (iron carrier protein):

- The level of transferrin is not measured directly, but it is quantified in terms of iron it will bind, i.e. total iron binding capacity (TIBC). In an average normal adult, serum transferrin can bind to 300 µg/dl (250–400 µg/dl) of iron (TIBC). But only 1/3rd of transferrin (33%) is bound to iron, i.e. percentage saturation of transferrin is 33%.
- The rate of synthesis of transferrin is inversely related to iron store.
- The serum iron level that is measured is actually the amount of iron bound to transferrin.

Serum transferrin receptor:

These are cell surface receptors present on cells (of mainly iron storing organ) for iron-transferrin complex. The number of receptors decrease when a person is replete with iron (adequate iron store) and increase with depletion of iron and increased erythroid activity (erythropoiesis).

Serum ferritin

Ferritin is a storage form of iron and is found in plasma in small amounts and the serum ferritin concentration correlates roughly with the amount of iron in stores.

Normal value: 15–300 µg/l

Total body iron: 3–5 gm

Average daily intake of iron: 10–20 mg; 10% of which is absorbed.

42. Difference between IDA and anemia of chronic disease (ACD) (2004, 07)

43. Difference between IDA and sideroblastic anemia

44. Comparative table of microcytic and hypochromic anemia

S. No.	Traits	IDA	β-thalassemia trait	Sideroblastic	ACD
1.	Serum iron (50–150 µg/dl)	↓	Normal	↑	↓
2.	TiBC (310–340 µg/dl)	↑	Normal	Normal	↓
3.	% Transferrin saturation	↓↓	Normal	↑	Normal/↑
4.	Serum ferritin (50–300 µg/l)	↓	Normal	↑	↑
5.	FEP*	↑	Normal	↑	↑
6.	Marrow iron stores	Absent/↓↓↓	Present	Present	Present
7.	Iron in normoblast	Absent/↓↓	Present	Ring sideroblast	Absent
8.	Hb electrophoresis HbA$_2$	Normal/↓	↑	↓	Normal
9.	MCV, MCH, MCHC	Reduced	Very low	Very low (MCV ↑ in acquired)	Low normal to reduced
10.	Hematocrit	↓	Mild ↓	↓ .	↓
11.	Special tests	↑ FEP, ↑ transferrin receptor	↑ HbA$_2$	↑ FEP, sideroblasts	CRP, fibrinogen, ↑ ESR
12.	% sideroblast	↓	Normal	↑	↓
13.	HbF	Normal	Normal/↑	Normal/↑	Normal
14.	Cause of anemia	Iron deficiency	Genetic	Hereditary/ acquired	Chronic disease

*FEP: Free erythrocyte porphyrin.

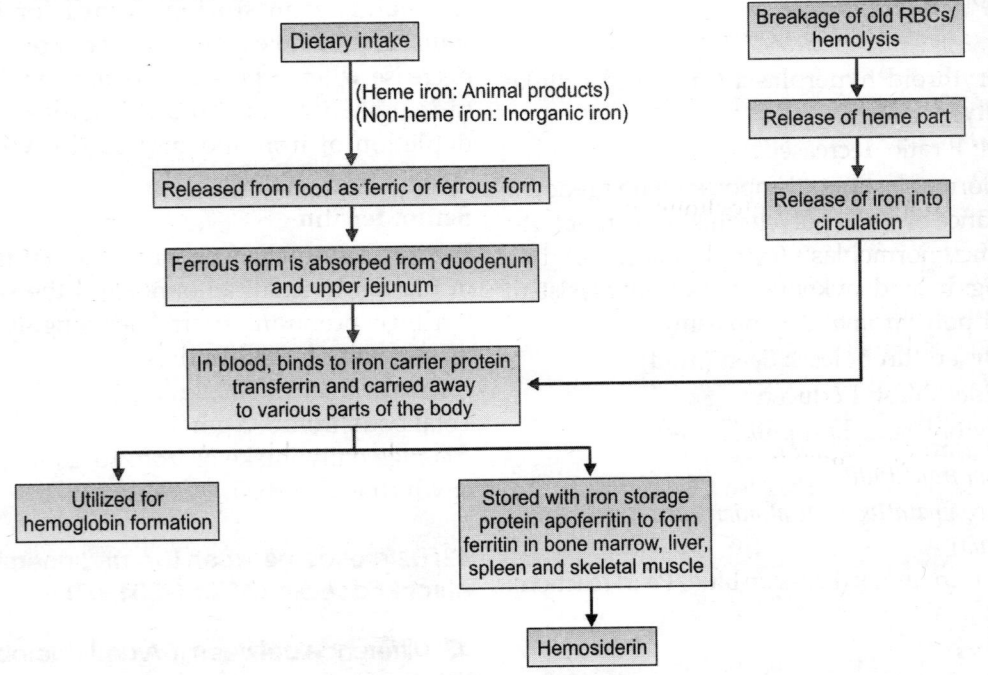

Fig. 10.11: Iron metabolism

45. Difference between thalassemia minor/traits (BTT) and iron deficiency anemia (IDA)

IDA and β-thalassemia major (2011)

S. No.	Traits	BTT	IDA
1.	Nature	Genetic	Acquired
2.	Deficient	Hb chain	Iron
3.	Anemia	Mild, usually asymptomatic	Moderate, symptomatic
4.	RBC	↑ed	↓ed
5.	Target cells	++ nt	+nt
6.	Anisocytosis	Less at same Hb level	More

Note: Other differences: See comparative table of microcytic hypochromic anemia.

46. Sideroblastic anemia

This is a type of anemia in which the body has adequate amount of iron but is unable to incorporate it into haemoglobin.

Causes

	Acquired	Hereditary
• *Hematological*	• *Drugs/chemicals*	X-linked
Myelofibrosis	Isoniazid	Mitochondrial
Polycythemia vera	Penicillamine	Autosomal dominant
Acute leukemia	Alcohol	
Myeloma	Pyridoxine deficiency	
Lymphoma	Chloramphenicol	
Hemolytic anemia	Lead poisoning	
• *Rheumatoid arthritis*	• *Myxoedema, carcinomatosis*	

Pathogenesis

The basic defect is a failure to completely form heme molecules, whose biosynthesis takes place partly in the mitochondria. The iron enters the mitochondria but cannot be utilized to synthesize heme. So, iron accumulates in mitochondria giving a ringed appearance: ringed sideroblast. Since these ringed sideroblast can develop poorly into mature red cells, so anemia ensues.

Laboratory diagnosis

- CBC
  - Hb: ↓ed
  - MCV, MCH: ↓ed
  - Reticulocyte count: ↓ed
- PBS
  - Dimorphic blood picture: Red cells are microcytic, hypochromic along with normocytic, macrocytic RBC.

- *Bone marrow*
  - Presence of ring sideroblast (partial or complete ring demonstrated by Prussian blue reaction in normoblast)
  - Ineffective erythropoiesis
  - Presence of siderotic granules (para-appendicular bodies in red cells)
  - Increased iron stores.

- *Biochemical analysis*
  - Iron stores: Increased iron load
  - Serum ferritin: Increased
  - Serum iron: Increased
  - Transferrin saturation: Increased

47. Causes of normocytic normochromic anemia

Decreased red cell production	*Increased red cell loss*
• Anemia of chronic illness	• Acute blood loss
• Marrow hypoplasia or aplasia	• Hypersplenism
• Myeloproliferative disorders	• Hemolytic disorders
• Myelofibrosis	• Hemoglobinopathies (sickle cell disease)
• Chronic renal disease	• Hereditary spherocytosis
• Chronic liver disease	• G6PD deficiency
• Sideroblastic anemia	• Microangiopathic anemias
• Hypothyroidism	• Autoimmune hemolytic anemia
• Adrenal insufficiency	• PNH

48. Red cell distribution width (RDW)

It is essentially an indication of the degree of anisocytosis (abnormal variation in size RBCs).

Reference value: 11.5–14.5 coefficient of variation (CV) of red cell size.

Helpful in differentiating uncomplicated heterozygous thalassemia from IDA (low MCV in both, RDW is normal in thalassemia but high in IDA); and anemia of chronic disease from early IDA (MCV is low normal in both, but RDW is normal in ACD but high in IDA).

Increased RDW	*Normal RDW (anemia with homogenous RBCs)*
Iron deficiency anemia (IDA)	Anemia of chronic disease
Vitamin B_{12} or folate deficiency	Acute blood loss
Acute blood loss	Aplastic anemia
Aplastic anemia	Hereditary spherocytosis
Immune hemolytic anemia	HbE
Marked reticulocytosis	Sickle cell disease
Fragmentation of RBCs	Thalassemia

49. Anemia of chronic disease (ACD)

Associated with broadly three categories
• Chronic microbial infections: Bacterial endocarditis, osteomyelitis, lung abscess, pneumonia.
• Chronic immune disorders: Rheumatoid arthritis, regional arteritis.
• Neoplasms: Hodgkin's disease, breast and lung carcinoma.

Pathogenesis
The key pathological feature is failure to mobilize stored iron (ferritin) and inhibition of erythropoietin synthesis (See Fig. 10.12).

Laboratory diagnosis
• *CBC*
  – Hb: ↓ (mild to moderate anemia)
  – Generally normocytic, normochromic (MCV and MCH are normal)
  – May be microcytic, hypochromic (MCV and MCH are ↓ed)
  – MCHC; slightly ↓ed (even in normocytic, normochromic)

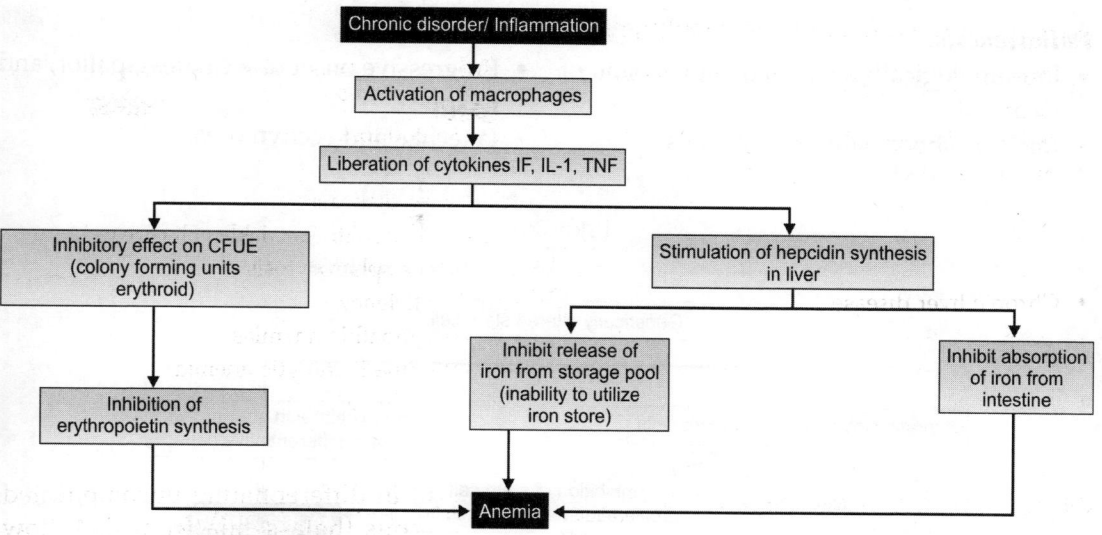

Fig. 10.12: Pathophysiology of ACD

– Reticulocyte count: ↓ed
– $t1/2$ RBC: ↓ed
• *PBS:*
– Generally normocytic, normochromic RBC; but microcytic, hypochromic RBC may be present.
– Anisocytosis and poikilocytosis may be present in renal failure.
• *Bone marrow:*
– Normal erythroid maturation
– Red cell precursors have decreased stainable iron than normal
– Macrophages: ↑ed iron
• *Biochemical analysis:*
– Serum iron and TiBC: ↓ed
– Serum ferritin level: ↑ed
– Phase reactant proteins are increased in chronic inflammation related anemia.
(*Also see comparative table of microcytic and hypochromic anemia*).

50. Aplastic anemia: Causes and pathogenesis

This is a condition characterized by pancytopenia due to failure or suppression of multipotent myeloid cells, with the net result of inadequate production or release of differentiated cell lines.

Causes:

Acquired
• Idiopathic   • Primary stem cell defect
• Immune mediated
• Drugs
– Cytotoxic drugs, idiosyncratic reaction
– Antibiotics: Chloramphenicol, sulphonamides
– Antirheumatic agents: Gold, penicillamine, indomethacin
– Antithyroid drugs
– Anticonvulsants
– Immunosuppressive: Azathioprine
– Antidiabetic (tolbutamide and chlorpropamide)
• Chemicals
– Benzene toluene solvent misuse—glue sniffing
– Insecticides: DDT, carbamates, organophosphates
• Physical agents: Whole body radiation
• Viral agents: Hepatitis, CMV, EBV
• Pregnancy • PNH • Pancreatitis
Inherited: Fanconi syndrome, Shwachman-Diamond syndrome.

Pathogenesis
- Immunologically mediated suppression of stem cells.
- Intrinsic abnormally of stem cells.

Clinical features
- Progressive onset of weakness, pallor, and dyspnea.
- Petechae and ecchymoses.

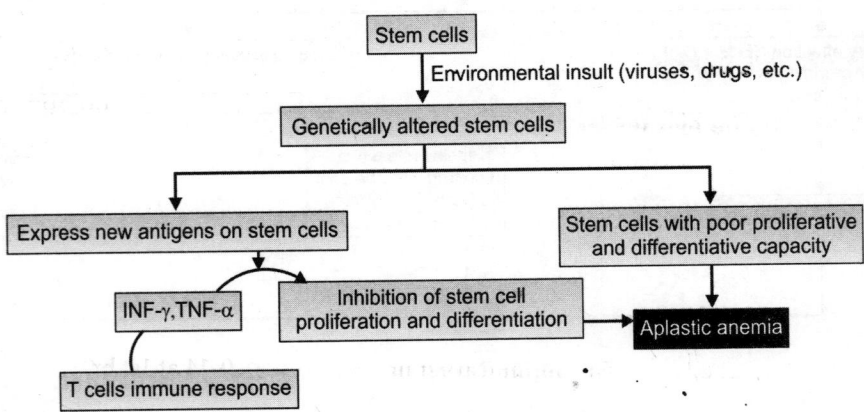

Fig. 10.13: Pathology of aplastic anemia

- Granulocytopenia (frequent and minor infection).
- Splenomegaly, if present, we should think twice before diagnosing it a case of aplastic anemia.

Laboratory diagnois
Aplastic anemia is diagnosed if any two of the following are present:
  i.   Hb ≤ 10 gl
  ii. Neutrophil count ≤ 1500/cc
  iii. Platelet count ≤ 50,000/cc

- *Complete blood count*
  - Hb: ↓ed
  - WBC: ↓ed
  - Platelet: ↓ed
  - RBC: ↓ed
  - MCV: Normal
  - MCH: Normal
  - MCHC: Normal
  - Reticulocyte count: ↓ed (it may be absent)
  - Hematocrit: ↓ed
  - DLC: Granulocyte count is decreased; relative lymphocytosis

- *PBS*
  - Normocytic, normochromic anemic picture
  - Some macrocytosis may be present
  - Decreased polychromatophilia (reticulocytes)
  - Neutrophils morphologically normal
  - No immature RBC or WBC.

- *BM*
  - BM aspirate is usually 'dry tap'
  - Trephine biopsy to be done
  - Hypocellular or aplastic marrow with decreased hematopoietic cells
  - Severe depression of myeloid cells, megakaryocytes and erythroid cells
  - Patchy cellular areas of hematopoiesis
  - Marrow has lymphocytes and plasma cells predominantly as blood cells
  - Replacement of marrow by fat (yellow gelatinous material)

- *Others*
  - HbF: ↑ed
  - BT: ↑ed
  - CT: Normal

- Neutrophil alkaline phosphatase (NAP/LAP): ↑ed
- S. iron: ↑ed
- Vitamin B_{12} and folate: Normal
- Erythropoietin: ↑ed

51. Erythrocytic sedimentation rate (ESR) and its significance (1994, 97, 2010)

52. Factors affecting ESR (2008)

ESR is the rate at which RBC settles down when blood (to which anticoagulant is added) is allowed to stand in a narrow tube for one hour undisturbed. It is expressed in mm of clear plasma at the end of 1st hour.

Mechanism of erythrocyte sedimentation
- Stage I: 10 minute, Rouleaux formation and aggregation of RBC.
- Stage II: 40 minutes, sinking of aggregates take place at constant speed.
- Stage III: 10 minutes, aggregated cells pack at the bottom of tube.
- Longer the tube, longer the stage II can last and greater will be ESR.

Normal values

Method	Male	Female
Wintrobe method (tube)	0–7 mm at 1st hr	0–14 at 1st hr
Westergren's method (pipette)	0–10 mm at 1st hr	0–20 at 1st hr

Pathological increase in ESR
- Anemia (decrease in cell to plasma ratio increases Rouleaux formation)
- Any toxic or infectious disease like TB
- Malignancies
- Nephrosis (↑ fibrinogen, ↓ albumin, marked lipidemia, ↑ globulin)
- Severe trauma

Pathological decrease in ESR
- Polycythemia
- Congestive heart failure
- Leukemia
- Severe allergic reaction
- Pernicious anemia
- Burns

Physiologic change of ESR
- *Age:* Lowest value in newborn (RBC count highest).
- *Sex:* Higher in female as RBC count lesser.
- *Pregnancy:* ESR increases as fibrinogen increases during pregnancy.
- *Temperature:* ESR is directly proportional to temperature, as viscosity increases with increase in temperature.

53. Reticulocyte count (1997, 98, 2002, 09, 11)

- Reticulocytes are newly formed RBCs released from bone marrow. These being immature, take 2–3 days to mature and are in circulation for about one day during which it can be detected in peripheral blood.
  - These are lager, and contain ribosomes and RNA, which stain with basic dyes like new methylene blue. Brilliant cresyl blue, demonstrating blue filamentous or granular material.
  - Reticulocytes stain *polychromatic* with Romanowsky stains.
  - *Polychromatophilia* indicates high reticulocytes count.
- Normal range: 0.5 – 2.0%
  - Reticulocyte count indicates the erythropoietic activity of bone marrow and red cell production (*see* table in next page)
- ***Reticulocyte count correction in anemia***
  Corrected reticulocyte count

$$= \frac{\text{Patient's Hb} \times \text{estimated reticulocyte count}}{\text{Normal Hb value for that age}}$$

	Decreased	Increased
Hypoproliferative disorders	**Maturation disorders**	**Hemolysis/hemorrhage**
• Marrow damage	• Cytoplasmic defect	• Blood loss
– Infiltration/fibrosis	– Iron deficiency	• Intravascular hemolysis
– Aplasia	– Thalassemia	• Metabolic defect (G6PD deficiency)
• Iron deficiency	– Sideroblastic anemia	• Membrane abnormality
• Decreased stimulation	• Nuclear defect	• Hemoglobinopathy
– Inflammation	– Folate/vit B_{12} deficiency	• Autoimmune defect
– Metabolic defect	– Drug toxicity	**Therapy response in anemics**
– Renal disease	– Refractory anemia	After iron/folate/vit B_{12} supplement

54. Various systems of blood grouping (for viva)

Major blood groups:	• ABO	• Rhesus (Rh)	
Minor blood groups:	• M and N	• P	
Familial blood groups	• Kell	• Duffy	
	• Lewis	• Kidd	• Deigo
	• Lutheran		

55. Difference between ABO and Rh blood group (2002)

S. No.	Traits	ABO	Rh
1.	Location	Found in many organs (like salivary gland, pancreas, kidney, liver lung), secretions like urine besides RBC	Only in RBC
2.	Landsteiner law	Follow both laws	Do not follow 2nd law, i.e. if Ag is absent then Ab must be present
3.	Antibody class	IgM	IgG
4.	Cross placenta	Do not cross	Cross placenta
5.	Ab properties	Cold Ab	Warm Ab
6.	Hemolytic disease	ABO blood incompatibility, rarely produces hemolytic disease of newborn	Common

56. Rh incompatibility (1990)

(*See disease of infancy and childhood*)

57. Mismatch blood transfusion, its effects (1996) and its lab diagnosis (2001)

58. Blood transfusion reactions (1990, 98, 2010)/hemolytic transfusion reaction (1998)

Immune mediated reaction

Acute hemolytic transfusion reactions: It occurs due to transfusion of incompatible blood usually due to ABO incompatibility.

The recipient has preformed antibodies that lyse donor erythrocytes. The ABO *isoagglutinins* are responsible for majority of these reactions, although *alloantibodies* directed against other RBC antigens like Rh, Kell, etc.

may also result in hemolysis. The transfused (donor) red cells are destroyed by antibody present in the recipient's plasma. The reaction occurs within minutes and produce severe intravascular hemolysis. These reactions involve complement fixations.

- **Clinical features:**
  - Hypotension
  - Fever
  - Hemoglobinuria
  - Tachycardia
  - Chills
  - Flank pain/discomfort at infusion site
  - Tachypnea
  - Hemoglobinemia

- **Laboratory test:**
  - Serum haptoglobin (intravascular hemolysis): ↓ed
  - Serum LDH: ↑ed
  - Serum indirect bilirubin level: ↑ed

- Coagulation studies (diagnosis for DIC) [PT, aPTT, fibrinogen, platelet count]
- Direct antiglobulin test (DAT, Coombs' test) for antibody detection
- Re-cross matching of blood of both recipient and donor.

- **Delayed hemolytic and serologic transfusion reaction:** Occurs in patient with previously sensitized RBC alloantigens who have a negative alloantibodies screen due to very low antibody levels. Such patients show anamnestic response with production of *alloantibodies* that coat RBC and hasten its removal in extravascular reticuloendothelial system (extravascular hemolysis). Mild reaction non-complement fixing antibodies are involved. It occurs 4 days to 2 weeks after transfusion.

- **Other reaction/complications:** (*see Harrison: transfusion biology and therapy*).

Immunologic reactions	Nonimmunologic reactions	Infectious complications
• Febrile nonhemolytic transfusion reaction • Allergic reactions • Anaphylactic reaction	• Fluid overload • Hypothermia • Electrolyte toxicity • Iron overload	• Viral: *HCV, HBV, HGV, HIV, Cytomegalovirus, HTLV-I HDV*

• Graft versus host reaction
• Transfusion related acute lung injury
• Post-transfusion purpura
• Allo-immunization
	• Hypotensive reactions
	• Immunomodulation
		Parvovirus B19
		• Bacterial contamination:
		  Pseudomonas
		  Yersinia
		• Parasites: Malaria

Massive blood transfusion		
• Coagulopathy • Citrate toxicity • Hypocalcemia • ARDS • Hypomagnesemia	• Hypothermia • Acid–base imbalance (Metabolic alkalosis) • Hyperkalemia • Decreased oxygen affinity	• Fluid overload • Cardiac failure (pulmonary edema)

59. Lab anticoagulants (1994, 95)

Anticoagulant	Mechanism of action	Uses
EDTA	Removes Ca^{2+} from blood by chelation, thus prevents coagulation	Hb, TLC, platelet count, eosinophil count, RBC count Used for HbF estimation and Hb electrophoresis
Sodium citrate	Binds loosely with Ca^{2+} and form complex	For coagulation studies (blood : anticoagulant = 9 : 1) ESR (by Westergren)—4 : 1 ratio (blood : anticoagulant)
Heparin	Antithrombin agent	Osmotic fragility test for spherocytes. Red cell enzyme like G6PD, pyruvate kinase deficiency study
Double oxalate	Mixture of K^+ and ammonium oxalate (2 : 3 ratio)	Was used as 2 mg/ml of blood instead EDTA
Sodium fluoride	It inhibits glycolytic enzymes	Used for blood sugar estimation

EDTA

- Tripotassium EDTA, being more soluble than trisodium EDTA, is preferred for cell counters.
- Such blood can be used for making peripheral smears till 4 hrs after collection of samples, because after that morphological changes start to appear.
- Not suitable for coagulation studies.

Heparin: Disadvantages—It causes clumping of platelets and leukocytes, so not used for cell counts.

Double oxalate: It has been replaced by EDTA. K^+ causes cell shrinkage while ammonium salt causes swelling therefore, double oxalate salts were preferred over single oxalate.

60. Blood component therapy (2007, 08)

Transfusion of specific parts of blood, rather than whole blood is called blood component therapy.

Blood is a precious and short supplied life saving resource that has limited self-life. So,

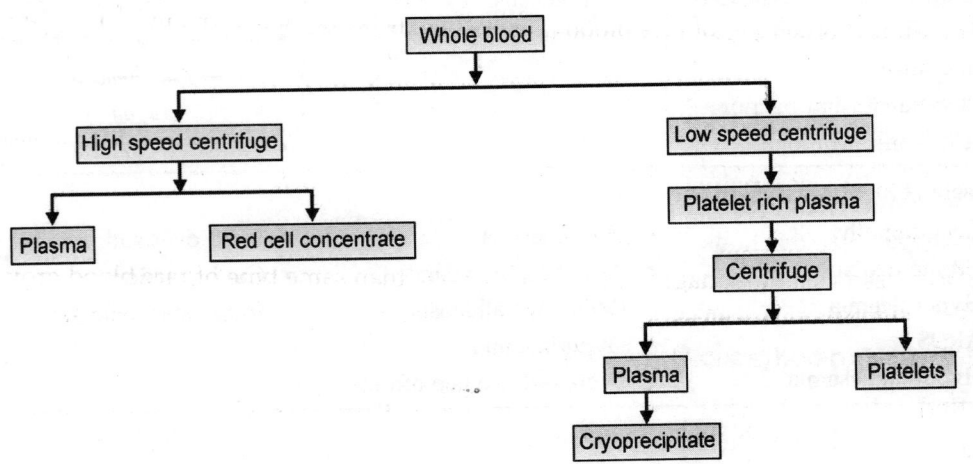

Fig. 10.14: Separation of whole blood into components

Component	Composition and uses
Whole blood	RBCs, plasma, non-functional WBCs and platelets
Packed RBCs	RBCs, some plasma, non-functional WBCs and platelets: treatment of anemia. Each unit of packed RBCs should raise Hb level by 1 g%
Leukocyte reduced RBCs	RBCs, minimal plasma; non-functional WBCs (filtering out of WBCs) and platelets. Used in cases where previous packed RBCs/WB has resulted in blood reaction
Platelets (single unit from whole blood)	Platelets, some non-functional WBCs, few RBCs; plasma, level of labile clotting factor depends on storage time
Platelet (apheresis from random donor)	As above; usually contains as many platelets as 6–10 single unit
Leukocyte concentrate	WBCs; may contain large number of platelets, some RBCs: reserved for patients with severe sepsis associated with absolute neutropenia < 500 cell/μl that has not responded to appropriate antibiotic therapy
Fresh frozen plasma	Plasma; all coagulation factor: used in cases of coagulation abnormality
Cryoprecipitate	Fibrinogen, factor VIII, VIIIR, XIII, fibronectin: used in treatment of mild von Willebrand's disease and fibrinogen deficiency
Factor VIII concentrate	Treatment of hemophilia A
Albumin	In severe hypoprotenemia
Immune serum globulin	Treatment of hypogammaglobulinemia.

transfusion of whole blood is being discouraged and blood component therapy is advocated. One unit of whole blood can be processed to give one unit FFP, one unit PRBC's and one random donor unit platelet.

Advantages of blood component therapy are:
- One donated unit can help multiple patients
  - Conserves resources
  - Make availability of rare blood components more convenient
- Give only what is needed
  - Optimal method for transfusing large amounts of a specific component
  - Avoid circulatory overload
  - Minimize reactions
- Decreased cost of management

61. Bombay blood group (1995, 2002, 04, 08)

- Red cells of all ABO groups possess a common antigen, the H antigen/substance.
- H antigen serves as precursor for the formation of A and B antigens.

- The amount of H antigen is related to the ABO group of the cell, group O cells have the most and AB cells have the least amount of H antigen.
- Ordinary H antigen is universally found and it does not pose any problem in blood grouping and blood transfusion.
- But in 1952, a rare situation was observed from Bombay by Dr Bhende in which A and B as well as H antigens were absent from red cells of some persons.
- Such blood group was called Bombay or OH blood group (or O⁺ Bombay group).
- These persons have anti-A, anti-B, anti-H antibodies; they cannot receive blood other than same type of rare blood group. When misdiagnosed, this Bombay blood group can cause fatal hemolytic transfusion reaction. It is very difficult to detect Bombay O⁺ group people, when routine blood group testing is done. There is serum grouping, also called reverse grouping. If this test is conducted, only then we can detect the

presence of H antibody, which indicate Bombay blood group. This test is done with the help of a reagent called H-lectin.

(Viva) Secretors are those person (75%) who have A, B, H antigens in secretion like saliva, gastric juice, sweat, besides RBC and all tissues; while those lacking antigens in secretions are *non-secretors*.

62. Indications for bone marrow aspiration (2002, 07)

• Red cell disorders: Megaloblastic anemia.
• White cell disorders: Aleukemic leukemia, neutropenia, all acute blastic leukemia for FAB typing.
• Megakaryocytic disorders: ITP and other thrombocytopenia.
• Pancytopenia
• Myeloproliferative disorders: Polycythemia vera, CML.
• Myelodysplastic syndromes.
• Storage diseases: Gaucher's disease, Niemann Pick's disease.
• Parasitic diseases: Kala-azar.

• Plasma cell disorders: Multiple myeloma.
• For iron stores studies.
• For metastatic deposits (carcinoma breast, prostate, lung, kidney, etc.).
• Unexplained enlargement of spleen, lymph nodes and liver.

63. Causes of polycythemia

Relative: Reduced plasma volume (hemoconcentration): Hypovolemia, dehydration.

Absolute: (there is real increase in RBC number)

• *Primary:*
Polycythemia vera (Abnormal proliferation of myeloid stem cells, normal or low erythropoietin level)
• *Secondary:* Increased erythropoietin level
 – Appropriate (in proportion to demand): Lung disease, high altitude living, and cyanotic heart disease.
 – Inappropriate: Erythropoietin-secreting tumors (RCC, hepatocellular carcinoma, cerebellar hemangioblastoma).

11

Bleeding Disorders

1. Investigation in a case of bleeding diathesis (2004)

2. Bleeding time (BT) (1994)

- **Definition:** It is the duration of bleeding from a standard puncture wound on skin, which is the measure of number and function of platelets as well as integrity of vessel walls.
- **Principle:** A small puncture is made on the skin (fingertips, ear lobules) and time for which it bleeds is noted. Bleeding stops when platelet plug is formed and breach in the vessel wall is sealed.
- **Methods:**
  - Fingertip method
  - Ivy method
  - Duke's method
  - Template method
- **Normal value:** 3–8 minutes (Ivy method)
- BT is **prolonged** in:
  - Thrombocytopenia
  - Platelet function disorders like vWD, thrombasthenia
  - Vascular abnormality
  - In uremic patients
  - Antiplatelet medications like aspirin
  - DIC

3. Clotting time (CT)

- Also called whole blood clotting time.
- Test for *Intrinsic + common* coagulation pathway.
- **Definition:** This is the time taken for blood to clot spontaneously in a glass tube.
- **Method:** Lee and White method.
- **Normal value:** 4–11 minutes at 37° C.
- **Significance:** Not a sensitive method, but simple test for controlling the dose of heparin in anticoagulant therapy.
- CT is **prolonged in:**
  - Severe deficiency of clotting factors
  - Afibrinogenemia
  - DIC
  - Administration of heparin

4. Thrombin time

- It is a time taken for clotting to occur when thrombin is added to plasma (normal <15 sec).
- It tests the conversion of fibrinogen to fibrin and depends on adequate fibrinogen levels.
- Those conditions associated with decreased fibrinogen level like afibrinogenemia, dysfibrinogenemia, heparin-like inhibitor or heparin administration, DIC are associated with increased thrombin time.

5. Prothrombin time (PT) (1993, 97, 2001, 04, 07, 08, 11)

- Tests for extrinsic + common coagulation pathway (V, VII, II, I).
- *Definition:* It is the time taken by plasma to clot after tissue factor (usually an extract of brain tissue) and Ca^{2+} are added.
- *Requirement:*
  - Citrated test plasma (anticoagulant: blood = 1:9)
  - $CaCl_2$ (0.025 M)
  - Water bath at 37° C
  - Citrated control plasma
  - Stopwatch
- *Method:*
  - Incubate all reagents and test tube at 37°C for 15 min.
  - Deliver 0.1 ml of plasma into one test tube and add 0.1 ml of thromboplastin suspension to it and keep the tube in 37°C water bath.
  - After 1 min, add 0.1 ml of $CaCl_2$ solution to the tube and start the stopwatch and submerge the lower end of the tube in water bath.
  - The tube is gently tilted to look for fibrin clot (gel formation). As soon as the fibrin strand appears, time is recorded.
- *Normal range:* 11–16 sec (PT exceeding 3 sec from normal control is significant)
- PT is *prolonged in:*
  - Oral anticoagulant therapy
  - Obstructive jaundice
  - Fibrinogen deficiency
  - Vitamin K deficiency

- DIC
- Factor VII deficiency
- Liver diseases
- Mild/severe factor V, X deficiency
- Hemorrhagic disease of newborn
- *Indication* of PT determination:
  - Before liver biopsy, since liver diseases are likely to impair the production of various clotting factors;
  - Monitoring of oral anticoagulant therapy;
  - As screening test while investigating the 'bleeding diathesis'.

6. Partial thromboplastin time with kaolin (PTTk) or activated PTT

- Test for *intrinsic + common* coagulation pathway.
- *Definition:* The time taken by plasma, previously incubated with kaolin or other contact factors (which activates the surface clotting factors XII), to clot in the presence of optimum level of platelet substitute and calcium.
- *Normal value:* 30–40 seconds; (PTTk exceeding 5 sec from normal control is significant).
- PTTk is *prolonged in:*
  - Hemophilia A and B
  - Liver diseases
  - Vitamin K deficiency
  - vWD
  - Heparin therapy
  - Oral anticoagulant therapy
  - DIC

7. Causes of thrombocytopenia (2004)

Megakaryocytic (increased destruction)	
Immune destruction	*Non immune destruction*
• ITP	• DIC
• Transplacental thrombocytopenia	• TTP
• Alloantibodies (transfusion or pregnancy)	• HUS
• Drugs	• Hypersplenism
• Other disease like SLE	• Liver disease

(Contd.)

(Contd.)

Amegakaryocytic (hypoplasia of megakaryocyte—decreased production)			
Decreased megakaryocyte proliferation	*Replacement of normal marrow*	*Ineffective thrombopoiesis*	*Hereditary thrombocytopenia*
• Aplastic anemia • Chemotherapy • Radiation therapy	• Leukemias • Fibrous tissue • Granulation tissue	• Megaloblastic anemia	• Wiskott-Aldrich syndrome • Bernard-Soulier syndrome • May-Hegglin anamoly

8. Causes of thrombophilia

(See Hemodynamic disorders, thrombosis and shock: Hypercoagulate state)

9. Idiopathic thrombocytopenic purpura (ITP): Mechanism of platelet destruction (2000) and clinical features

Acute and chronic ITP are autoimmune disorder in which platelet destruction results from formation of antiplatelet antibodies.

Mechanism
- Platelet membrane has glycoproteins like IIb–IIIa, Ib–IX.
- Autoantibodies (mainly IgG type) against these glycoproteins lead to opsonization of platelets.
- Opsonized platelets are more susceptible to phagocytosis by cells of the mononuclear phagocyte system like spleen, and they are removed in the same fashion as RBC in autoimmune hemolytic anemia (AIHA).
- Destruction of megakaryocytes may add to platelet destruction, but not significant.

Clinical features (Chronic ITP)
- Patient presents with pinpoint hemorrhage (petechiae) or ecchymoses.
- Have long history of easy bruising, nose-bleeds, bleeding from gums, extensive bleeding into soft tissues from relatively minor trauma, melena, hematuria and excessive menstrual flow.
- We should suspect causes other than ITP, if splenomegaly and lymphadenopathy are present.

- Diagnosis of ITP should be made by exclusion method excluding all other causes.

10. Lab diagnosis of ITP (including bone marrow finding; 1994, 98) (2000, 09, 11)

- *Platelet count:* Acute ($< 20,000/\mu l$), Chronic ($20,000–1,00,000/\mu l$)
- *BT:* ↑ed
- *CT:* Normal
- *PT:* Normal
- *PTTk:* Normal
- *Anemia:* Present only in severe blood loss (normochromic, normocytic anemia may be present).
- *ESR:* Normal
- *PBS:* Lymphocytosis and eosinophilia are common. ↓ed platelet, which is abnormally large in size.
- *BM:*
  - Normal or ↑ed number of megakaryocytes, which have large non-lobulated single nucleus, may have reduced cytoplasmic granularity and presence of vacuoles. Increased percentage of immature cells (precursors of megakaryocytes);
  - Cellularity normal;
  - M : E ratio normal (3:1).
- *Immunochemistry:* Anti-platelet IgG auto-antibodies can be demonstrated.
- *Platelet survival studies:* ↓ed platelet life.
- *Tourniquet test:* Positive
- Impaired clot retraction.

11. Difference between acute and chronic ITP (2007)

S. No.	Traits	Acute ITP	Chronic ITP
1.	Age	2–9 yrs, children	20–40 yrs; Adult
2.	Sex ratio (F: M)	1:1	3:1
3.	Antecedent infection	Common; viral	Uncommon
4.	Platelet count	<20,000/µl	20,000–1,00,000/µl
5.	Onset	Abrupt	Gradual
6.	Hemorrhagic bullae	Common	Uncommon
7.	Duration	2–6 wks	Years
8.	Spontaneous remission	80% cases	Uncommon
9.	Progression	Self limiting	Not so
10.	Eosinophilia and lymphocytosis	Common	Rare
11.	Response to corticosteroids	Variable	Common
12.	Response to splenectomy	Variable	Common

12. von Willebrand disease (vWD) (1995, 2011)

- Autosomal dominant hereditary disorder (gene located on chromosome 12).
- Most common hereditary coagulation disorder.
- vWD is due to qualitative or quantitative defect in vWF.
- *vWF synthesis:* Endothelial cells, megakaryocytes and platelets.

- *Functions of vWF*
  - It binds with clotting factor VIII in circulation and form a complex, increasing its t1/2.
  - It binds with collagen exposed after endothelial injury and helps in platelet adhesion to subendothelial collagen and also, platelet to platelet sticking (adhesion).
  - It can also bind heparin, platelet membrane glycoproteins—involved in hemostasis.

- *Clinical features of vWD*
  - Platelet adhesion defect resulting in impaired hemostatic plug: mucosal and cutaneous bleeding (epistaxis); menorrhagia and GIT bleeding.
  - Coagulation defect due to decreased t1/2 of factor VIIIc. Hemarthroses and intramuscular hematoma.

Types of disease
- Type I: Most common, mild to moderate ↓ in plasma vWF.
- Type II: Less common, functional defect though vWF level normal/slightly ↓ed.
- Type III: Extremely rare, most severe form of disease, no detectable vWF activity.

Laboratory diagnosis
CBC
- Platelet count: Normal
Screening test
- BT: Prolonged
- CT: Normal
- PTTk: Prolonged (due to factor VIIIc deficiency)
- PT: Normal
Confirmatory tests
- Plasma VIII level: ↓ed (↓ed t1/2);
- Ristocetin aggregation test delayed. Ristocetin is an antibiotic which causes platelet aggregation. If there is deficiency of von Willebrand factor, ristocetin induced platelet aggregation does not take place.
- Functional state of vWF: Normal/↓ed (depends on type of defect—qualitative or quantitative).

- Immunoassay for von Willebrand factor: It is one of the most sensitive methods available for the diagnosis of von Willebrand disease.

13. Hemophilia A/clinical feature of hemophilia (2002, 11)

- Second most common hereditary coagulation disorder.
- *Pathogenesis*
  - Sex (X) linked recessive disease.
  - There is quantitative reduction (90% cases) or qualitative dysfunction (10% cases) of factor VIII.
  - These clinical hemophilics have less than 5% of normal level even though 25% factor VIII activity may take care of normal hemostasis.
  - It produces clinical manifestation of disease mostly in males, while females are carrier.
  - Even some carrier females may show VIII level below 50% of normal (mild hemophilics).

- Homozygous female hemophilics may arise from consanguinity.
- *Clinical features*
  - Patients have tendency for easy bruising, massive bleeding after trauma or surgery.
  - Spontaneous hemorrhage is seen in parts subjected to trauma like joints (hemarthrosis; recurrent, painful).
  - *Petechiae are characteristically absent.*
- *Laboratory diagnosis*
  CBC:
  - Platelet count: Normal; Hb: May be low
  Screening tests:
  - Whole blood clotting time: Prolonged only in severe cases
  - PT: Usually normal
  - BT: Normal
  - PTTk: Prolonged
  Confirmatory tests:
  - Factor VIII assay: ↓ed plasma level and (or) ↓ed function
  - Cytogenetics: Mutations like deletion, nonsense, mutation creating stop codons, inversion, splicing defect in X chromosome.

14. Difference between hemophilia A and von Willebrand disease (2008)

S. No.	Traits	Hemophilia A	von Willebrand disease
1.	Deficiency	Factor VIII (quantitative or qualitative)	vWF (quantitative or qualitative)
2.	Inheritance	X linked	Somatic, autosomal dominant
3.	Synthesis of factor	Liver parenchymal cells	Endothelial cells, platelet cells
4.	Defect	Intrinsic pathway of coagulation	Platelet adhesion and aggregation, decreased factor VIII half life
5.	Skin, mucosal bleeding	−nt	+nt
6.	Petechiae	Absent	Present
7.	Haemarthrosis	++	+
8.	Bleeding time	Normal	↑
9.	Hess test	−nt	+nt
10.	F VIII assay	↓	Normal or ↓
11.	vWF ristocetin factor assay	Normal	↓
12.	Clotting time	↑	↑
13.	APTT	↑	↑
14.	PT	Normal	Normal

15. Disseminated intravascular coagulation (DIC) (2000, 02, 08), laboratory diagnosis (1999) (2004)

- *Definition:* This is an acute, subacute, chronic thrombohemorrhagic disorder secondary to some diseases characterized by activation of the coagulation pathway leading to the formation of microthrombi throughout the microcirculation of body.

Thrombus formation activates fibrinolytic mechanism, thus leading to consumption of platelets, fibrin, and coagulation factors.

Obstetrics complications	Infections	Massive tissue injury	Neoplasm
• Retained placenta	• Gram negative sepsis	• Trauma	• Acute promyelocytic leukemia
• Retained dead fetus	• Meningococcemia	• Extensive surgery	
• Septic abortion	• Rocky Mountain spotted fever	• Burns	• Pancreatic, lung, prostate, stomach carcinoma
• Abruptio placentae		*Others*	
• Toxemia (Eclampsia)	• Malaria	• Snakebite • Shock • Heat stroke	
	• Aspergillosis	• Acute intravascular hemolysis	

- *Pathophysiology*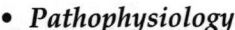

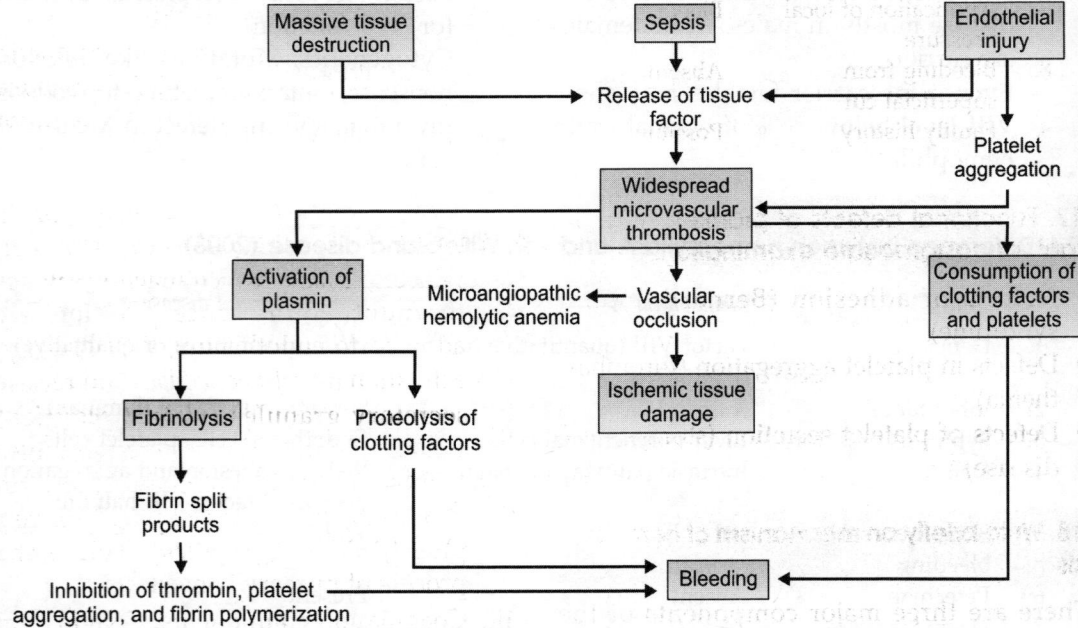

Fig. 11.1: Pathophysiology of DIC

- *Laboratory diagnosis:*
  CBC:
  – Platelet count: ↓ed
  – Hb: ↓ed (microangiopathic intravascular hemolysis)
  PBS: Presence of *schistocytes*.

Screening test:
  – BT: ↑ed
  – TT: ↑ed
  – CT: ↑ed
  – Thrombin-antithrombin (TAT) complex: ↑ed

- PT: ↑ed
- Plasmin-antiplasmin (PAP) complex: ↑ed
- PTTk: ↑ed

Confirmatory tests:
- Plasma fibrinogen level: ↓ed
- Fibrin degradation products (FDPs): +
  (D-dimer: It is a parameter of activation

of coagulation. It measures degraded fragments of polymerized fibrin).
- Fibrinopeptides: ↑↑ed
- Clotting factors like, V, VIII, II, etc.: ↓ed

Other tests:
- LDH: ↑ed
- Hemoglobinuria: Present
- Hemoglobinemia: Present

16. Difference between bleeding in platelet and coagulative disorder (2001)

S. No.	Traits	Coagulation defect	Platelet defect
1.	Petechiae	Absent	Present
2.	Ecchymosis	Large and solitary	Small and multiple
3.	Bleeding after trauma	Delayed, persistent > 48 hrs, voluminous	Immediate, for short time < 48 hrs, less
4.	Hemarthrosis	Characteristics	Absent
5.	Deep hematoma	Present	Rare
6.	Spontaneous bleeding	Uncommon	Common
7.	Application of local pressure	Bleeding stops quickly	Does not stop quickly
8.	Bleeding from superficial cut	Absent	Present
9.	Family history	Possible	Absent

17. Functional defects of platelets (Important for postgraduate examinations)

- Defects of adhesion (Bernard-Soulier syndrome)
- Defects in platelet aggregation (thrombasthenia)
- Defects of platelet secretion (storage pool disease)

18. Write briefly on mechanism of hemostasis

There are three major components of the normal hemostatic mechanism:

i. *Vascular component*: Whenever the blood vessel is injured, there is intense local vasoconstriction to prevent the blood loss.

ii. *Platelet component*: Endothelial injury exposes highly thrombogenic subendothelial extracellular matrix which allows platelets to adhere to endothelium

(*Platelet adhesion*). This adhesion is brought about by the action of von Willebrand factor which attaches platelets to endothelium. Once platelets are adhered to endothelium, they undergo activation (*platelet activation*) and release secretory granules (*platelet secretion*) within minutes. The secreted granules will recruit additional platelets to form hemostatic plug/platelet plug/primary plug (*platelet aggregation*). This is the process of primary hemostasis.

iii. Coagulation components: Coagulation component involves three pathway—intrinsic (contact of factor XII and platelets with collagen in the vascular wall initiates the intrinsic pathway), extrinsic (tissue thromboplastin released from damaged cells in the vascular endothelium activates extrinsic pathway) and common pathway.

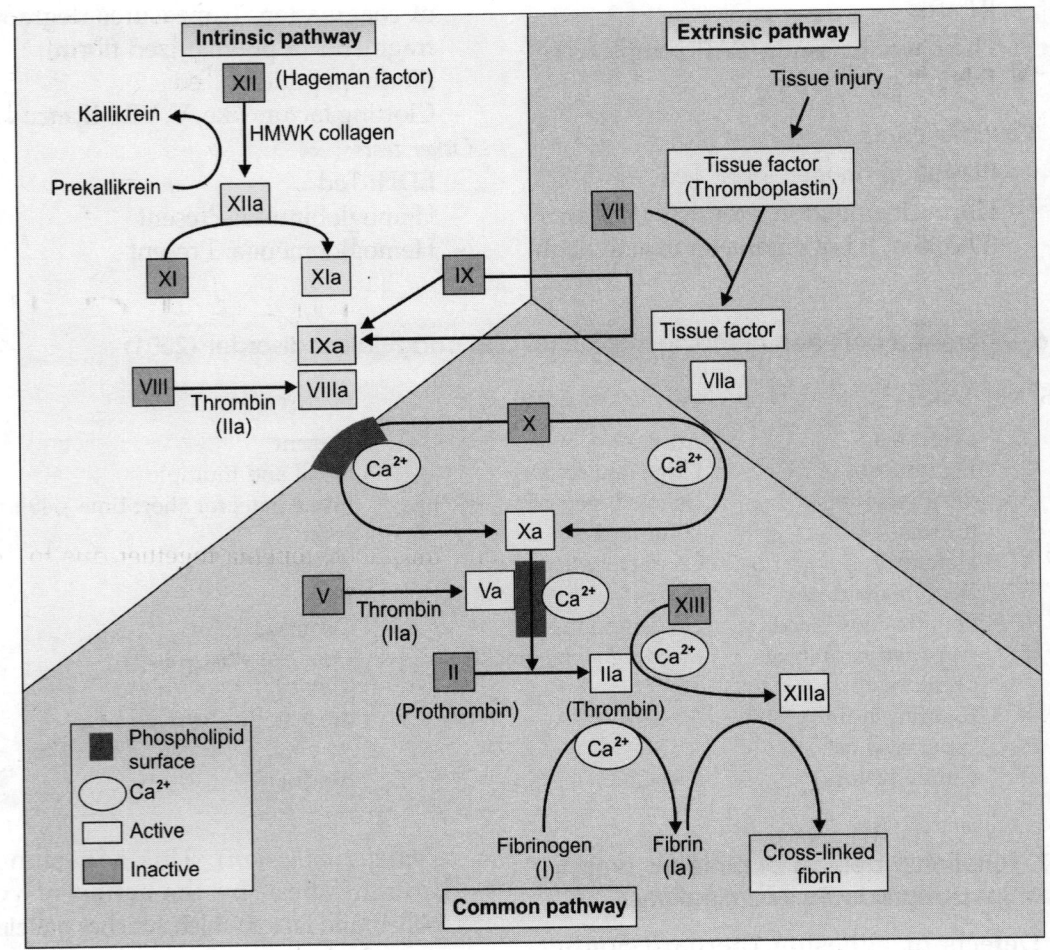

Fig. 11.2: Coagulation pathway

(Factor I: Fibrinogen, II: Prothrombin, Factor III: Tissue thromboplastin (tissue factor), Factor IV: Ionized calcium (Ca⁺⁺), Factor V: Labile factor or proaccelerin, Factor VI: Unassigned, Factor VII: Stable factor or proconvertin, Factor VIII: Antihemophilic factor, Factor IX: Plasma thromboplastin component, Christmas factor, Factor X: Stuart-Prower factor, Factor XI: Plasma thromboplastin antecedent, Factor XII: Hageman factor, Factor XIII: Fibrin-stabilizing factor).

12

Disorders of White Blood Cells

1. Pancytopenia (1990, 2001, 07, 09, 11)

This is a condition having anemia, leukopenia and thrombocytopenia together due to ↓ed erythrocytes, ↓ed leukocytes, and ↓ed platelets.

- *Aplastic anemia*
- *Pancytopenia with normal or ↑ed marrow cellularity:*
  - Myelodysplastic syndromes
  - Hypersplenism
  - Megaloblastic anemia

- *Infectious diseases:*
  - Kala-azar, miliary tuberculosis, syphilis

- *Paroxysmal nocturnal hemoglobinuria*
- *Bone marrow infiltration:*
  - Hematologic malignancies like leukemia, lymphomas, myeloma
  - Non-hematologic metastatic malignancies
  - Storage disease like Gaucher's disease
  - Osteoporosis
  - Myelofibrosis
  - AIDS

2. Difference between lymphoblast and myeloblast (1995, 99, 2003, 08)

S. No.	Traits	Lymphoblast (ALL)	Myeloblast (AML)
1.	Blast size	Smaller; variable	Larger and uniform
2.	Nuclear chromatin	Slightly clumped, condensed, finely stippled	Fine meshwork
3.	Nuclear membrane	Fairly dense	Very fine
4.	Nucleoli	Indistinct, absent or 1 or 2	Prominent, 1–4
5.	Cytoplasm	Scanty, agranular	Moderate, granular
6.	Auer rods	Absent	Present (60–70% cases)
7.	PAS	+ve (75%)	−ve
8.	Acid phosphatase	+ve	−ve
9.	Non-specific esterase (NSE)	±ve (M_4 and M_5, focal)	+ve; (monocytic, diffuse)
10.	Myeloperoxidase (MPO)	−ve	+ve
11.	Sudan black (B)	−ve	+ve

3. Classify leukemia (1996)

Acute lymphoblastic
- Common type (Pre-B)
- T cell
- B cell
- Undifferentiated

Acute myeloid
  (See FAB classification)

Chronic myeloid
- Ph +ve
- Ph –ve, bcr-abl +ve
- Ph –ve, bcr-abl –ve
- Eosinophilic leukemia

Chronic lymphocytic
  B cell (common)
  T cell (rare)

4. Write briefly on etiopathogenesis and clinical features of leukemia

Etiopathogenesis of leukemia
- Familial and genetic: Down syndrome, ataxia telangiectasia, Fanconi's anemia, Bloom syndrome.
- Drugs and toxins: Cytotoxic drugs like alkylating agents, and exposure to benzene.

- Retroviruses: Human T-cell leukemia—lymphoma virus.
- Ionizing radiation: Therapeutic irradiation, diagnostic X-ray.
- Immunological: Immunodeficiency states.

Acute leukemia
It is characterised by the replacement of normal marrow elements by immature cells, called leukemic blasts, which may or may not spill over to involve peripheral blood.

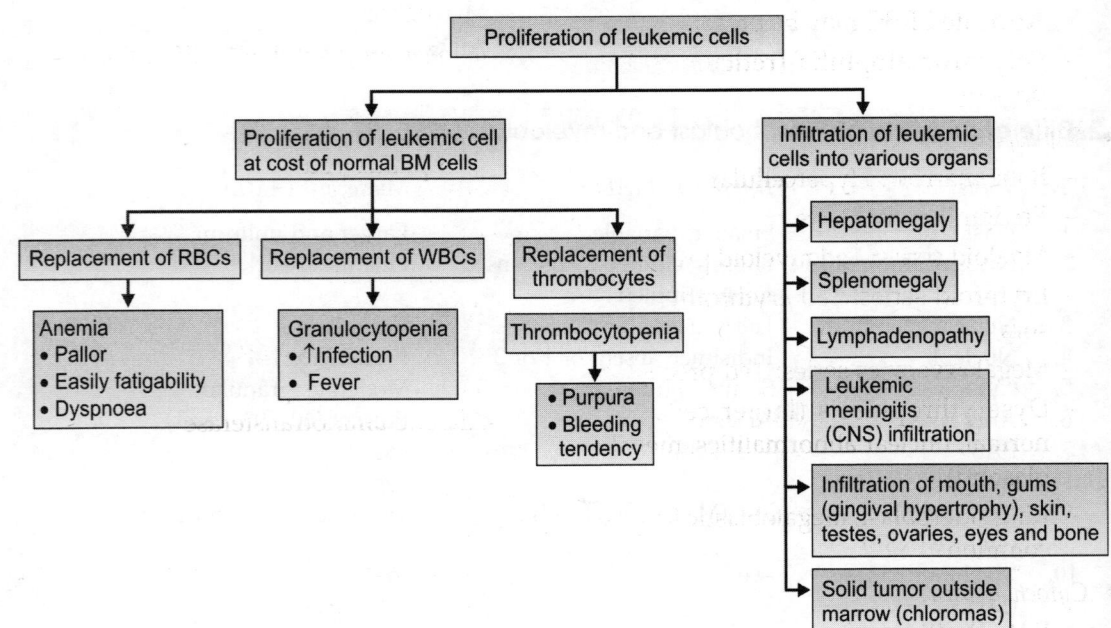

Fig. 12.1: Clinical features of leukemia

5. ALL: Clinical features, PBS, BM findings (1995, 2011)

Clinical features: See previous question and difference table.

Laboratory diagnosis

- *CBC:* Presence of leukemic cells in blood and BM with reduction of normal hemopoietic cells.
  - Hb: ↓ed
  - Hematocrit: ↓ed
  - Platelet count: ↓ed
  - ESR: may ↑
  - TLC: ↑↑ed
  - RBC counts: ↓ed
  - A moderate increase in reticulocytes up to 5% is common
- *PBS*
  - Marked leukocytosis—blast cells
  - Blast cells twice the size of lymphocytes (Clumped chromatin, nucleoli seen)
  - Normocytic normochromic red cells
  - Mild to moderate anisocytosis and poikilocytosis
  - Nucleated RBC may be present
  - Polychromatophilia (reticulocytosis) present
- *BM aspiration*
  - Bone marrow: Hypercellular
  - Predominantly blasts
  - Myeloid series: ↓ed myeloid precursors
  - Erythroid series: ↓ed erythroid precursors
  - Megakaryocytes series: ↓ed precursors
  - Dyserythropoiesis (larger cells than normal, nuclear abnormalities, megaloblastoid)
  - Ring sideroblast, megaloblastic features common
- *Cytochemistry*
  - PAS: Positive
  - MPO and Sudan black negative

- Immunophenotyping
  - B cell markers
    - ➤ B cell progenitor: CD34 +ve, DR +ve, TdT +ve
    - ➤ Early pre B cell: CD10, 19 and 34 +ve, DR +ve, TdT + ve
    - ➤ Pre B cell: CD10, 19 and 20 +ve, cytoplasmic IgM present, DR +ve, TdT +ve
    - ➤ B cell: Surface Ig present, CD19, 20 21 and 22 +ve, DR +ve, TdT –ve
    - ➤ Plasma cells: CD38, 56 +ve
  - T cell markers:
    - ➤ T cell progenitor: CD34 +ve, TdT +ve
    - ➤ Early thymocyte: CD1, 2, 5, 7, and 34 +ve, TdT +ve
    - ➤ Common thymocyte: CD1, 2, 4, 5, 7 and 8 +ve, TdT +ve
    - ➤ Mature T cell: T helper cell: CD2, 3 and 4 +ve, TdT –ve
      T cytotoxic cell: CD2, 3 and 8 +ve, TdT –ve
- *Cytogenetics*
  - Hyperploidy, translocation (12, 21), t(9, 22), t(8, 14)
- *Serum markers:* (cellular proliferation)
  - LDH: ↑ed
  - Uric acid: ↑ed
  - Phosphate: ↑ed
  - Calcium: ↓ed
- *Hepatic function tests (also in AML)*
  - Total protein
  - Albumin
  - Alkaline phosphatase
  - Bilirubin
  - Alanine aminotransferase
- *Renal function test (also in AML)*
  - Plasma urea and creatinine
- Radiology
  - Long bones: Leukemic lines
  - Mediastinal mass
- *Lumber puncture:* CSF cytology
- *Others:* BT ↑ed

6. Prognostic factors in ALL (2001, 02, 04, 08, 11)

S. No.	Traits	Poor	Good
1.	Age	<2 yr, >7 yr, Adult	2–8 yr
2.	Sex	Male	Female
3.	TCL	>50 × 10⁹/L	<20 × 10⁹/L
4.	Ploidy	Hypoploidy, pseudodiploidy	Hyperploidy > 50 chromosomes
5.	Race	Black	White
6.	Organomegaly	++nt	Nil
7.	CNS manifestation	++nt	Nil
8.	Testicular involvement	+nt	Nil
9.	FAB	L2–L3	L1
10.	Hb	<7 gm/dl	>10 gm/dl
11.	Platelet	<30,000/mm³	>1,00,000/mm³
12.	Cell type	Pre B, pre T, B-cells; T-All in children	CALLA* +ve, B-All, CD10, early pre B cell
13.	Cytochemistry	PAS negative	PAS positive
14.	Chromosome abnormality	Philadelphia chromosome present	Absent

*CALLA/CD10: Common acute lymphoblastic leukemia antigen.

7. Difference between ALL and AML (2001)

S. No.	Traits	ALL	AML
1.	Age	<10 yr mostly (<15 yr)	15–39 yr
2.	Occurrence	80% of childhood leukemia	20%
3.	Clinical finding		
	Splenomegaly	++nt	+nt
	Hepatomegaly	++nt	+nt
	Lymphadenopathy	++nt	+nt
	Bony tenderness	++nt	+nt
	Gum hypertrophy	–nt	++nt (M₅)
	Meningeal involvement	+nt	–nt
	Testicular involvement	in 10–20%	Not seen
	Eye involvement	More common	Less common
	Bleeding manifestation	Less common	More common
4.	Laboratory finding		
	Cell type PBS	Lymphoblasts	Myeloblast and promyelocytes
	Cell type BM	Lymphoblasts	Myeloblast and promyelocytes
5.	Cytochemistry	PAS +ve, acid phosphatase (focal) +ve	Myeloperoxidase +ve, Sudan black +ve; NSE and acid phosphatase (diffuse) +ve in M₄ and M₅
6.	Therapy	Vincrystine, anthracycline, prednisolone, L-asparaginase	Cytosine arabinoside, anthracycline, 6-thioguanine
7.	Response to therapy	High remission rate, prolonged remission duration	Remission rate low, duration of remission shorter
8.	Median survival	Children (with CNS prophylaxis) 60 months, adults 12–18 months	12–18 months

Note: Leukocyte count ranging from low to high and moderate to severe thrombocytopenia might occur in both cases.

8. CLL: Clinical features, PBS, BM findings

This is a disease of neoplastic proliferation of mature looking lymphocytes.

B-CLL is the the commonest type having prolymphocytes less than 10%.

- *Causes*
  - Common in asbestos worker
  - Genetic factors
  - Older age: 6th decade (but remain asymptomatic)
- *Clinical features*
  - Asymptomatic in early stage. Symptoms are mainly due to massive splenomegaly, anemia and hypermetabolic state.
  - Generalized lymphadenopathy, splenomegaly
  - Easily fatigability (due to anemia)
  - Bacterial infection (deranged immune function due to hypogammaglobinemia)
  - Autoimmune hemolytic anemia or thrombocytopenia due to autoantibodies by non-neoplastic cells
  - Fever, weight loss, night sweats, heat intolerance (hypermetabolic state)
  - Bleeding tendency: Later
- *Laboratory diagnosis*
  CBC
  - TLC: 20,000–1,00,000/m^3 or more
  - Hb: Normal/↓ed
  - RBC: ↓ed/normal
  - Reticulocyte count: ↑ed
  - Platelet count: Normal/↓ed
  - Absolute lymphocytic count: ↑ed

  PBS
  - Normocytic normochromic anemia
  - Mature lymphocytes (70–80%), a few prolymphocytes.
  - More than 95% of cells are small and mature—appearing lymphocytes with scanty, fragile cytoplasm.
  - *Smudge cells* (lymphocytes that are fragile and are broken during smear preparation)/basket/smear cells.

  BM
  - Hypercellular
  - Replacement by mature lymphocytes
  - Erythroid and myeloid precursors are seen
  - Occasional megakaryocytes are seen
  - Lymph node biopsy: Well differentiated, small, non-cleaved lymphocytes

  Immunophenotype
  - CD5 +ve
  - CD19, CD20 and CD21 +ve
  - Surface Ig: –ve

  Cytogenetics
  - Trisomy 12 and 14 q
  - t (11; 14)

  Serum uric acid, protein and LDH: ↑ed
  Serum folate levels: Low
  Direct Coombs' test: +ve (autoimmune hemolytic process)

9. FAB (French, American and British) classification of ALL

FAB classification of ALL

Features	L$_1$	L$_2$	L$_3$
Occurrence	Most common (80–85%) type	14%	Least common (1%)
Type	Childhood ALL (B-ALL and T-ALL)	Adult ALL (mostly T-ALL)	Burkitt type ALL (B-ALL)
Cell size	Small cells, homogenous	Large heterogenous in size	Large homogenous
Amount of cytoplasm	Scant	Variable	Moderately abundant
Nucleoli	Small and inconspicuous	One or more, often large	One or more, often prominent

(Contd.)

FAB classification of ALL (*Contd.*)			
Features	L_1	L_2	L_3
Nuclear chromatin	Homogenous	Heterogenous	Finely stippled and homogenous
Nuclear shape	Regular	Irregular clefting and indentation	Regular
Basophilia of cytoplasm	Variable	Variable	Intensely basophilic
Cytoplasmic vacuolation	Variable	Variable	Prominent
PAS	+/–ve	+/–ve	–ve
Acid phosphatase	+/–ve	+/–ve	–ve
MPO	–ve	–ve	–ve

10. Burkitt lymphoma (BL) (1990, 91, 95, 2004, 11)

This is a high grade non-Hodgkin's lymphoma having small noncleaved cells.

- *It includes*
  - African (endemic) BL
  - Sporadic (non-endemic) BL
  - HIV-associated aggressive lymphoma
- *Pathogenesis*
  (*See neoplasm: Burkitt lymphoma and EBV*)
- *Morphology*
  - Diffuse infiltration of involved organ by intermediate sized lymphoid tumor cells.
  - These cells are 10–25 μm in size, having round to oval nuclei (approximately size of nuclei of macrophages) with coarse chromatin, several nucleoli (2–5), and a moderate amount of faint basophilic or amphophilic cytoplasm.
  - High mitotic index and high rate of apoptotic death of these tumor cells are characteristics. It leads to numerous tissue macrophages with ingested nuclear debris.
  - *Starry sky pattern:* Macrophages are surrounded by a clear space give rise to a special appearance.

- In some cases there is leukemic picture showing slightly clumped chromatin, 2–5 distinct nucleoli, and royal blue cytoplasm having multiple, clear cytoplasmic vacuole.
- *Clinical features*
  - Mostly at extra nodal site
  - Age: Children and young adults
  - African type present as mass in mandible, while nonendemic type present as abdominal mass involving ileocecum, peritoneum.

11. Multiple myeloma (MM): Lab diagnosis (1990, 93, 97, 99, 2001, 04, 10)/Bence-Jones protein (1994, 2000)

- This is a neoplastic proliferation of plasma cell with characteristic involvement of skeleton at multiple sites.
- Normally plasma cells secrete several different immunoglobulins (polyclonal), but in multiple myeloma, the neoplastic plasma cell arises from single clone of lymphocytes (monoclonal proliferation). These neoplastic plasma cells secrete monoclonal immunoglobin, this in blood is called M component.
- Pathophysiology of MM.

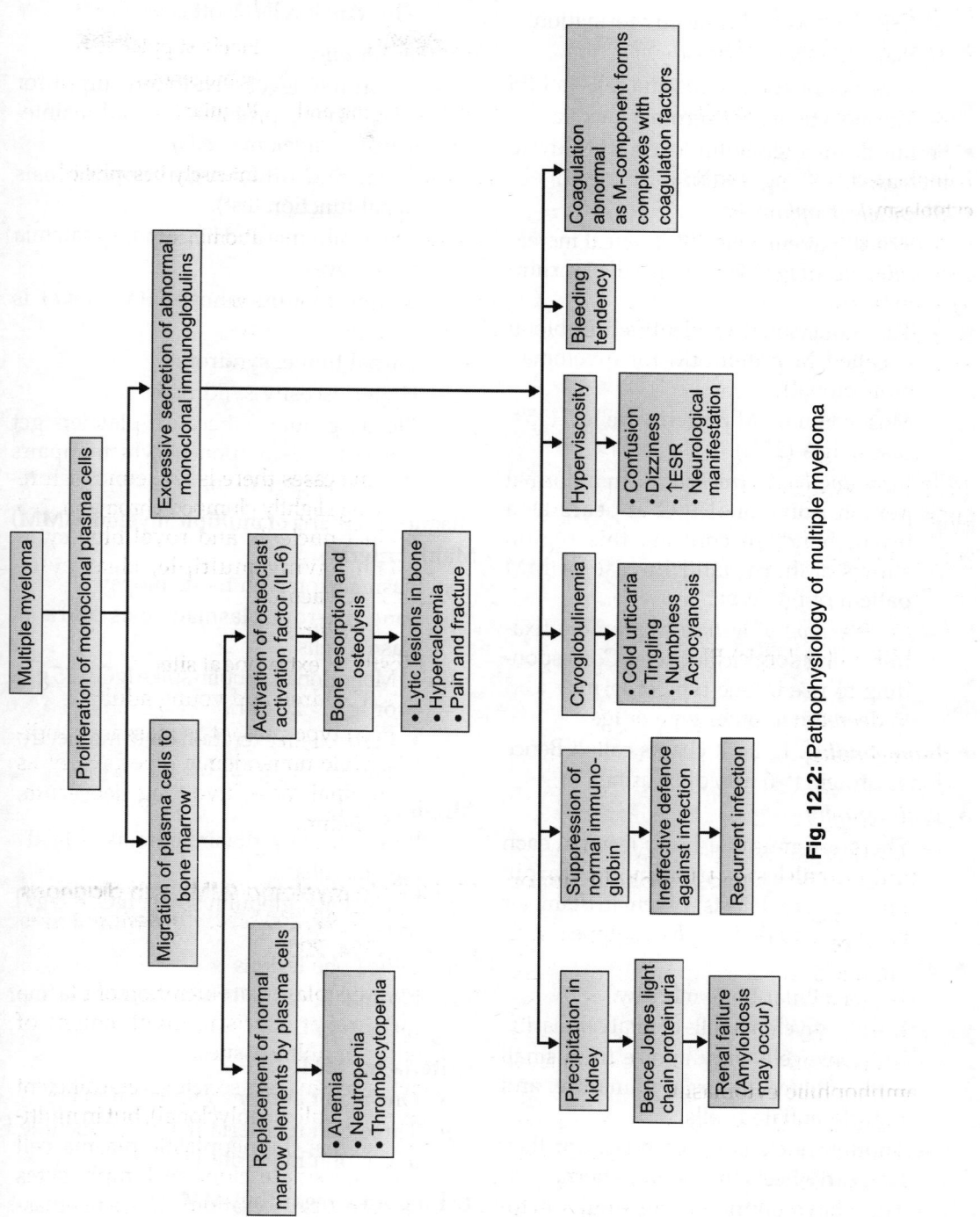

Fig. 12.2: Pathophysiology of multiple myeloma

- *Blood finding*
  - Hb: ↓ed
  - ESR: ↑ed (as ↑ed rouleaux formation)
  - Platelets: May decrease
  - Presence of atypical plasma cells in PBS
  - Normocytic normochromic anemia
- Serum β_2 microglobulin levels in MM are increased (4–9 mg/L) (N: 1–2.5 mg/L)
- *Blood electrophoresis*
  - 99% of patients with MM reveal increased level of Ig (> 3 gm of Ig/dl of serum) in blood.
  - The monoclonal Ig identified in blood is called M protein (M for myeloma/monoclonal).
  - Most common M proteins are IgG (55% cases), IgA (25%).
  - *Screening by electrophoresis:* In a normal person polyclonal IgG appears as a broad band, in contrast this region shows a sharp band in case of MM patient of IgG type.
  - *Confirmation of Ig type* by immunofixation using specific antisera. Corresponding to rise in one type of Ig may lead to decrease in other type of Ig.
- *Urine finding:* Ig light chains called Bence Jones protein (> 6 mg/dl of urine).
- *Radiography*
  - There are multiple bony lesions, each individual lesion appears as sharply punched out defects, 1–4 cm in diameter having a rounded *soap-bubble* appearance.
- *BM*
  - Hypercellular bone marrow.
  - 15–30% myeloma cells of total cellularity.
  - Myeloma cells vary in size from small differentiated to large, immature, and undifferentiated cells.
  - Though nucleus is eccentric, but they lack cartwheel chromatin pattern.
  - They have abundant basophilic cytoplasm with perinuclear hof and may contain Russell bodies and their intranuclear counterpart Dutcher bodies.
  - Variants of myeloma cells include plasmablast, bizarre multinucleated cells, flame cells, Mott cells, etc.
- *Other findings*
  - Serum IL-6 level: ↑ed (main culprit for bony lesions, proliferation and maintenance of myeloma cells).
  - Renal and other organ amyloidosis (renal function test).
  - Hypercalcemia and hyperphosphatemia
  - Panda eyes
  - Serum alkaline phosphatase level is normal
  - Carpal tunnel syndrome
  - Hyperviscosity syndrome
  - Bleeding time: ↑ because platelets get coated by M-component which impairs platelet aggregation.

Diagnostic criteria of multiple myeloma (MM)

Major criteria

i. Plasmacytoma on tissue biopsy

ii. Bone marrow plasmacytosis >30% of plasma cells

iii. • Monoclonal globulin spike IgG > 35 g/L or IgA > 20 g/L.
   • Light chain excretion on urine electrophoresis ≥ 1g/24 hr.

Minor criteria

i. Bone marrow plasmacytosis, 10–30% plasma cells

ii. Monoclonal globulin spike, IgG <35 g/L or IgA < 20 g/L

iii. Lytic bone lesions

iv. Normal IgM < 500 mg/L, IgA < 1 g/L or IgG < 6 g/L

Criteria for MM

i. One major and one minor criteria or

ii. Three minor criteria that must include i and ii of minor criteria.

Extra points regarding MM

- Plasma cells produce immunoglobulins in dysregulated manner and sometimes result in intracellular accumulation of intact or partially degraded immunoglobulins. This produces certain variants of plasma cells: Flame cells (presence of fiery red cytoplasm), Mott cell (presence of multiple blue grape-like cytoplasmic droplets). Besides these there are cells containing variety of other inclusions: Fibrils, crystalline rods, Russel bodies (cytoplasmic inclusion), Dutcher bodies (nuclear inclusion).

12. Reed-Sternberg cells (RS cells) and its variants

- "Identification of RS cells and their variants in an appropriate background of non-neoplastic inflammatory cells is essential for histologic diagnosis of HD (Hodgkin disease)".
  - In difficult cases immunohistochemical, molecular methods are used.
  - RS cells are tumor giant cells.
- *Classic RS cell* is large (15–45 μ in diameter), binucleated or bilobed, with the two halves often appearing as mirror image of each other.
  - The nucleus has large, inclusion like, owl-eye nucleoli having size of small T lymphocytes and surrounded by a clear halo.
  - The nucleus is enclosed by abundant, amphophilic cytoplasm.
- *Variants*
  - Mononuclear variants: Round or oblong single nucleus with large inclusion like nucleoli.
  - Lacunar cells: Multilobed or folded nuclei surrounded by abundant pale cytoplasm.
  - L and H (lymphocytic and histiocytic) variants: Popcorn appearance.

13. Hodgkin disease: Classification (2004), pathology (1990, 93, 96, 2002)

14. Nodular sclerosis HD (2001, 08)

15. Mixed cellularity HD (1994, 2011)

Hodgkin disease

Subtype	Morphology	Immunophenotype	Clinical features
Nodular sclerosis (65–75%)	Lacunar cells—frequent, RS cells—less frequent. BG*: T lymphocytes, eosinophils, macrophages, and plasma cells. Collagen fibrous septa divide cellular area into nodules	RS cells: CD15+ve, CD30+ve, EBV–ve	Female predominance, stages I and II more common; mediastinal, lower cervical, supra-clavicular involvement common
Mixed cellularity (25%)	Mononuclear and RS cells frequent, BG*: T lympho-cytes, eosinophils, macro-phages, plasma cells	RS cells: CD15+ve, CD30+ve, 70% EBV–ve	Male predominance, Stages III and IV (>50%), Biphasic peak (young adults and >55 yr)
Lymphocyte rich	Frequent mononuclear and diagnostic RS cells. Background infiltrate rich in T-lymphocytes	RS cells: CD15+ CD30+ 40% EBV+	Uncommon, male >F, Older adults
Lymphocyte predominance (6%)	L and H (popcorn cells) frequent, BG*: follicular	RS cells: CD20+ve,	Males, young; cervial and axillary

(Contd.)

Hodgkin disease (Contd.)

Subtype	Morphology	Immunophenotype	Clinical features
	dendritic cells and reactive B cells	CD15 –ve, CD30 –ve EBV–ve	lymphadenopathy, mediastinum uncommon
Lymphocyte depletion (rare)	Frequent RS cells; controversial and most cases seem to be large cell lymphoma, reticular variant, paucity of background reactive cells	RS cells: CD15 +ve, CD30 +ve Most EBV +ve	Male, older age, associated with HIV, developing countreis, disseminated diseases

*BG: background

Pathology

- Infections: EBV (most important), HTLV–I and II, HIV, and hepresvirus-6.
- Genetic: Some familial predisposition.
- Cytokines: IL-4, IL-5 (by RS cells—eosinophils accumulation), TNF-α, GM-CSF; TGF-β (by eosinophils, fibroblasts).
- It is proposed that RS cells are monoclonal lymphoid cells originating from B cells.

Clinical features

- Painless encouragement of lymph nodes, which are discrete, non-tender and rubbery.
- Constitutional symptoms (fever, night sweats, unexplain weight loss of greater than 10% body weight) in advanced stage.
- Classical "Pel-Ebstein fever" (fever showing cyclical pattern, several days to weeks of fever alternating with afebrile periods) is rare.
- Cutaneous allergy due to depressed cell-mediated immunity may be seen.

16. Causes of lymphadenopathy (1993)

Infective	Neoplastic
Bacterial: *Streptococcus, M. tuberculosis, Brucellosis* Viral: *EBV, HIV* Protozoal: Toxoplasmosis Fungal: Histoplasmosis, Coccidioidomycosis **Sarcoidosis**	Primary: Leukemias, Lymphomas Secondary: Lung, Breast, Thyroid, Stomach *Connective tissue disorders:* Rheumatoid arthritis, SLE *Drugs:* Phenytoin **Amyloidosis**

17. Difference between Hodgkin disease (HD) and non-Hodgkin disease (NHD)

S. No.	Traits	HD	NHD
1.	Cell derivation	Mostly B cells	90% B cells, 10% T cells
2.	LN involvement	Localized to a single axial group of nodes like cervical, mediastinum, para-aortic	Frequently involve multiple peripheral nodes

(Contd.)

Difference between Hodgkin disease (HD) and non-Hodgkin disease *(Contd.)*

S. No.	Traits	HD	NHD
3.	Involvement of Mesenteric group and Waldeyer ring	Rare	Common
4.	Extranodal involvement	Uncommon	Common
5.	Spread of tumor	Orderly spread by contiguity	Non-contiguous spread
6.	Spread to blood	Never	May be
7.	LN architecture	Not deranged	Deranged
8.	Bone marrow involvement	Common	Uncommon
9.	Pathognomic cell types	RS cells and its variants	Histiocytes and lymphocytes
10.	Other autoimmune diseases	Less common	Common
11.	Constitutional symptoms	Common	Uncommon
12.	Chromosomal defects	Aneuploidy	Translocations, deletion
13.	Frequency	Less common	More common
14.	Prognosis	Good	Poor

18. Acute myelogenous leukemia (AML): Clinical features, PBS, BM findings (1998)

(See ALL, almost same kind of picture except cell type)

Clinical features: *(See table)*

- *CBC:*
  - Hb: ↓ed
  - RBC: ↓ed
  - Platelet: ↓ed
  - WBC: ↑↑ed
- *PBS:*
  - Normocytic normochromic red cells
  - Nucleated RBC may be seen
  - Myeloblasts or related cells
- *BM:*
  - Marrow hypercellular
  - M: E ratio = 80:1
  - Megakaryocyte: ↓ed
  - Blasts > 30%, other cell type
  - Lymphoid and erythroid precursors: ↓ed
- *Cytochemistry: (see difference table)*
- *Immunophenotyping:*
  - Myeloid: CD13 and 33 +ve
  - Monocytes: CD14 +ve
  - Megakaryocytes: CD61, 41 and 26 +ve
- *Cytogenetics:*
  - M_2: $t(8, 21)$
  - M_2 (with basophilia): $t(6, 9)$
  - M_3: $t(15, 17)$
  - M_4: Inversion 16q
  - M_5: Translocation or deletion of chromosome 11

19. Prognosis of AML

S. No.	Traits	Poor	Good
1.	Age	<2 yr, >60 yr	<45 yr
2.	Cause	Therapy induced or myelodysplastic syndrome associated	de novo

(Contd.)

Prognosis of AML (*Contd.*)

S. No.	Traits	Poor	Good
3.	Infection	Present	Absent
4.	Leukocyte count	>1,00,000/mm^3 (very high)	<25,000/mm^3 (low)
5.	Serum LDH	Increased	Normal
6.	Extramedullary involvement	Present	Absent
7.	CNS involvement	Present	Absent
8.	Sex	Male	Female
9.	Other hematological disorders	Present	Absent
10.	Cytogenetics	M_2 with basophilia: $t(6, 9)$ M_5: Translocation or deletion of chromosome 11	M_2: $t(8, 21)$ M_3: $t(15, 17)$ M_4: inversion (16) del (16q)
11.	Response to therapy	Delayed/Incomplete	Rapid
12.	Auer rod	Absent	Present
13.	FAB type	M_5, M_6, M_7	M_2, B_3, M_4, E_0
14.	Cell marker	CD13; CD14, CD33	CD2, CD19

20. FAB classification of AML (1998, 2003, 08)

21. Acute promyelocytic leukemia (2004)

22. Laboratory diagnosis of AML–M$_3$ (2009)

Class and incidence	Marrow morphology	Cytochemistry/clinical features
M_0: Minimally differentiated AML (2–3%)	Blasts lack definitive cytologic and cytochemical markers of myelo-blasts, but express myeloid lineage Ag and resemble myeloblast ultra-structurally	Myeloperoxidase (MPO): –ve
M_1: AML without differentiation (20%)	Very immature but >3% are MPO +ve, granules or Auer rods are few, a little maturation beyond myeloblast	MPO: May +ve
M_2: AML with maturation (30–40%)	Full range of maturation through granulation. Auer rods present in most cells	MPO: +++ve; presence of $t(8:21)$ defines prognostically favorable subgroup
M_3: Acute promyelocytic leukemia (5–10%)	Hypergranular promyelocytes (most cells), many Auer rods per cells	MPO: +++ve, younger with median age of 35–40 yr, development of DIC, $t(15:17)$ characteristics
M_4: Acute myelomonocytic leukemia (15–20%)	Myelocytic and monocytic differentiation present, myeloid cells resemble M_2	MPO: ++ve, NSE: +ve, if chromosomal abnormality of 16 present: marrow eosinophilia and good prognosis

(Contd.)

FAB classification of AML *(Contd.)*

Class and incidence	Marrow morphology	Cytochemistry/clinical features
M_5: Acute monocytic leukemia (10%) Older age	M_{5a}: Monoblasts and promonocytes predominates in blood and bone marrow M_{5b}: Mature monocytes in peripheral blood	Monoblasts: MPO +ve and NSE ++ve, high incidence of organomegaly, lymphadenopathy and tissue infiltration
M_6: Acute erythroleukemia (5–10%)	Dysplatic erythroid precursors (some megaloblastoid, others with giant or multiple nuclei) are predominant; non erythroid cells of which > 30% are myeloblast	Seen in advanced age, 1% of de novo AML, 20% of therapy related AML Erythroblast: PAS +ve Myeloblast: MPO +ve
M_7: Acute megakaryocytic leukemia	Blasts of megakaryocytic lineage predominate, which reacts with specific antiplatelet Ab against GPIIb/IIIa or vWF; Myelofibrosis/ ↑ed marrow reticulin present	Platelet peroxidase +ve

23. WHO classification of AML (2011)

(See textbook for details)

Class
I. AML with genetic aberrations
II. AML with MDS-like features
III. AML, therapy related
IV. AML, not otherwise specified

24. CML (1993, 96): Clinical features, PBS, BM findings (1990), chromosomal abnormality (role of Philadelphia chromosome) (2000), pathogenesis of CML (2002)

25. Laboratory diagnosis of CML (2004, 08, 11)

CML is a myeloproliferative disease characterised by excessive proliferation of myeloid cells with near normal maturation.

Clinical features
- Age: 25–55 yr, child <5% and infants
- Triphasic
  i. Initial chronic phase: 3–5 yr
  ii. Accelerated phase: A few months
  iii. Blast crisis: AML/ALL
- Splenomegaly (massive)
- Weight loss, fever, sweats (hypermetabolic state)
- Bone tenderness (hyperplastic marrow)
- Hyper-viscosity of blood due to high leukocytes
- Lethargy, fatigue (due to anemia)
- Bleeding present or absent
- Visual disturbances
- Priaprism

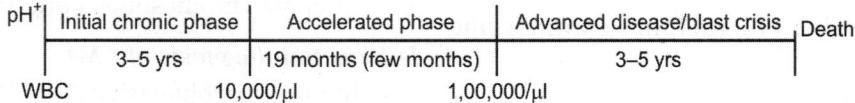

Fig. 12.3

Laboratory diagnosis

Initial phase

- *CBC:*
  - TLC: ↑ed (100 – 300 × 10^9/L)
  - Platelet count: ↑ed/Normal
  - Hb: ↓↓
  - *DLC:*
    - ➢ Blasts: <5%
    - ➢ Myelocytes: 6–10%
    - ➢ Stab cells, neutrophils, eosinophils: 30–40%
    - ➢ Promyelocytes: Few
    - ➢ Metamyelocytes: 6–10%
    - ➢ Basophils: >2%

(*Differentiate it from AML-blasts ++nt, platelet ↑↑ed, and other immature cells <10%)

- *PBS*
  - Nucleated RBC
  - Leukocytosis
  - Thrombocytosis
  - Granulocyte precursors ranging from myeloblasts, myelocytes and metamyelocytes to mature neutrophils are seen.
  - Segmented neutrophils and myelocytes predominate.
  - Normocytic normochromic anemia.

- *BM*
  - Hypercellular: (>70%; normal 50% cellularity and 50% fat)
  - M: E ratio = ↑↑ed
  - Megakaryocytes: ↑ed, ↑ed small dysplastic form
  - Erythroid progenitor: N/↓ed
  - Blasts and promyelocytes: <20%
  - Blasts: <5%
  - *Sea blue histiocytes* +nt (scattered storage histiocytes with wrinkled, sea blue cytoplasm)

- *Cytochemistry*
  - LAP: ↓↓↓ed or absent

- *Cytogenetics:* Philadelphia chromosome present

- *Other findings*
  - Serum vitamin B$_{12}$: ↑ed;
  - Vitamin B$_{12}$ binding proteins: ↑ed (due to transcobalmin I synthesis by myeloid cells);
  - Serum alkaline phosphatase and serum uric acid: ↑ed (due to proliferation).

Accelerated phase

- TLC: ↑ed despite treatment
- ↑ed blasts and promyelocytes > 20% in BM
- ↑ed blasts > 15% in PBS
- ↑ed basophils and eosinophils in PBS >10%
- Thrombocytopenia/thrombocytosis
- Progressive anemia: ↑↑ing
- Marrow fibrosis
- ↑ in splenic size

Acute leukemic phase (blast crisis)

- In 50% cases of CML
- Most resistant to treatment
- Changes to de novo AML (70%) or ALL (30%)
- No intermediate accelerated phase

Blast crisis is characterised by

- Sudden increase in splenic size
- Anemia and thrombocytopenia
- Generalised lymphadenopathy
- Peripheral smear and bone marrow showing numerous blast cells (>20%) simulating acute leukemia.
- Refractoriness to treatment

Atypical CML

- Philadelphia chromosome absent
- Lower % of basophils
- Larger % of immature precursors of erythroblast in BM
- Organomegaly present
- Dysplastic features of granulocytes
- Old age group
- Lower TLC
- Additional chromosomal abnormality

Differential diagnosis of CML

- Other myeloproliferative disorders
- Leukamoid reaction

26. Philadelphia chromosome (1994, 95, 2001, 07)

- This is an example of oncogenes formed by fusion of two separate genes.
- Present in CML and certain ALL (total of 20%; adult type).
- *Chromosomal abnormality:* There is reciprocal translocation (part of chromosomes is exchanged between two chromosomes—'give and take') between chromosome 9 (*abl* oncogene) and 22 (*bcr* oncogene). The hybrid gene *abl-bcr* is formed on chromosome 22. It codes for a chimeric protein having tyrosine kinase activity.
  - This chimeric protein have molecular weight of 210 kD in CML, whereas 190 kD in ALL.
  - These gene products dysregulate the mechanism of controlling the proliferation of hematopoietic stem cells.

bcr (break cluster region), *abl* (protooncogene).

- Variants of Ph chromosome are present in 5–10% cases.
  - Simple: 22q is translocated other than chromosome 9.
  - Complex: 3 or more chromosomes are involved in translocation.
- *Identification of Ph chromosome:*
  Molecular technique (*also see diagram in textbook*):
  - RT-PCR: Detects bcr-abl gene products [190 kD: ALL, 210 kD: CML, 230 kD: CNL]
  - Southern Blotting
  - FISH (fluorescent in situ hybridization)

27. The cytogenetic abnormalities associated with hematological malignancies

(*See all hematological malignancies and cytogenetic abnormalities given above*).

28. Cytochemistry of acute leukemia (1994, 95, 98)

29. Role of cytochemistry in diagnosis of leukemia (2000)

(*See from difference table of ALL and AML, lab diagnosis of all leukemia*).

30. Leukemoid reaction (1995, 97, 2002)

- Leukocytosis (excessive) in response of some infections or other stimulus; may be confused with leukemia.
- Myeloid leukemoid reaction is more common than lymphoid leukemoid reaction.
- *Causes of myeloid leukemoid reaction*
  Infections
  - *Staphylococcus pneumoniae*
  - Endocarditis
  - Meningitis
  - Disseminated TB
  Intoxication
  - Eclampsia
  - Severe burn
  Malignant tumors
  - Multiple myeloma
  - Hodgkin's disease
  Severe hemorrhage and hemolysis
- *Causes of lymphoid leukemoid reaction*
  Infections
  - Infectious mononucleosis
  - CMV infection
  - Measles
  - Tuberculosis
  - Pertusis

31. Difference between CML and leukemoid reaction (1995, 97, 99, 2000, 01, 02, 07, 08, 10)

S. No.	Traits	CML	Leukemoid reaction
1.	Age	25–60 yr; peak—30–40 yr	Any age
2.	Etiology	Clonal disorder	Infections
3.	TLC	>50,000/cc	<50,000/cc

(*Contd.*)

Difference between CML and leukemoid reaction (Contd.)

S. No.	Traits	CML	Leukemoid reaction
4.	Anemia	+nt, progressive	+/−nt
5.	Immature cells	+++nt, >30%	+nt, <5–10%
6.	LAP	Low or absent	High
7.	Toxic granules	Absent	Present
8.	Dohle's bodies	Absent	Present
9.	Cytogenetics	Philadelphia chromosome is present	Absent
10.	Splenomegaly	Present	Absent
11.	Eosinophilia and basophilia	Present	Absent
12.	Platelet	Increased	Normal or increased

32. Difference between CML and CLL

S. No.	Traits	CML	CLL
1.	Age	20–60 yr, <3 yr juvenile CML	>50–60 yr
2.	M: F	1:1	2:1
3.	Cytogenetics	Philadelphia chromosome (70–90%)	Trisomy of 12, 14 (30%)
4.	Organomegaly	Hepatosplenomegaly, lymph node enlargement in juvenile CML	Massive splenomegaly, lymphadenopathy
5.	Presentation	Bone tenderness, hypermetabolism, dragging sensation, left upper quadrant pain (acute splenic infarct)	Found to be CLL in routine examination of other diseases. Mainly asymptomatic.
6.	Cell type	Increased myeloid cells	Increased lymphocytes
7.	LAP	Decreased/absent	Normal range
8.	Other features	Vitamin B_{12} is increased	Immunoglobin decreased

33. Leukocytic alkaline phosphatase (LAP) or Neutrophilic alkaline phosphatase (NAP)

- Its level increases in:
  - Leukamoid reaction
  - Essential thrombocytosis
  - Polycythemia vera
  - Myelofibrosis with myeloid metaplasia
- Its level decreases in:
  - CML (almost absent)
  - PNH

34. Causes of splenomegaly/hypersplenism (2003, 08, 11)

- *Hypersplenism is characterized by three features:*
  - Splenomegaly;
  - Reduction of one or more of cellular elements of blood (anemia, leukopenia, thrombocytopenia, or its combination) in association with hyperplasia of marrow precursors of the deficient cell type;
  - Correction of the blood cytopenia(s) by splenectomy.

- *Causes of splenomegaly:*

Lymphohematogenous disorders	Infections	Congestive state related to portal hypertension
Hodgkin disease	*Bacteria:*	Cirrhosis of liver, Portal or splenic
Non-Hodgkin lymphoma	Tuberculosis, Typhoid fever,	vein thrombosis,
Multiple myeloma	Brucellosis, Syphilis	Cardiac failure
Myeloproliferative disorders	*Viral:*	*Others*
Hemolytic anemia	Cytomegalovirus	Amyloidosis
Thrombocytopenic purpura	Infectious mononucleosis	Primary neoplasm and cysts
Immunologic-inflammatory	*Parasites:*	Secondary neoplasm
conditions	Malaria, Histoplasmosis	
Rheumatoid arthritis	Toxoplasmosis, Kala-azar	
SLE	Trypanosomiasis,	
Storage diseases	Schistosomiasis	
Gaucher disease	Echinococcosis	
Niemann-Pick disease	Nonspecific splenitis	
Mucopolysaccharidoses		

35. Peripheral blood finding in infectious mononucleosis/glandular fever (1998)

- This is a benign, self-limiting lymphoproliferative disease caused by EBV.
- *Age:* Teenagers and young adults
- *Laboratory diagnosis*
  Blood count and PBS
  - TLC: ↑ed (10,000–20,000/µl)
  - Leukocytosis with absolute lymphocytosis
  - Normal as well as atypical T lymphocytes
  - Diagnostic feature is presence of at least 10–12% of atypical/mononucleosis cells of total lymphocytes in PBS.
  - Size of atypical T cells is that of large lymphocytes.
  - Appearance of mononucleosis cells are variable and classified as Downey type I (most frequent), type II, type III.

Serology
- To demonstrate antibodies against virus by methods:
  - Paul-Bunnell test: Heterophile Abs against sheep RBC are found in serum at high titre (80–90% of patients, peak at 2nd–3rd wks)
  - Detection of specific Ab for EBV antigen
  - Monospot test: Simple slide test for antibody detection
- Detection of *EBV* antigens:
  Acute infectious mononucleosis is characterized by:
  - Antiviral capsid (VCA) antibodies of IgM type
  - Antibodies to *EBV* early antigen (EA)
  - Absent antibodies to *EBV* nuclear antigen (anti-EBNA)

36. Agranulocytosis (1988)

- When neutropenia reaches to the extent that it predisposes to infections, it is called agranulocytosis.

Leukocytosis	Leucopenia
- Leukemia	- Aplastic anemia
- Leukamoid reaction	- Hypersplenism
- Bacterial and viral infections	- Typhoid and paratyphoid fever
- Infectious mononucleosis	- Drug induced

(Contd.)

Leukocytosis	Leucopenia
• Diabetic and uremic coma • Pregnancy • Exercise	• Radiation and cytotoxic therapy • Megaloblastic anemia • Subleukemic leukemia

Neutrophilia	Neutropenia	Eosinophilia

Infection
  Acute bacterial, fungal
Trauma (acute stress)
  Surgery, Burns
Infarction
  MI, Pulmonary embolism
  Sickle cell crisis
Inflammation
  Gout, Rheumatoid arthritis
	Infection
	  Viral
	  Bacterial: Typhoid
	  Protozoa: Malaria
	  Chemical: Benzene
	Drugs
	  Chloroquine
	  Phenytoin
	  Sulphonamides
		Parasitic infection
		Allergy
		  Hay fever, Eczema, Asthma
		Skin disease
		Connective tissue (CT) disease
		  Polyarteritis nodosa
		Malignancies
		  Solid tumors, Lymphoma
		Drug hypersensitivity

		Basophilia

Ulcerative colitis (UC)
  Crohn's disease
Malignancy
  Solid tumors, HD
Myeloproliferative disease
  Polycythemia, CML
Physiological
  Exercise, Pregnancy
	Autoimmune
	  CT disorders
	Alcohol
	Congenital
	  Kostmann's syndrome
		Myeloproliferative disease
		  Polycythemia, CML
		Inflammation
		  Acute hypersensitivity
		  UC, Crohn's disease
		Iron deficiency

Lymphocytosis	Lymphopenia	Monocytosis

Infection
  Viral; Bacterial TB, syphilis
  Bordetella pertusis
Lymphoproliferative disease
  CLL, Lymphoma
Postsplenectomy
	Inflammation: CT diseases
	Lymphoma
	Renal failure
	Sarcoidosis
	Drugs: Steroids, Cytotoxic
	Congenital: SCID
		Infection: Bacterial tuberculosis,
		Syphilis
		Inflammation: CT disease, UC
		Crohn's disease
		Malignancy: AML–M5, M4, Solid
		tumors

37. Difference between CML and myelofibrosis

S. No.	Traits	CML	Myelofibrosis
1.	Splenomegaly	Moderate to marked	Marked
2.	Fever	Common	Uncommon
3.	RBCs	• Marked anemia • Mild poikilocytosis	• Slight to moderate anemia • Prominent poikilocytosis with tear drop cells

4.	WBCs	• Marked increase;
		  $20–50 \times 10^9/L$
			• N/$\uparrow$/$\downarrow$; when raised not more
			  than $50 \times 10^9/L$

5.	Nucleated RBC	Few if any	Numerous
6.	LAP	Low	• N/$\uparrow$/$\downarrow$
7.	BM Aspiration	Hyperplastic marrow with absence of fat spaces	Dry tap without marrow fragments
8.	Chromosomal analysis	Philadelphia: Positive	Philadelphia: Negative

13

Miscellaneous Questions for Paper I

1. Significance of microscopic examination of urine (2002)

2. Laboratory diagnosis of chronic renal failure (2001, 04)

3. Blood and urinary finding of chronic renal failure (1999)

4. Difference between nephrotic and nephritic syndrome (1995)

5. Significance of creatinine clearance test (1994)

6. Urinary casts (1993)

7. Giant cells (2001)

8. Pathogenesis of Rh hemolytic disease of newborn (2000)

9. Hemolytic diseases of newborn (1993)

10. Glucose tolerance test (1993, 99, 2002, 04)

11. Ketoacidosis (1993)

12. Difference between melanin and hemosiderin (1997)

13. Difference between CSF in tuberculosis and pyogenic meningitis (1995, 2002)

14. Laboratory diagnosis of tubercular meningitis (2008)

15. CSF in tubercular meningitis (1994)

16. Mallory hyaline (1994)

17. Difference between obstructive and hemolytic jaundice (1993)

18. Lab finding of hepatocellular jaundice (2002)

19. Rodent ulcer (1993)

20. Hemoglobin estimation (1993)

21. Component therapy of blood (2007, 08)

22. Laboratory diagnosis of diabetes mellitus (2008)

Miscellaneous Questions for Paper 1

PART II

Heart and Blood Vessels

14

1. What is atherosclerosis? Describe the etiopathogenesis, morphology and clinical consequences of atherosclerosis (1994, 97)

2. Pathogenesis of atherosclerosis and its clinical manifestation (2001, 10)

3. Atheroma aorta (1997)

4. Sequelae of aortic atherosclerosis (1995, 98)

5. Complications of atheromatous plaque (1994, 2008)

6. Morphology and complications of atheromatous plaque (2004), 2011)

Atherosclerosis is characterized by formation of fibrous plaque with lipid-rich core in the tunica intima of arteries leading to *thickening and loss of elasticity of arterial walls*.

Pathogenesis

Following stages occur in the pathogenesis of atherosclerosis

i. Endothelial injury
   - Earliest stages of development of atherosclerosis mediated by inflammatory cascade, which results in endothelial injury.
   - After injury, endothelium is activated and there is increased expression of adhesion molecule VCAM-1 and there is increased permeability to endothelium (major role of TNF).

ii. Migration of leukocytes
   - When VCAM-1 is expressed on endothelium, leukocytes adhere to the endothelium. Leukocytes cross the endothelial barrier and begin to accumulate in "subendothelial intimal space".
   - Macrophages engulf LDL cholesterol and form foam cells—formation of earliest lesion, i.e. fatty streak.
   - Macrophages also form oxygen free radicals that cause oxidation of LDL to yield 'oxidized LDL' (modified LDL). Oxidized LDL increases monocyte accumulation in lesion, stimulates release of growth factors and cytokines and is cytotoxic to smooth muscle cells and endothelial cells.

iii. Smooth muscle cell migration and proliferation
   - Inflammatory cells in subendothelial intimal space secrete cytokines (PDGF, TGF-α and FGF) which cause migration of smooth muscle cells from media to subendothelial intimal space as well as their proliferation.

iv. Maturation of plaque
   - Smooth muscle cells synthesize extracellular matrix (especially collagen) and convert a fatty streak into a mature

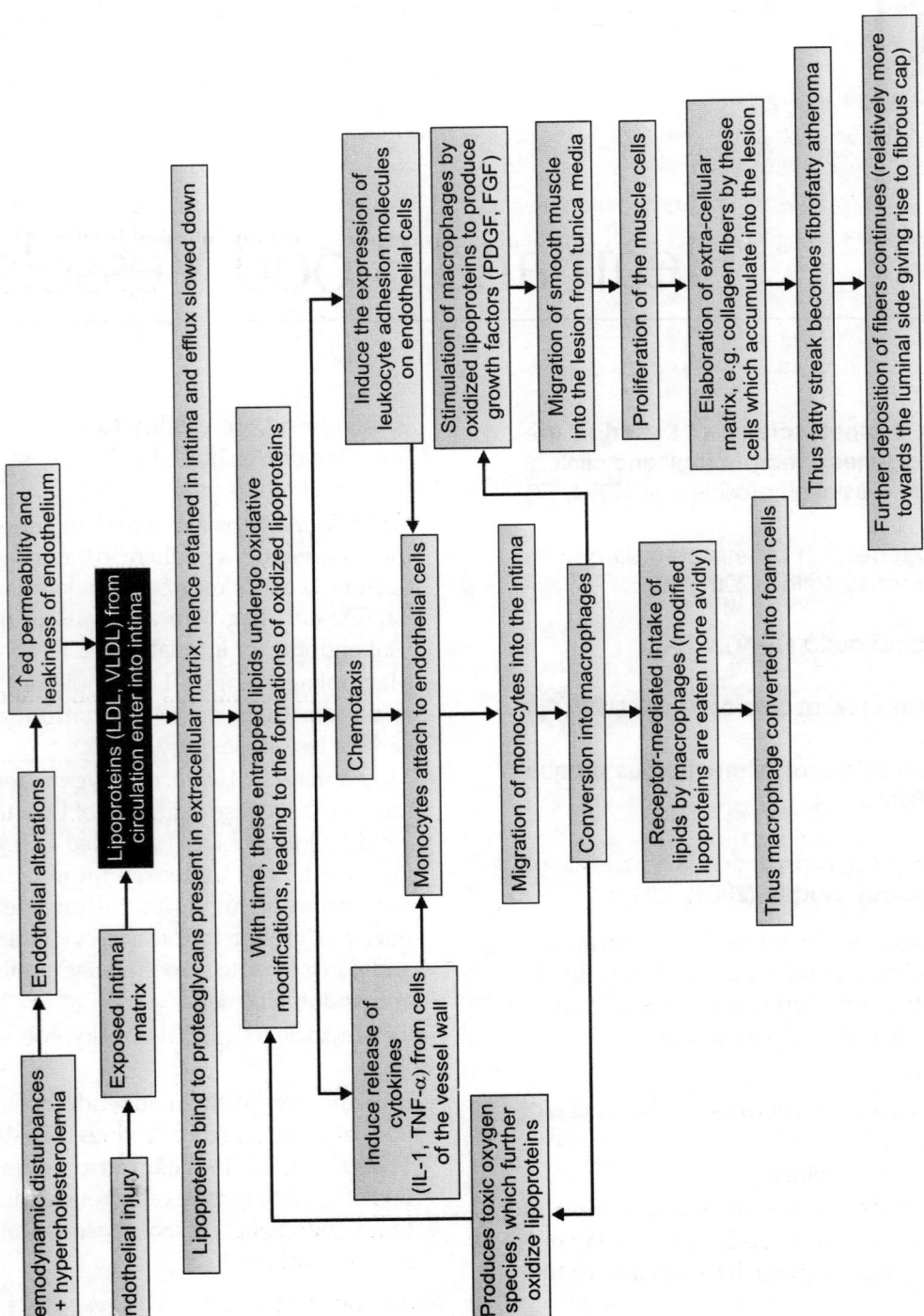

Fig. 14.1: Pathogenesis of atherosclerosis

fibrofatty atheroma, and contribute to the progressive growth of atherosclerotic lesions.

The disease starts with the formation of fatty streak (focal ↑ in contents of lipoproteins within the region of intima).

Risk Factors

(Major) Important risk factors		Others
Non-modifiable (constitutional): • Age: Risk ↑es with age • Sex: More in male than premenopausal women • Positive family history • Genetic factors of lipoprotein metabolism derangement	*Modifiable (acquired):* • Hyperlipidemia (particularly serum LDL level) • Hypertension (both systolic and diastolic BP) • Cigarette smoking • Diabetes mellitus	• Lifestyle factors: For example, obesity, physical inactivity, stress, atherogenic diet, metabolic syndrome • Postmenopausal deficiency of estrogen • Lipoprotein a (Lp a) level • Homocysteine (↑ed level) • Inflammation

Morphology of atheromatous plaque

These are focal lesions formed within the intima of involved arteries in atherosclerosis.

Gross

• Whitish-yellow in color
• Small sized (0.3–1.5 cm in diameter); may sometimes coalesce to form larger masses.
• Distribution: Any arteries of body may be involved, but arteries most heavily involved (↓ing order) are:
  i. Lower abdominal aorta
  ii. Coronary artery
  iii. Popliteal artery
  iv. Descending thoracic aorta
  v. Internal carotid artery
  vi. Circle of Willis
• Composition: Composed of a deeper, whitish-yellow, soft core, and a firm white fibrous cap covering the core from the luminal side.

Microscopic features

• The central core is composed of abundant lipid material (mainly cholesterol and its esters), foam cells, a few smooth muscle cells, cellular debris, and also may be thrombus in various stages of organization.

• Superficial (luminal) part of fibrous cap is covered by endothelium, composed of smooth muscle cells, dense connective tissue and extracellular matrix.
• Cellular area under fibrous cap (shoulder of lesion) is composed of macrophages, foam cells, lymphocytes, and a few smooth muscle cells, which may contain lipid.
• A network of proliferating small blood vessels (neovascularization) is usually seen around the periphery of lesion.

Sequelae of atherosclerosis

Clinical features

• Symptomatic plaques most often involve arteries supplying the heart, brain, kidney and lower extremities.
• Major clinical consequences are:
  – Myocardial infarction
  – Cerebral infarction (stroke)
  – Peripheral vascular disease of lower limbs
  – Ischemic bowel disease, infarction and ischemic strictures of intestine
  – Renovascular hypertension

Complications

During the initial stage of the development of an atheroma, the growth is often outward and does not encroach upon the lumen. Only late in its history does the plaque growth may encroach upon the lumen and produce clinically significant narrowing.

So the complications that are of more clinical significance than the plaque itself:

1. *Thrombosis*
   - The most feared complication
   - May lead to ischemia and infarction
   - Rupture, erosion or ulceration of the fibrous cap of plaque permits contact between coagulation factors in blood and thrombogenic substances in the plaque core.

2. *Rupture of plaque ulceration:* May lead to thrombosis or embolism

3. *Embolism*

4. *Hemorrhage:* Abundant new microvascular network formed in the plaque are prone to rupture and may produce intraplaque hemorrhage. Hematoma, thus produced may either leak into blood vessel or rupture the plaque.

5. *Wall weakening and aneurysmal dilatation* (major complication in aorta)

6. Calcification in advanced plaque

7. Progressive plaque growth: It causes critical stenosis and obstruction of vessels.

7. Difference between fatty streak and an atheroma (2008)

S. No.	Trait	Fatty streak	Atheroma
1.	Age affected	Starts in child as young as <1yr	Affects older individual
2.	Composition	Lipid accumulation is mainly intracellular (lipid filled foam cell); T-lymphocytes and extra-cellular lipids are present in small amounts.	Large core of extracellular lipid
3.	Gross appearance	• Multiple yellow flat lesions less than 1 mm in diameter • Do not encroach upon the union	• Whitish-yellow, raised, usually eccentric lesions, measuring 0.5 to 1.5 cm in diameter • Encroch upon the lumen
4.	Vasculative involved	May be distributed in areas other than those affected by atherosclerosis	Primarily affects elastic as well as large and medium size muscular arteries
5.	Geographic distribution	May be seen in geographic areas, which have low incidence of atherosclerosis	Common in western world and developed countries
6.	Clinical consequences	Do not generally cause obstruction to blood flow	May cause symptomatic obstruction/complications

8. American Heart Association (AHA) classification (1995) of human atherosclerosis

Type	Sequence in progression	Main growth mechanism	Earliest onset	Clinical correlation
Type I (initial lesion, isolated foam cells and macrophages)	I	Growth mainly by lipid accumulation	From 1st decade	Clinically silent

(Contd.)

American Heart Association (AHA) classification (1995) of human atherosclerosis (Contd.)

Type	Sequence in progression	Main growth mechanism	Earliest onset	Clinical correlation
Type II (fatty streaks) mainly intracellular lipid accumulation	II	Growth mainly by lipid accumulation	From 1st decade	Clinically silent
Type III (intermediate lesion) Type II changes plus small extracellular lipid pool	III	Growth mainly by lipid accumulation	From 3rd decade	Clinically silent
Type IV (atheroma lesion) Type II lesion plus core of extracellular lipid	IV	Growth mainly by lipid accumulation	From 3rd decade	Clinically silent or overt
Type V (fibroatheroma lesion) lipid core plus fibrotic layer/multiple lipid cores plus fibrotic layer/mainly calcific/ mainly fibrotic	V	Accelerated smooth muscle and collagen synthesis	From 4th decade	Clinically silent or overt
Type VI (complicated lesion) surface defect, hematoma, hemorrhage and thrombus	VI	Thrombosis, hematoma	From 4th decade	Clinically silent or overt

9. Classification of vasculitis based on vessel size

Large vessel vasculitis	Medium vessel vasculitis	Small vessel vasculitis	
		ANCA positive	ANCA negative
• Giant cell arteritis • Takayasu's arteritis • Cogan's syndrome	• Polyarteritis nodosa • Kawasaki disease • Buerger's disease	• Wegener's granu-lomatosis • Microscopic poly-angiitis • Churg-Strauss syndrome • Drug induced	• Behçet's syndrome • Hypersensitivity • Urticarial vasculitis

10. Classification of vasculitis based on type of inflammation

Vasculitis with granulomatous inflammation	Vasculitis with necrotising inflammation
• Giant cell arteritis • Takayasu's disease • Wegener's granulomatosis • Churg-Strauss syndrome	• Polyarteritis nodosa • Churg-Strauss syndrome • Wegener's granulomatosis • Microscopic polyangiitis

11. Takayasu's arteritis (1998)

- This is an *inflammatory and stenotic* disorder affecting large- and medium-sized arteries.
- It has strong predilection for arch of aorta and its branches. Specially involves in the origin of the arterial branches from aorta. Fibrous thickening of the aortic arch leads to narrowing or obliteration of the origin of the great vessels resulting in marked weakening of pulses in the upper extremities. Hence also called *Pulseless disease*.
- Cause and pathogenesis are unknown. Most common in women < 35 yr.
- *Morphology:* Involves mainly aortic arch and its branches, but may involve the remaining aorta with its branches, and the pulmonary arteries.
  Gross
  - Marked intimal thickening, fibrosis, and scarring of the tunica media.
  - It leads to irregular thickening and narrowing of the involved arteries.
  Microscopic features
  - Panarteritis (involving all three layers)
  - Initially there is adventitial mononuclear infiltration with prominent perivascular cuffing of vasa vasorum.
  - Later: Marked mononuclear infiltration in media. Also in some cases, granuloma formation with necrosis and abundant giant cells (granulomatous inflammation).

- *Clinical features*
  - Weakening of pulse, marked lowering of BP in upper extremities with coldness or numbness of fingers.

12. Polyarteritis nodosa (PAN) (1996, 2009)

A *systemic* necrotizing vasculitis disease, involving small- and medium-sized muscular arteries.

Arteries involved
- Typically focal, episodic and random involvement of small- and medium-sized muscular arteries in any organ.

- Involvement of renal visceral vessels in most cases (but no glomerulonephritis, as PAN does not involve arterioles or capillaries).
- Never involves pulmonary arteries.

Morphology
- Gross
  Segmental lesion
  - Tend to occur at sites of branching or bifurcation
  - Usually cause segmental erosion and, hence weakening of arterial walls at some places (perceived clinically as *palpable nodule*) or even rupture.
  - May impair perfusion leading to *ulceration, infarction* and *ischemic atrophy* in the areas supplied.
- Microscopic
  Inflammation
  - Necrotizing type
  - No granuloma formation
  - Often transmural
- Sequence of events
  Acute stage
  - Heavy infiltrate of neutrophils, some eosinophils and few mononuclear cells
  - Proliferation of tunica media
  - Fibrinoid necrosis of inner half of vessel wall (ongoing inflammation and tunical proliferation compromise the lumen leading to increased intraluminal pressure and exudation of plasma in the vessel wall)

Chronic inflammatory stage: Increased mononuclear infiltrate and fibrosis
Healing stage: Marked fibrotic thickening of affected vessel. No inflammatory cells
Particularly important in PAN is that all the three stages may coexist in different vessels or even within the same vessel.

Clinical features
- Non-specific constitutional symptoms (fatigue, malaise, fever, weight loss, anorexia).

- Renal manifestation (hypertension, renal failure)
- Peripheral nervous system (neuropathy)
- GIT (abdominal pain, nausea, vomiting, hepatic and pancreatic infarct)
- Skin (rash, Raynaud's phenomenon)
- Cardiac (CHF, MI)
- CNS (CVA, seizures)

13. Wegener's granulomatosis (2009)

Three important features of the disease are:
1. Necrotizing and granulomatous vasculitis
   - Most prominent in vessels of lungs and upper airways.
2. Necrotizing and granulomatous inflammation of upper and lower respiratory tracts.
3. Glomerulonephritis: Only necrotizing; granulomas very rare.
   - Initially focal and segmental; later on rapidly proliferative and crescentic.
- *Etiology:* Unknown
- *Pathogenesis:* May involve cell-mediated immune mechanism.
- Most patients have circulating c-ANCA.
- *Morphology:* Typically shows necrotizing vasculitis (segmental or circumferential) of small and sometimes large vessels.
  - *Upper respiratory tract:* Range from simple granulomatous inflammation of mucosa to ulcerative lesions.
  - *Lungs:* Foci of necrotizing granulomas dispersed in lung and blood vessels.
  - *Kidney:* Focal and segmental necrotizing glomerulonephritis, diffuse necrosis in advanced cases.

Clinical features
- It usually effects adult males in the 5th decade; multiple organ involvement
- Non-specific constitutional symptoms
- Respiratory system: It is first to involve
- Kidney involvement: It is most dangerous: Hematuria and non-nephrotic range proteinuria.

- Eye, joint, skin, git and peripheral nervous system involvement

14. Buerger's disease (thromboangiitis obliterans)

- "An *inflammatory* and *occlusive* vascular disorder of small- and medium-sized arteries and veins in the distal upper and lower extremities".
- It mainly involves tibial and radial arteries.
- Predominance in male <35 yr.
- *Cause:* Unknown, but strong relation with heavy smoking (99%)

  'Cessation of smoking at early stage may bring dramatic relief, but once the disease progresses there is little relief even after cessation of smoking'. It is associated with HLA-B5 and HLA-A9.
- *Morphology:* Segmental lesions in the involved arteries.

Initial stage
- Polymorphonuclear infiltrate permeating the arterial wall.
- Later on, polymorphonuclear infiltrate is replaced by mononuclear cells, fibroblasts and giant cells.
- *Thrombus formation* in the lumen
- Thrombus has characteristically small microabscesses formed by a central focus of neutrophils, surrounded by granulomatous inflammations.

Later stage
- Inflammation heals with perivascular fibrosis, and thrombus may undergo organization and recanalization.
- Complication: May be digital ischemia, atrophic changes in nails, etc.
- *Clinical features:* Triad
  - Migratory superficial vein thrombophlebitis
  - Features of Raynaud's phenomenon
  - Pain in the instep of foot by exercise (instep claudication)

15. Raynaud's disease and phenomenon

"A disease of digits of the hands or feet, characterized by episodic development of pallor or cyanosis. The episode occurs after exposure to cold, and on subsequent re-warming color changes from white to blue to red."

- *Morphology:* No organic change in arterial wall
- *Cause:* Not known

- *Mechanism* (proposed): Exaggeration of *central and local reflex vasoconstriction* in response to cold.
- *Raynaud's phenomenon:* This is the appearance of the similar features in extremities. But it is not idiopathic rather 2° to certain diseases like SLE, scleroderma, atherosclerosis, Buerger's disease, which induce arterial narrowing or vasospasm, thus causing arterial insufficiency.

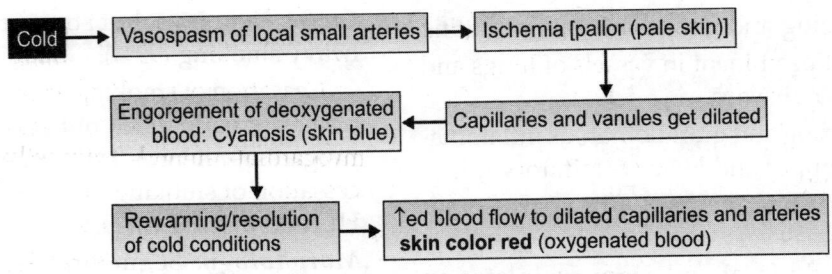

Fig. 14.2: Pathogenesis of Raynaud's disease

16. Aneurysm of aorta (1995)

An aneurysm is a permanent abnormal dilatation of a blood vessel occurring due to congenital or acquired weakening or destruction of the vessel wall. It is generally seen in large elastic arteries especially aorta and its major branches.

- The two most important causes of aortic aneurysm are atherosclerosis and cystic medial degeneration of arterial media.
- It most commonly affects old person (> 50 yr), male > female.
- The most common location is abdominal aorta, others are thoracic (ascending and arch of aorta), iliac artery and large systemic arteries.

Pathogenesis

Severe atherosclerosis
↓
Thinning and destruction of the medial elastic tissue
↓
Atrophy and weakening of the wall
↓
Aneurysm formation

Complications
- Rupture into the peritoneal cavity and retroperitoneal tissues with massive potentially fatal hemorrhage. Risk of rupture is directly related to the size of aneurysm
- Obstruction of iliac, renal, mesenteric or vertebral branches due to direct pressure or narrowing of ostia → ischemic damage
- Impingement on adjacent structures, e.g. compression of ureter or vertebral erosion
- Embolism from atheroma or mural thrombus.

17. Dissecting aneurysm of aorta (1998)

- Aortic dissection is a catastrophic illness characterized by forceful separation of the planes of media with the formation of a intramural hematoma within the vessel wall, which may rupture outside causing massive hemorrhage.
- There is intimal tear, within 10 cm of aortic valve, through which blood enters into media. The dissecting hematoma spreads characteristically along the laminar plane

of aorta, usually between the middle and outer third. Sometimes, blood reruptures into the lumen distally, i.e. there is second tear distally, so that a complete new vascular channel is formed inside the media of aortic wall. Blood enters from proximal tear into the media and comes out into the lumen from distal tear. This is called "double-barrel aorta with false-channel" in media. Later on, this false channel becomes endothelialized—chronic dissection.

Classification of aortic dissection

* Risk of serious complication depends strongly on the level of aorta affected, with the most serious complications occurring from the aortic valve to the arch.
  i. Proximal lesion (Type A)
     - More common and more dangerous
     - Involves either the ascending portion only or both ascending and descending portions of aorta.
  ii. Distal lesion (Type B)
     - Involves only descending part distal to subclavian artery.

18. Etiopathogenesis of ischemic heart disease (IHD) (2011)

It is a group of pathophysiologically related syndrome resulting from myocardial ischemia—an imbalance between the supply (perfusion) and demand of the heart for oxygenated blood. Ischemia brings not only an insufficiency of oxygen, but also reduces the availability of nutrients and removal of metabolites.

Pathogenesis

The dominant cause of IHD syndrome is the insufficient coronary perfusion relative to myocardial demand. It is mostly due to chronic, progressive atherosclerotic narrowing of epicardial coronary arteries, and variable degree of superimposed acute plaque change, thrombosis, and vasospasm (Fig. 14.3).

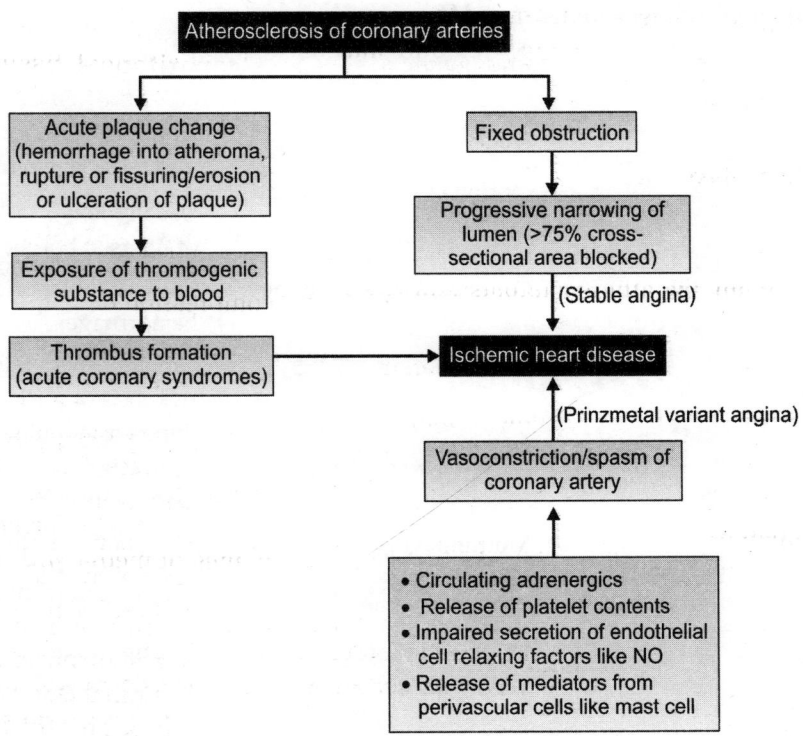

Fig. 14.3: Pathogenesis of IHD

19. Differentiated among different types of angina

S. No.	Traits	Stable angina	Prinzmetal variant angina	Unstable/Crescendo angina
1.	Cause	Fixed coronary atherosclerotic narrowing	Due to coronary artery spasm	Induced by acute plaque change, embolization or vasospasm or both
2.	Precipitating factors	Heart vulnerable to ischemia whenever O_2 demand increases	Occurs at rest, not related to O_2 demand	Often occurs at rest and tends to be of prolonged duration
3.	Relieving factors	Relieved by rest/decreased demand and nitroglycerin	Responds promptly to vasodilators like nitroglycerin and calcium channel blocker	May responds to vasodilator like nitroglycerin and calcium channel blockers
4.	Outcome	Responds to medication	Transmural ischemia, which generally responds to medication.	Harbinger of subsequent acute MI (also called pre-infarction angina)

20. Describe the morphological changes in the heart in acute MI in chronological order and discuss its laboratory findings (2000)

21. Laboratory findings in MI (1993, 98, 2001, 06, 10)

Morphological changes in heart in MI

Time	Gross feature	Light microscope
Reversible injury		
0–½ hr	None	None
Irreversible injury		
½–4 hr	None	Usually none, variable waviness of fibers at border
4–12 hr	Occasional dark mottling	Early coagulation necrosis, edema, hemorrhage
12–24 hr	Dark mottling	Ongoing coagulation necrosis, pyknosis of nuclei, myocyte hypereosinophilia, marginal contraction band necrosis; early neutrophilic infiltration
1–3 days	Mottling with yellow-tan infarct center	Coagulation necrosis with loss of nuclei and striations, interstitial infiltrate of neutrophils
3–7 days	Hyperemic border, central yellow-tan softening	Beginning disintegration of dead myofibers, with dying neutrophils, early phagocytosis of dead cells by macrophages at intact border

(Contd.)

Morphological changes in heart in MI (Contd.)

Time	Gross feature	Light microscope
7–10 days	Maximally yellow-tan and soft, with depressed red-tan margins	Well-developed phagocytosis of dead cells; early formation of fibrovascular granulation tissue at margins.
10–14 days	Red-gray depressed infarct borders	Well-established granulation tissue with new blood vessels and collagen deposition.
2–8 wk	Gray-white scar, progressive from border to core of infarct	Increased collagen deposition, with decreased cellularity.
>2 months	Scarring complete	Dense collagenous scar

Electron microscopic finding: Very early changes:
0–½ hr of MI: Relaxation of myofibrils, glycogen loss, mitochondrial swelling.
½–4 hr of MI: Sarcolemmal disruption, mitochondrial amorphous densities.

Laboratory diagnosis of MI

It may be divided into four groups
- ECG
- Serum cardiac biomarkers
- Cardiac imaging
- Non-specific indexes of tissue necrosis and inflammation
- *ECG:*
  - In asymptomatic cases of MI, ECG changes mostly consist of new Q waves.
  - In symptomatic cases, ECG shows generally ST elevation (STEMI showing complete occlusion of an epicardial artery): Some will show ST depression.
  - In some symptomatic, no ST elevation appears on ECG. Such cases can be diagnosed only by cardiac biomarkers.

- *Serum cardiac biomarkers*
  These are intracellular macromolecules that leak out of several injured myocardial cells.
- *Creatinine kinase (CK, total)*
  - Sensitive, but not specific marker
  - Also ↑ed in conditions like skeletal muscle trauma, skeletal muscle diseases like muscular dystrophy, myopathies, etc., electrical cardioversion, stroke, hypothyroidism, etc.
- *Creatinine kinase MB*
  - A cardiac specific isoenzyme of CK
  - More specific for heart
  - Absence in change in levels of CPK and CPK-MB during first two days essentially exclude the diagnosis of MI.

Biomarkers	Begin to rise	Peak	Return to normal
Creatinine kinase (total)	2–4 hr	24 hr	72 hr
CK-MB	4–8 hr	18 hr	48–72 hr
Troponin-t	4–6 hr	48 hr	7–14 days
Troponin-I	4–6 hr	48 hr	7–10 days
LDH	24 hr	3–6 days	14 days
AST/SGOT	Within 12 hr	48 hr	4–5 days
Myoglobin	One of the 1st markers to ↑ after MI	–	48 hr

- *Cardiac specific troponin-t and troponin-I*
  - Cardiac specific isomers of troponin
  - Not normally detectable in blood of healthy individuals, but may increase after MI to very high level.
  - Now marker of choice for MI, sensitivity is similar to CPK, but more specific.
  - Levels remain ↑ed for 7–10 days after MI, helping in detecting MI even after CK-MB level has returned to normal.

- *Myoglobin*
  - One of the first cardiac markers to rise after MI, but returns to normal within 24–48 hr.
  - Also not specific so not used now.

- *Non-specific indexes*
  - Polymorphonuclear leukocytosis: Appears within a few hour and persists for 3–7 days.
  - ESR: Raised slowly, peaks during first week, may remain elevated for 1–2 wk.

- *Cardiac imaging*
  To point out additional anatomic, biochemical and functional data.
  - Echocardiography
  - Radioisotope studies
  - MRI
  - Perfusion scintigraphy

22. Complications of MI (2002, 04, 08, 09)

(Mnemonic—CAMP P²RIMItiVe)

1. Contractile dysfunction: Abnormality of left ventricular function is proportional to the size and location of infarct. It may lead to left ventricular failure, hypotension and pulmonary vascular congestion.
2. Arrhythmias: Due to myocardial ischemia (conduction system ischemia) may lead to conduction disturbances and heart blocks.
3. Myocardial rupture:
   - Myocardial rupture may cause hemopericardium and cardiac tamponade.

- Complete interventricular/interatrial wall rupture lead to formation of a left to right shunt.
- Papillary muscle rupture may lead to valvular dysfunction.
- Incomplete rupture leads to formation of a pseudoaneurysm.

4. Pericarditis: Fibrinous or fibrinohemorrhagic (Dressler's syndrome).
5. Papillary muscle dysfunction: Mitral or aortic regurgitation.
6. Progressive late heart failure: Chronic ischemic heart disease (ischemic cardiomyopathy) is caused by postinfarction cardiac decompensation due to exhaustion of compensatory hypertrophy of noninfarcted myocardium.
7. Right ventricular infarction: Isolated RV infarction is rare.
8. Infarct expansion: New necrosis/weakening and disproportionate stretching, thinning or dilatation of infarct, lead to its expansion.
9. Mural thrombus: Abnormal myocardial contractility and endocardial damage lead to mural thrombosis. Thrombi can lead to systemic embolism.
10. Infarct extension
11. Ventricular aneurysm formation

23. Etiopathogenesis, clinical features, laboratory diagnosis of RHD (1990, 93, 95)

24. Complications of rheumatic heart diseases (2000)

25. Sequelae of RHD (2006)

26. MacCallum plaques (1998)

27. Morphology of heart in acute rheumatic fever (ARF)

- Rheumatic fever is an acute immune-mediated multisystem disease, which primarily involves the heart, joints, CNS, skin and subcutaneous tissues.

- Its peak incidence is between 5 and 15 yr.
- It is a delayed inflammatory response to pharyngeal infection with Group A Streptococci.
- The latent period between pharyngeal infection and onset of rheumatic fever ranges from 1–5 wk.
- Antibodies develop against streptococcal antigen, but cross reacts with cardiac myosin and sarcolemmal membrane protein.

Clinical manifestations
- Sore throat

- Polyarthritis (acute migratory or fleeting polyarthritis of large joints of extremities)
- Carditis (pancarditis involving all three layers)
- Subcutaneous nodules (small painless nodule over extensor surface and bony prominence)
- Erythema marginatum (erythematous macules with a clear center and serpiginous margins, most commonly seen on trunk and proximal parts of extremities)
- Chorea (Sydenham's chorea, chorea minor, saint vitus chorea)

Diagnosis: (Jones criteria for rheumatic fever)

Major criteria	*Minor criteria*
• Carditis	• Clinical
• Migratory polyarthritis	– Fever
• Sydenham's chorea	– Arthralgia
• Subcutaneous nodule	• Laboratory
• Erythema marginatum	– Elevated acute phase reactant (ESR, CRP)
	– Prolonged PR interval

PLUS

Supporting evidence of a recent Gr A Streptococci infection (e.g. positive throat culture or rapid antigen detection test, and/or elevated or increasing streptococcal antibody test)

To fulfill Jones criteria either two major criteria or one major and two minor criteria plus evidence of antecedent streptococcal infection are required.
- Isolation of group A *Streptococci* (throat swab)
- Streptococcal antibody test (serological test)
  - ASO level
  - Anti-DNAase level
  - Anti-Streptozyme test
- Acute phase reactants (ESR and CRP)
- Hematologic abnormalities
  - Neutrophilic leukocytosis
  - ↑ complement level
  - Anemia
- ECG
- Chest X-ray (cardiomegaly, pulmonary congestion)
- ECHO (myocardial, valvular dysfunction and pericardial effusion)

Key points of heart morphology
- Diffuse inflammation of all the three layers of heart (pancarditis)
- Aschoff bodies
- Bread and butter pericarditis—pericardial inflammation in ARF is accompanied by a fibrinous or serofibrinous exudates sandwitched between visceral and perietal pericardium, hence called bread and butter pericarditis. It often resolves without producing any complications.

Valvulitis
- Particularly mitral valve followed by aortic valve.
- Fibrinoid necrosis in the cusps and (or) tendinous chords; small vegetations called 'verrucae' sit on these lesions.
- MacCallum plaques

28. Aschoff bodies (1998, 2000, 04)

Widely disseminated, but focal inflammatory lesions are formed in various sites of body in ARF. They are most extensive within the heart and are known as Aschoff bodies.

Morphology

These are areas of *fibrinoid degeneration* surrounded by:
- Mainly lymphocytes (mostly T cells)
- Plasma cells (occasional);
- Aschoff giant cells (macrophages of RF)
- *Anitschkow cells:*
  - Not always found, but if present they are pathognomonic for rheumatic fever.
  - They are modified macrophages with:
    a. Abundant amphophilic cytoplasm
    b. Central round to ovoid nuclei and
    c. Chromatin material spread in the center of nuclei in thin and wavy ribbon-like fashion (hence also called Caterpillar cells).

Location
- Present in all three layers of the heart along with diffuse inflammation of all layers (pancarditis).
- Within myocardium, Aschoff bodies are present largely in the perivascular interstitial tissue.

29. Describe etiopathogenesis, pathology and complications of bacterial endocarditis (1996, 2000).

30. Embolic complication of bacterial endocarditis (2003)

31. Sequelae of bacterial endocarditis (1990)

or

Diagnostic criteria and complications of infective endocarditis (2008)

"Invasion and proliferation of microorganisms on the endothelium of the heart leading to formation of bulky, friable vegetations". Most commonly involves heart valves (but may also occur on mural endocardium of other sides of the heart).

The vegetations is composed of—platelets, fibrin, microcolonies of microorganisms and few inflammatory cells.

Etiology
- Bacterial, fungal, etc., but mostly bacterial (Hence IE is also known as bacterial endocarditis)
- Most bacterial cases are also caused by a limited number of species: *Staphylococci, Streptococci, Enterococci* and oral cavity commensals HACEK (*Hemophilus, Actinobacillus, Cardiobacterium, Eikenella* and *Kingella*).
- About 10% cases are culture negative.
- IE of abnormal valves or previously damaged valves, most commonly caused by *Streptococcus viridans.*
- Attack on normal valves by organisms of high virulence (most commonly *Staphylococcus aureus*)
- IE in drug abusers—mostly by *Staphylococcus aureus* (because it is commonly found on the skin)
- Prosthetic valve endocarditis—mostly by coagulase negative Streptococci.

Predisposing factors
1. Presence of cardiovascular abnormalities, e.g. valvular deformities, prosthetic valves, vascualr grafts.
2. Factors causing bacteremia: Foci of infection anywhere in the body, tooth extraction, surgical procedures, IV drug users, trivial injuries, etc.
3. ↓ed host defense: Neutropenia, immunodeficiency disorders, diabetes mellitus, etc.

Pathogenesis
- The normal intact endothelium is resistant to infection by most bacteria and also to thrombus formation. So IE mainly occurs at sites of pre-existing endocardial damage.

The aberrant flow at the sites of valvular defects usually leads to endothelial injuries. These areas allow either direct infection by virulent organisms or the thrombus formation, which then serves as site for bacterial attachment.

- Organisms enter the blood stream usually through injured skin, mucosal surfaces or from the sites of focal infection.
- More virulent bacteria like *S. aureus* can then attack even intact endothelium. Other bacteria usually adhere to thrombi. They proliferate in the thrombus and elicit the release of tissue factors from adherent monocytes. This leads to activation of coagulation and deposition of fibrin over the thrombus and platelet aggregation, thus forming vegetations.

Morphology
- *Gross appearance*
  1. Formation of vegetation: Most commonly on the heart valves, particularly mitral and aortic valves
  2. Vegetations: Large and bulky, friable, single or multiple, and potentially destructive
     Usually present on the valve cusps (and, may extend into and destroy chordae tendinae).
  3. Ring abscesses: The vegetation sometimes erodes into the underlying myocardium and produce abscess cavity.
  4. Septic infarct: May result in infarction of organs like heart, kidney, brain, etc. due to emboli formation.
  5. Metastatic abscesses at various sites

- *Microscopic features*
  1. Vegetations have platelets, fibrin, few inflammatory cells and the causative organisms.
  2. In case of subacute IE, vegetations have often granulation tissues at their bases.
  3. *In older vegetations:* Signs of calcification, fibrosis, and chronic inflammatory infiltrate

Diagnostic criteria of IE (Duke's criteria)

Diagnosis of IE by Duke's criteria requires either pathological or clinical criteria. If clinical criteria are used, 2 major, 1 major + 3 minor or 5 minor criteria are required for diagnosis.

Pathological criteria
1. Micro-organisms demonstrated by culture or histologic examination, in a vegetation, embolus from a vegetation or intracardiac abscess.
2. Histologic confirmation of active endocarditis in vegetation or intracardiac abscess.

Clinical criteria
Major
1. Blood culture(s) positive for a characteristic organism or persistently positive for an unusual organism
2. Echocardiographic identification of a valve-related or implant-related mass or abscess, or partial separation of artificial valve
3. New valvular regurgitation

Minor
1. Predisposing heart lesion or intravenous drug use
2. Fever
3. Vascular lesions, including arterial petechiae, sublingual splinter hemorrhage, emboli, septic infarcts, mycotic aneurysm intracranial hemorrhage and Janeway lesion
4. Immunological phenomenon: Glomerulonephritis, Osler nodes, Roth spots, rheumatoid factors
5. Microbiologic evidence: A single culture positive for unusual organism
6. Echocardiographic finding consistent with, but not diagnostic of endocarditis, including worsening or changing of a pre-existing murmur.

Complications
- Cardiac complications
  - Valvular insufficiency or stenosis with cardiac failure
  - Perforation, rupture or aneurysm formation

- Myocardial ring abscess
- Suppurative pericarditis
- Extracardiac complications:
  - Embolic complication
- Osler's nodes: Painful, tender nodule seen in pulps of fingers due to immune complex deposition.
- Roth's spots (circular retinal hemorrhages with pale centers)
- Janeway spots (on palms and soles due to septic emboli in skin)

- Sublingual splinter hemorrhages (due to embolic damage to cutaneous capillaries)
- Renal complications:
  - Embolic phenomenon
  - Focal and diffuse glomerulonephritis due to trapping of Ag-Ab complex which may lead to hematuria, albuminuria or renal failure.

Causes of death:
- Cardiac failure
- Renal failure
- Rupture of mycotic aneurysms in vital organs

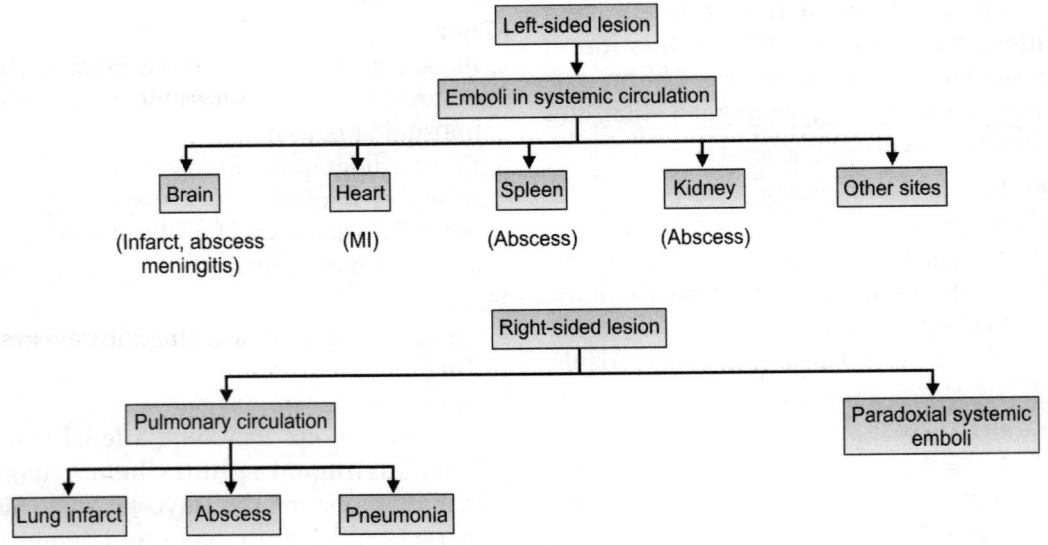

Fig. 14.4: Embolic complications

32. Difference between acute and subacute infective endocarditis

S. No.	Traits	Acute IE	Subacute IE
1.	Causative organisms	More virulent organisms like *Staphylococcus aureus*	Relatively less virulent ones like *Streptococcus viridans*
2.	Pre-existing pathology	Normal	Previously deformed valves
3.	Onset	Acute (< 6 wk)	Insidious (> 6 wk)
4.	Clinical severity	Very severe; more than 50% of patients die within days to weeks despite antibiotics and surgery.	Mild; event if untreated, the disease runs a protracted course of weeks to months. Also most patients recover after appropriate antibiotic therapy.
5.	Damage to valves	Necrotizing, ulcerative and invasive lesion of the valve.	Relatively less destructive vegetations; often show evidence of healing.
6.	Prognosis	Poor, rapid deterioration	Good

33. Difference between acute rheumatic (RHD) and bacterial endocarditis (IE) (1998, 2001, 06, 08, 11)

34. Difference between vegetation of rheumatic heart disease and bacterial endocarditis (1995, 2001)

35. Difference between vegetation of RHD and IE

36. Libman Sack's endocarditis (1993, 1997)

37. Difference between bacterial and Libman Sack's endocarditis

38. Non-bacterial thrombotic endocarditis (NBTE)

39. Difference between vegetation in SLE (Libman Sack's endocarditis, LSE) and rheumatic endocarditis (2004)

Traits	IE (bacterial)	RHD	NBTE	LSE
Valves affected	Most commonly mitral and aortic valve	Left-sided valves (usually mitral)	Any valve	Atrioventricular valves (mitral and tricuspid)
Location	On valve cusps (on one side); may extend onto the chordae	Along the line of closure (on one side)	Usually along the line of closure (on one side)	On the leaflets (on either or both sides). Additionally, may be scattered on valvular endocardium, on the chords and also on endocardium of atrial and ventricular surfaces.
Gross:				
I. Size	Bulky	Small and warty	Small (but larger than RHD)	Small or medium-sized; granular; pink
II. Number	Single or multiple	Multiple	Single or multiple	Multiple
III. Attachment	Loosely attached; friable	Firmly attached; friable (less)	Very loosely attached; friable	—
IV. Extent of damage to valve	Potentially destructive; usually damage the underlying endocardium. Sometimes even erode into the myocardium to produce an abscess cavity. In still more severe cases, may perforate the cusps.	Generally produce thickening and shorten-ing of leaflets. Also fusion of valve commissure (commissural fusion may convert tricuspid aortic vlave into bicuspid)	Usually no damage to valve	Generally not much deformity

(Contd.)

(Contd.)

Traits	IE (bacterial)	RHD	NBTE	LSE
Composition	Deposition of fibrin and platelet. Bacterial colonies into deeper parts of vegetation (Non-sterile). Extensive acute inflammatory cells. Granulation tissue at the bases (in case of subacute IE)	Fibrin and platelets; no bacteria. (Inflammation fibrinoid degeneration of endocardium erosion vegetaion formed over erosion)	Deposition of small masses of fibrin, platelets and other blood components on valve leaflets. No micro-organisms (i.e. sterile, non-inflammatory and non-destructive thrombus)	Sterile; composed of finely granular and fibrinous eosinophilic material. Vegetation may contain hematoxy-lin bodies which are equivalent to LE cells.
Chances of emboli	High (friable vegetation)	Low	Very high	Less common

40. Hypertrophic (obstructive) cardiomyopathy (2000)

41. Difference between hypertrophied and congestive (dilated) cardiomyopathy (1996, 2007)

or

Restrictive (Obliterative or infiltrative cardiomyopathy (RCM)

A group of diseases that result from a primary abnormality in the myocardium and not the result of other diseases (e.g. hypertension, CVDs, etc.) which indirectly lead to myociardial injury.

Divided into: DCM (dilated CM or congestive CM), HCM (hypertrophic CM), and RCM (restrictive CM) on the basis of morphological and functional characteristics.

S. No.	Traits	DCM	HCM	RCM
1.	Definition	Characterized by progressive *hypertrophy* of myocardium along with *dilation* of heart chambers, and *contractile dysfunction*	Characterized by myocardial hypertrophy of left ventricle, but without dilation, and leads to diastolic dysfunction	Diastolic dysfunction (restriction in ventricular filling due to reduction in the volume of ventricles)
2.	Occurrence	More common (90% cases of CM)	Less common	Less common
3.	Age	Mostly middle-aged men (20–60 yr)	Mostly adolescent and young adults	Variable
4.	Causes	Mostly unknown (causes are known only in a fraction of cases, e.g. pregnancy associated, alcoholism, chemotherapeutic agents, familial, etc.)	Genetic (inherited mutations in sarcomere proteins); other contributory factors	• Idiopathic • Associated with amyloidosis, sarcoidosis and radiation induced

(Contd.)

(Contd.)

S. No.	Traits	DCM	HCM	RCM
5.	Functional impairment	Systolic dysfunction; the heart becomes hypocontractile and, thus there is reduced ejection fraction	Diastolic dysfunction; there is no hypo-contractility and reduction of ejection fraction; rather the left ventricle is hyperdynamic. ↑ed stiffness of hyper-trophied muscle leads to elevated diastolic filling pressure and, hence impaired left ventricular filling.	Dystolic dysfunction
6.	Sub-aortic stenosis	Absent	Present	Absent
7.	Clinical features	Because of systolic dysfunction symptoms of progressive CHF appears slowly in most patients	Many patients are asymptomatic. In symptomatic patients the most common complaint is dyspnea	Presentation depends upon the specific type. It may manifest with dyspnea, angina, CHF or sudden death
8.	Gross	Heart: Heavy, large, and flabby, hypocontract-ing heart. Dilation of all chambers. Hypertrophy is symmetrical ↑ed cavity size.	Heavy and musclular, hypercontracting heart No dilation Most patients develop asymmetrical hyper-trophy mainly of interventricular septum compared to free wall of left ventricle ↓ed (loss of ovoid shape and reduced into a 'banana-like confirma-tion' by bulging of ven-tricularly septum towards lumen) cavity size	• Ventricles normal or slightly enlarged • Cavities not dilated • Myocardium is firm
9.	Histology	Most muscle cells are hypertrophied with enlarged nuclei. Variable degree of interstitial and endocardial fibrosis	Relatively more extensive hypertrophy. There is a bizarre and disorganized arrangement of myocytes and also disarray of contractile elements in the sarcomere. Variable degree of myocardial fibrosis.	• Patchy or diffuse interstitial fibrosis, which vary from minimal to extensive
10.	Outcome	Arrhythmia may be observed. Average survival from onset to death is 5 yr.	Medical treatment to relax ventricles and surgical reduction of septum can be undertaken.	Gradually progressive cardiac failure

42. Difference between causes and sequelae of constrictive and fibrinous pericarditis (2002)

43. Constrictive pericarditis (1994)

S. No.	Traits	Fibrinous	Constrictive
1.	General feature	An acute form of pericarditis, usually caused in cases of acute MI, post-MI syndrome, uremia, chest radiation, SLE, etc.	A chronic form of pericarditis, usually a sequelae to acute fibrinous or serofibrinous pericarditis, or to a caseous pericarditis. May also follow trauma, cardiac operation of any type, mediastinal irradiation, SLE, etc.
2.	Occurrence	Relatively more common	Less common
3.	Character	Pericardial space is filled with thick mixture of serous fluid with fibrinous exudate.	Pericardial space is obliterated due to the organization of the underlying acute pericardial lesion, producing dense fibrosis.
4.	Fate	Fibrinous exudates may resolve without sequelae or may undergo organization.	Fibrotic scar may undergo calcification.
5.	Functional derangement	Usually no functional compromise	As heart gets encased in a dense fibrotic or fibrocalcific scar, it limits diastolic expansion, thus inability of ventricular filling, ↓ed ventricular end-diastolic volume, stroke volume, and cardiac output.
6.	Pericardial friction rub	Pathognomonic	Absent

44. Difference between syphilitic and atherosclerotic aneurysm (1995)

45. Brown atrophy of heart (2000)

46. Difference between pathophysiology of left- and right-sided heart failures (2009)

Left-sided heart failure
- There is reduction in left ventricular output, increase in left atrial pressure and increase in pulmonary venous pressure due to left-sided heart failure.
- Acute increase in left atrial pressure causes pulmonary edema and congestion (wet lung). Hemosiderin containing macrophages in alveoli (siderophages, heart failure cells) denotes previous episodes of pulmonary edema. Patient presents with dyspnea, orthopnea and paroxysmal nocturnal dyspnea. Kidney and brain show ischemic sign and symptoms.

Right-sided heart failure
- There is reduction in right ventricular output, which results in systemic vascular congestion leading to accumulation of fluid in the body, resulting in swelling and edema.
- Most common cause of RVF is secondary to LVF.
- Isolated right-sided failures are most often occur with chronic severe pulmonary hypertension (cor pulmonale).
- Dilatation and hypertrophy are confined to right atrium and ventricle.
- Peripheral edema of dependent portion (ankle, pretibial), hepatic enlargement (congestion), congestive splenomegaly, pleural effusion, ascites.

15

Lung

1. Atelectasis: Definition and its types (1994)

- **Definition:** Incomplete expansion of the lung or collapse of previously inflated lung substance, producing airless pulmonary parenchymal areas; resulting in diminished oxygenation and increased chances of infections.
- **Types**
  1. *Reabsorption* or *obstruction atelectasis*: Some obstruction in bronchi or bronchioles causes reabsorption of air trapped in dependent alveoli, leading to lung part(s) collapse. Mediastinum shifts towards it and blood flow may be normal.
  2. *Compression atelectasis*: Pleural cavity filled with fluid exudates, blood or air, or a mass (tumor) of a part of lung press on lung and mediastinum. It may result in compression atelectasis. Mediastinum shifts away from it.
  3. *Contraction atelectasis*: Generalized/local fibrotic changes of lung/pleura, prevents its full expansion resulting in atelectasis of that part of the lung.

2. Define COPD (Chronic obstructive pulmonary disease)

COPD, a common preventable and treatable disease, is characterized by persistent airflow limitation that is usually progressive and associated with an enhanced chronic inflammatory response in the airways and the lung to noxious particles or gases. Spirometry is required to make the clinical diagnosis of COPD; the presence of a post-bronchodilator FEV1/FVC < 0.70 confirms the presence of persistent airflow limitation and, thus COPD. This definition does not use the term chronic bronchitis and emphysema and excludes asthma (reversible airflow limitation). Patient present with dyspnea, chronic cough and chronic sputum production.

(*Global Initiative for Chronic Obstructive Lung Disease, GOLD*).

3. α_1 Antitrypsin (AT) deficiency (1986, 88, 95)

4. Emphysema (1986, 2007, 08)

- "Abnormal permanent enlargement of the airspaces distal to the terminal bronchiole; accompanied by destruction of their wall, without any fibrosis or little fibrosis."

Types of emphysema:
  i. *Centriacinar (centrilobular) emphysema*
  - Only central or proximal part of acini is affected, leaving distal part spared.
  - Predominantly seen in heavy smokers. Smoke particles are predominantly impacted in small bronchi and bronchioles—recruiting macrophages and

neutrophils in the small bronchi to cause centriacinar emphysema.
- More common in upper lobe.
- Wall of emphysematous spaces contain large amount of pigments associated with coal workers' pneumoconiosis or smoker.

ii. *Panacinar (panlobular) emphysema*
- Acini are uniformly enlarged from the level of respiratory bronchioles to terminal blind alveolar sac.
- It is associated with α_1 AT deficiency. In α_1 AT deficiency, antiprotease activity is absent throughout the acinus producing chonic low level proteolysis involving whole acinus during lung circulation by neutrophil elastase, producing panacinar emphysema. There is no role of macrophages. Also, perfusion and number of neutrophils are greater in lower parts of lung, so panacinar emphysema involves lower zone more than other zones.

iii. *Paraseptal (distal acinar) emphysema*
- Proximal part of acinar is normal, only distal part is involved.
- Localized along pleura and perilobular septa. Usually seen in upper part of lungs, adjacent to areas of fibrosis and atelectasis.
- Characteristic finding is presence of multiple, continuous, and enlarged spaces 0.5–2 c, forming cyst-like structures. It is one of the causes of spontaneous pneumothorax in young person.

iv. *Irregular (paracicatricial) emphysema*
- Acini are irregularly involved, associated with scarring.

iv. Other forms of emphysema: Compensatory hyperinflation (emphysema), obstructive hyperinflation, bullous emphysema and interstitial emphysema.

Pathogenesis: Protease-antiprotease theory: Due to imbalance between protease (elastase) and antiprotease activity in lung.

- *Protease:*
  - Neutrophil elastase (main assault), cellular proteases (proteinase 3 and cathepsin) and matrix metalloproteinases.
  - Oxygen free radicals (produced by activated neutrophils)—*inactivates α_1 AT* activity.
  - Macrophage elastase (not inhibited by α_1 AT).
- *Antiprotease:*
  - α_1 antitrypsin (α_1 AT)—in blood and interstitium (main)
  - Secretory leukoprotease inhibitor (in bronchial muscles)
  - α_1 microglobulin in blood
- Neutrophils are present more in lower zone of lung, so lower zone is more involved.
- Role of smoking in emphysema: Smoking enhances elastase activity of macrophages. Macrophage elastage is not inhibited by α_1 AT, and macrophage can digest α_1 AT.
- *Factors* promoting emphysema: Any stimulus that increases number of neutrophils or increases release of granules containing elastase.

Morphology
- *Gross:* See difference
- *Microscopic examination*
  - Complete destruction of the alveolar septal wall
  - Enlargement airspaces
  - Location varies according to type
- **Complications**
  - Respiratory distress
  - Secondary pulmonary vascular hypertension
  - Barrel chest
  - Cor pulmonale
  - Congestive heart failure
- **Death** in COPD is due to
  - Respiratory acidosis and coma
  - Right-sided heart failure
  - Massive collapse of the lung secondary to pneumonia

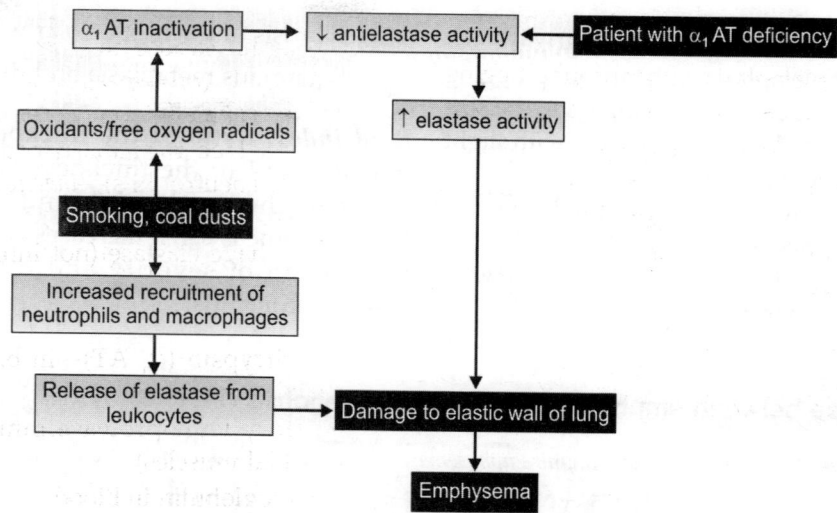

Fig. 15.1: Pathogenesis of emphysema

5. Difference between centriacinar and panacinar emphysema (1998) (1995, 97, 99, 2001)

S. No.	Traits	Centriacinar	Panacinar
1.	Sites	Central or proximal parts of the acini; (respiratory bronchiole) are affected.	Acini are uniformly affected from respiratory bronchiole to terminal alveoli.
2.	Lobes	Upper lobe more involved	Lower part of the lung more involved
3.	Parts severely affected	Apical segments of the lung more severely affected	Basal zone of the lung more severely affected
4.	Risk factors	Tobacco smoking, coal workers	α_1 AT deficiency
5.	Gross features	Not much impressive	Voluminous lung overlapping heart, and hiding it when anterior chest wall is removed.
6.	Occurrence	More common	Less

6. Chronic bronchitis

- Clinically defined as the presence of persistent cough with sputum production for at least 3 months for at least two consecutive years.

Pathogenesis: (Refer to Fig. 15.2).

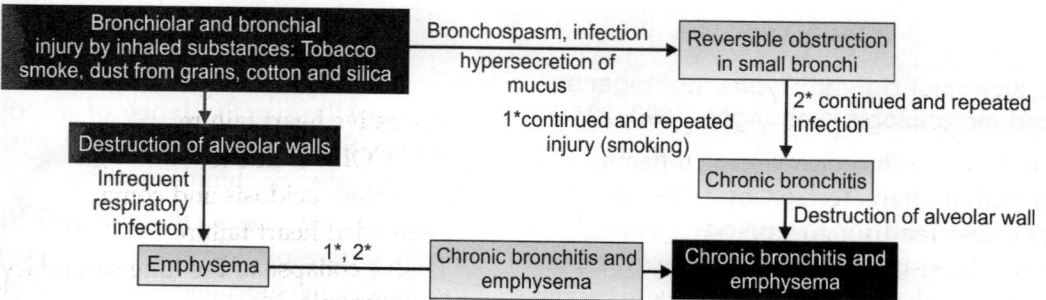

Fig. 15.2: Pathogenesis of chronic bronchitis and emphysema

- *Histological* features of small airways
  - Goblet metaplasia with mucous plugging of the lumen, major change is in the size of mucus gland (hyperplasia) with slight increase in number of goblet cells
  - Clustering of the pigmented alveolar macrophages
  - Inflammatory infiltration of airway predominantly lymphocytic
  - Fibrosis of the bronchiolar walls
  - Squamous metaplasia and dysplasia

Reid index: Ratio of the thickness of the mucus gland to the thickness of the wall between the epithelium and cartilage. Normal value is 0.4; it increases according to proportion of severity and duration of chronic bronchitis.

7. Difference between emphysema and chronic bronchitis (1998, 2009)

S. No.	Traits	Predominant emphysema	Predominant bronchitis
1.	Age	50–75 yr	40–50 yr
2.	Underlying pathology	Destruction of alveolar septal wall and narrowing of bronchiole due to inflammation	Hypertrophy of mucus producing cells
3.	Dyspnea	Severe; early	Late; mild
4.	Cough	After dyspnea starts	Before dyspnea starts
5.	Sputum	Scanty, mucoid, less frequent; late	Copious, purulent; early
6.	Infections	Occasional	More frequent
7.	Respiratory insufficiency	Terminal	Repeated
8.	Cor pulmonale	Rare, terminal	Common
9.	Airways resistance	Normal or slightly increased	Increased
10.	Elastic recoil	Low due to loss of elastic fibers	Normal
11.	Lung capacity	Increased; barrel chest	Normal
12.	Blood gas value	Hyperventilation; pO_2, pCO_2 almost normal	$\downarrow pO_2$, $\downarrow pCO_2$; compensatory hyperventilation absent
13.	Chest radiograph	Hyperinflation, small heart	Prominent vessels, large heart
14.	Appearance	Pink puffer	Blue bloater
15.	Cyanosis	Rare	Common
16.	Diffusion capacity	Decreased	Normal
17.	Hematocrit	Normal	Increased
18.	Prognosis	Good	Poor

8. Bronchial asthma: Types, pathogenesis and morphological changes (1990, 2011)

"Asthma is a chronic relapsing inflammatory condition characterized by hyper-reactive airways, leading to episodic, reversible bronchoconstriction, due to increased responsiveness of the tracheobronchial tree to various stimuli".

Types

1. Atopic/Allergic: Evidence of allergen sensitization, often in a patient with a history of allergic rhinitis, eczema.

2. *Non-atopic/non-reaginic (intrinsic type):* Viral infection of respiratory mucosa lowers the threshold of the subepithelial vagal receptors to irritants, resulting in exaggerated response.

S. No.	Traits	Extrinsic asthma	Intrinsic asthma
1.	Definition	Initiated by type I hyper sensitivity reaction induced by exposure to an extrinsic antigen	Initiated by diverse, nonimmune mechanism. Stimuli are intrinsic to body
2.	Age of presentation	Childhood	Adult
3.	Family history	Present	Absent
4.	Preceding allergic reactions	Present in form of rhinitis, urticaria, eczema	Absent
5.	Allergens	Present	Absent
6.	Drug hypersensitivity	Absent	Present; aspirin
7.	Serum IgE level	Increased	Normal
8.	Skin test	Positive	Negative
9.	Emphysema	Unusual	Common
10.	Associated bronchitis	Absent	Present
11.	Examples	Atopic/allergic asthma, occupational asthma, allergic bronchopulmonary aspergillosis	Aspirin ingestion, pulmonary infection especially viral, cold, inhaled irritants, stress, exercise, etc.

3. *Drugs induced:* Aspirin induced

4. *Occupational:* Repeated exposure, mechanism varies; type I IgG-mediated hypersensitivity reaction

Pathogenesis of Atopic Asthma

- An example of extrinsic asthma
- IgE-mediated reaction
- Type I hypersensitivity (genetic predisposition)

"The inheritance of susceptibility genes makes individuals prone to develop strong Th2 reactions against environmental antigens that are ignored or elicit harmless response in most individuals".

Steps in pathogenesis

1. *Sensitization* to allergen: APC (Antigen presenting cells) present antigens with MHC II to T helper cells to form predominantly Th2 cells.

   Th2 cells produce cytokines IL-4 and IL-5 to stimulate B-cells to produce IgE (humoral immunity); eosinophil recruitment (through IL-5), mucus secretion from submucosal gland (IL-3).

2. *Allergen* triggered asthma: On reexposure of it or related Ag, IgE bound to eosinophils cross-link and release preformed mediators to induce early and late phase reactions.

Immediate phase reaction: (Within minutes)

- Due to mediators released, opening of the tight junction between epithelial cells.
- Ag enter mucosa to activate mucosal mast cells and eosinophils releasing additional mediators.
- Results in *direct/neuronal transmission* → **bronchospasm**, ↑ed vascular permeability, ↑ed mucus production and recruitment of additional inflammatory cells.

Late phase reaction: (Neutrophils, eosinophils, basophils; lymphocytes, monocytes). Eosinophil cationic protein, major basic protein and other mediators cause damage to epithelium.

- Repeated episodes of asthmatic attack may result in "Airway remodelling".

Morphology

- *Gross*
  - Lung overdistended (overinflation)
  - Small areas of atelectasis
  - Obstruction of bronchi and bronchioles by thick, tenacious mucus plugs
- *Microscopic examination*
  - Mucus-plugs contain whorls of shed epithelium (Curschmann's spiral)

– Charcot-Leyden crystals (crystalloids made up of eosinophil lysophospholipase-binding protein, galectin-10) are present.
– Mucus layer thickness increase on the epithelium
– Eosinophils in the mucus layers
– Goblet cells hyperplasia; overall thickening of airway wall
– Thickness of basement membrane of bronchial epithelium
– Edema and inflammatory infiltrate in the bronchial wall; eosinophils dominate; macrophages, neutrophils, mast cells, lymphocytes are also present.
– Increase in size of submucosal glands, and mucous metaplasia of airway epithelial cells
– Hypertrophy/hyperplasia of bronchial wall muscles
– Subbasement membrane fibrosis (due to deposition of type I and III collagens beneath the classical basement membrane composed of type IV collagen and laminin)

9. Bronchiectasis: Define, predisposing factors, pathogenesis, gross, microscopic appearance and complications (1999, 2001), (1990, 95, 97, 98, 2003, 2006)

• *Defined* as the chronic necrotizing infection of the bronchi and bronchioles leading to or associated with *abnormal permanent dilatation* of these airways.
• *Predisposing factors*
  1. *Bronchial obstruction*
     – Tumor
     – Mucus impaction
     – Foreign bodies
     – Diffuse obstruction of airways
  2. *Congenital/hereditary conditions*
     – Congenital bronchiectasis
     – Kartagener's syndrome
     – Immunodeficiency states
     – Immotile cilia
     – Cystic fibrosis

3. *Necrotizing pneumonia*
   – *Mycobacterium tuberculosis*
   – *Haemophilus influenzae*
   – Adenovirus, influenza virus, HIV
   – Fungi (Aspergillus)
   – *Staphylococcus aureus*
   – Pseudomonas
4. *Other conditions*
   – Rheumatoid arthritis, SLE, inflammatory bowel disease, post-transplantation
• *Pathogenesis:* Obstruction and infection (see Fig. 15.3)
   – Lower lobe is more involved
   – Bilaterally
   – Vertical airways; distant bronchi and bronchioles more severely affected
• *Morphology*
  Gross
   – Cystic pattern/honeycomb appearance on the cut surface
   – The bronchi and bronchioles are sufficiently dilated that they can be followed almost to the pleural surfaces in contrast to normal lung where bronchioles cannot be followed beyond a point 2–3 cm from pleural surfaces by gross dissection.
  Microscopic examination: (vary with activity and chronicity of disease)
   – Acute and chronic inflammatory exudate within walls of bronchi and bronchioles
   – Desquamation of epithelium
   – Necrotizing ulcers
   – Pseudostratification of columnar cells or squamous cells
   – Sometimes necrosis and destruction of bronchial and bronchiolar walls
• *Clinical features*
   – Persistent cough with expectoration of copious amounts of foul-smelling, purulent sputum; sometimes with blood

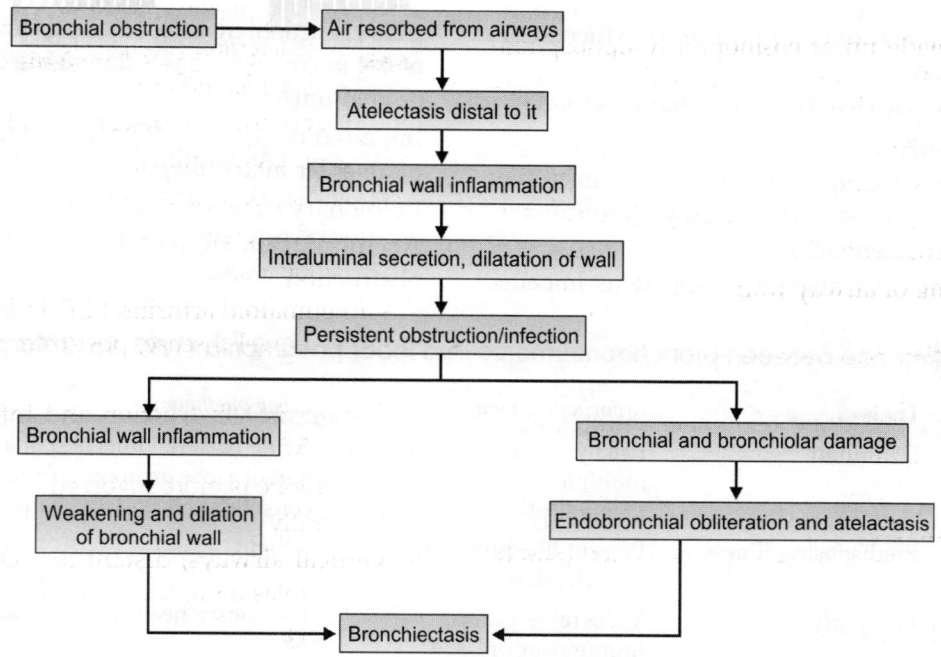

Fig. 15.3: Pathogenesis of bronchiectasis

- Dyspnea
- Orthopnea
- **Complications: (*very important*) (1995, 97, 2001, 03)**
  - Lung abscess
  - Peribronchiolar fibrosis
  - Metastatic brain abscess
  - Fibrosis of the bronchial and bronchiolar walls
  - Obstructive ventilatory insufficiency—cyanosis, dyspnea (respiratory failure)
  - Amyloidosis
  - Cor pulmonale
  - Recurrent bronchopneumonia
  - Empyema of thorax

10. Classify pneumonia and pathogenesis

"Pneumonia may be defined as the acute inflammation of lung parenchyma distal to the terminal bronchioles mostly resulting in consolidation of lung part(s)".

Classification
Etiological
1. Bacterial pneumonia: (see difference)
2. Viral and *mycoplasmal* pneumonia
3. *Other types*
   - *Pneumocystis carinii* pneumonia
   - Hypostatic pneumonia
   - Aspiration (inhalation) pneumonia
   - Lipid pneumonia

Anatomical distribution
1. Lobular/bronchopneumonia
2. Lobar pneumonia

Pathogenesis
"Pneumonia can result whenever defense mechanisms of respiratory system are impaired or immunity of host is decreased".

Defense mechanism
1. Nasal clearance: Anterior part: Non-ciliated epithelium (sneezing, blowing)
   Posterior part: Mucus lined ciliated epithelium

2. Tracheobronchial clearance: Mucociliary action

3. Alveolar clearance: Alveolar macrophages

Risk factors

1. Loss or suppression of the cough reflex: Coma, anesthesia and drugs (aspiration of gastric contents)

2. Injury to the mucociliary apparatus: Impaired

ciliary function; cigarette smoking, inhalation of hot or corrosive gases damaging ciliated epithelium

3. Impaired phagocytic or bactericidal action of alveolar macrophages

4. Pulmonary congestion and edema

5. Accumulation of secretions: Bronchial obstruction

11. Difference between bronchopneumonia and lobar pneumonia (1993, 95, 2000, 07, 10)

S. No.	Traits	Bronchopneumonia	Lobar pneumonia
1.	Definition	Patchy consolidation of multiple lobes and bilateral (generally)	Acute bacterial infection of a large part of a lobe or an entire lobe, diffuse consolidation
2.	Predisposing illness	Present like bronchitis/bronchiolitis	Absent
3.	Immunity status	Vulnerable group, immunosuppressed	Previously healthy individual
4.	Parts affected	Basal area more affected as secretion gravitates into lower lobe	No such characteristics, may involve any lobe
5.	Stages of inflammation	Not clear cut division	Divided into 4 stages
6.	Organisms	Staphylococci, Streptococci, Pneumococci, H. influenzae, Pseudomonas aeruginosa, Coliforms	Pneumococci/Streptococcus pneumoniae (95%), Klebsiella pneumoniae, H. influenzae
7.	Opportunistic infection	May be present	Absent
8.	Exudation	Less	Extensive, more
9.	Severity	Less	More
10.	Sputum	Purulent, non-hemorrhagic	Initially scanty, watery. Later on thick, purulent, hemorrhagic

12. Changes in lung in lobar pneumonia (1994)

Fibrinosuppurative consolidation

Four stages

1. *Stage of congestion:* Acute inflammatory response to bacterial infection

   Gross
   - Lung/its parts are heavy, boggy and red-congested
   - Cut surface—blood stained frothy fluid exudates

Microscopic features
- Vascular engorgement, intra-alveolar fluid
- A few neutrophils
- A few red cells
- Numerous bacteria
- Pale fluid in airspaces

2. *Red hepatization/early consolidation* Liver-like consistency

   Gross
   - Red firm consolidated

- Fibrinosuppurative exudates
- Cut surface: Lobe is airless, red-pink, dry and granular

Microscopic features
- Fibrin filling alveolar spaces
- Neutrophilic infiltration
- Red cells in large number
- Neutrophils containing bacteria

3. Gray hepatization/late consolidation

Gross
- Liver-like consistency
- Grayish-brown color
- Dry, granular surface

Microscopic features:
- Fibrin exudates in alveoli
- Neutrophils decreased
- Macrophages appear
- Number of bacteria decreased
- Red cells lyse

4. Resolution:
- Consolidate exudates within alveolar space undergoes progressive enzymatic digestion to form granular, semisolid debris.
- Debris is either coughed up or reabsorbed and ingested by macrophages.
- Exudates may undergo organization leaving fibrous thickening or permanent adhesion.

13. Complications of pneumonia (1996)

1. *Abscess formation:* Due to tissue destruction and necrosis; more in case of *Klebsiella* or type III *pneumococci* infections.
2. *Empyema:* Spread and involvement of pleural cavity—intrapleural fibrinosuppurative reaction.
3. *Organization of intra-alveolar exudate:* May convert a part of lung into solid fibrous tissue.
4. *Bacteremic dissemination:* Heart valves (endocarditis), pericardium (pericarditis), brain (meningitis), kidney, spleen, joints (suppurative arthritis) or metastatic abscesses

14. Primary atypical pneumonia/viral (1986, 91) and mycoplasmal pneumonia/interstitial pneumonitis (1993)

- Acute febrile respiratory disease with patchy inflammatory changes confined to alveolar septa and pulmonary interstitium of lung.

Causative organisms
- *Mycoplasma pneumoniae*
- Influenza virus type A and type B
- Respiratory syncytial viruses
- Rhinovirus
- Varicella virus
- Coxiella burnetii
- Adenovirus
- Rubeola
- Chlamydia

- Conditions favoring: Malnutrition, alcohol intake and other diseases decreasing immunity.

- *Morphology*

Gross
- Patchy or whole lobe involved
- Unilateral or bilateral
- Red-blue
- Subcrepitant
- Congested
- Pleural involvement is rare

Microscopic examination
- Inflammation is confined to interstitium (within the walls of alveoli).
- Mononuclear inflammatory infiltrate—lymphocytes, histiocytes, plasma cells in interstitium
- Alveolar space free from exudates (so atypical pneumonia), but intra-alveolar proteinaceous material, cellular exudates and pink hyaline membranes lining the alveolar septal wall may be seen.
- Superimposed bacterial infections may be present.
- In *cytomegalovirus* infection, epithelial giant cells with intranuclear or intracytoplasmic inclusion may be seen.

Clinical features
- Upper respiratory tract infection
- Headache
- Cold chest
- Muscle pain in legs, etc.
- Fever

15. Lung abscess and its complications (1993, 2007)

"A local suppurative process within the lung producing necrosis of lung tissue".

Risk factors
- Oropharyngeal surgical procedures
- Dental sepsis
- Bronchiectasis

Organisms
- Aerobic and anaerobic *streptococci*
- *Bacteroides*
- *Staphylococcus aureus*
- *Fusobacterium*
- *Peptococcus*

Ways of entry
1. *Aspiration of infective materials* (most common cause): Gastric contents (acid and food particles; mouth organisms) aspirated in conditions of coma, alcoholic persons, anesthesia, sinusitis and depressed cough reflex.
2. *Antecedent primary bacterial infection:* Immunosuppressive patients; *S. aureus, K. pneumoniae*, etc. infection of lung.
3. *Septic embolism:* From thrombophlebitis (systemic veins) or infective bacterial endocarditis vegetation in right side of the heart.
4. *Neoplasia:* Secondary infection common in that part/segment
5. Other conditions: Direct trauma, infection from other organs (direct and hematogenous spread)
6. Idiopathic/*primary cryptogenic* lung abscess: No cause is found

Morphology
- Characterized by suppurative destruction of lung parenchyma with a central area of cavity.

- May be solitary or multiple
- Pulmonary abscess due to aspiration is more common to right side as right bronchus is more vertical.
- Abscess secondary to pneumonia and bronchiectasis are usually multiple, basal and diffusely scattered.
- Abscess due to septic emboli and pyemia are multiple and in any part.
- Superimposed saprophytic infections lead to a large, ill-defined, foul smelling and multilocular cavity (gangrene of lung).

Complications (*very important*) (1992, 93)
- Involvement of pleural cavity by extension of the infections
- Hemorrhage
- Meningitis from septic emboli
- Clubbing of the fingers and toes
- Metastatic brain abscess
- Secondary amyloidosis (AA type)
- Carcinoma (Rule out hidden carcinoma)

16. Ghon's complex/primary complex (1989, 91, 2004, 07, 08, 11)

17. Etiopathogenesis of secondary pulmonary TB and its sequelae (2001)

18. Complications of pulmonary TB (2000)

19. Autopsy findings in a 45-year male who died on pulmonary TB (2000)

- *Sites for primary TB*
  - Lung
  - Skin
  - Intestine
  - Oropharynx
  - Lymphoid tissues
- *Pathogenic factors*
  "Due to escape from killing by macrophages and induce type IV hypersensitivity reaction".
- Cord factor
- LAM (lipoarabinomannan)

- Complements are activated on the surface of *Mycobacterium* and opsonize the organism. It facilitates the uptake of organism by macrophages by an alternative way (through complement receptor CR3).

   No triggering of respiratory burst to kill bacteria. Normal uptake is through Fc portion of Ig.
- Mycobacteria replicate within the macrophage and block the formation of phagolysosome by inhibition of calcium signals as well as blocking recruitment and assembly of proteins, which cause formation of phagolysosomes.

Primary tuberculosis

- 1st time exposure to TB bacteria
- Initially non-specific inflammatory reaction
- 2–3 wk later, skin test becomes positive and reaction becomes specific, granulomatous: center of the granuloma is caseous (soft tubercle) or without caseation.

Pathogenesis

Ghon's complex or primary complex: It consists of

1. A parenchymal subpleural lesion, often just above or just below the interlobar fissure between the upper and lower lobes, called Ghon's focus; and

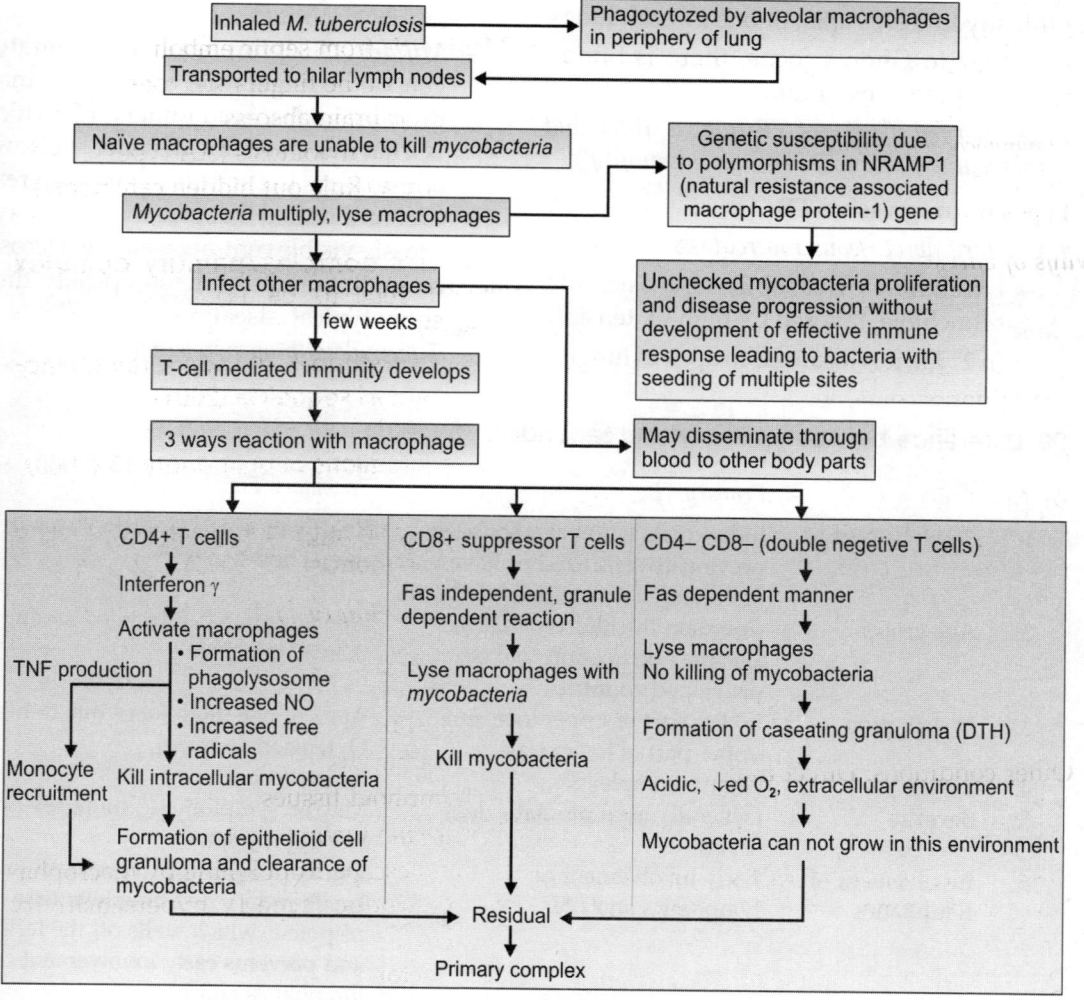

Fig. 15.4: Pathogenesis of primary complex

2. Enlarged caseous lymph nodes and lymphatics draining the parenchymal focus.

- *Fate of primary infection*
  - Mostly asymptomatic (lesion undergoes fibrosis and calcificaion)
  - In infants, children and immunodeficients may progress to:
    - ➢ Progressive spread with cavitation (progressive primary tuberculosis)
    - ➢ Tuberculous pneumonia
    - ➢ Miliary tuberculosis

Secondary tuberculosis

- *Cause:* Reinfection or reactivation of silent primary TB focus
- Mostly involves apex of one or both lungs
- Similar to Ghon's focus, there is Simon focus at the apex of lung
  (*See normal history of TB from textbook and tuberculin reaction/DTH from 'Immunity'*)

Types of progressive TB

- *Cavitary fibrocaseous tuberculosis:*
  - Extension of caseous necrosis into bronchiole, favored by high O_2 tension.
  - In 2° TB, it is localized to apex of lung(s).

- Cavity is lined and walled off by yellow-gray caseous materials.
- Arteries crossing the cavities are thrombosed (hemoptysis).
- Cavitation opens new pathways for spread through airways to outside (infectivity) and inside to other part of the same or opposite lung, hematogenous spread to other organ, lymphatic spread and contiguous spread.
- Pleura may be involved to produce serosal pleural effusion.
- If bacilli are implanted on the mucosal lining of the upper respiratory tract, it produces *endobronchial* and *endotracheal* TB. *Laryngeal* and *intestinal* TB may follow endotracheal TB.
- *Miliary TB:* Lymphatic and hematogenous dissemination from 1° site may produce widespread miliary TB, which is characterized by distinct, yellow-white, firm 1–2 mm (millet-like) areas of consolidation that usually do not have grossly visible central caseation necrosis or cavitation, but microscopically they show typical caseation.
- *Tuberculous bronchopneumonia*

20. Difference between primary and secondary TB (2007)

S. No.	Traits	Primary TB	Secondary TB
1.	Previous contact	Individuals who have not been previously sensitized or have not not suffered due to tubercle bacilli	Reactivation of a primary focus or reinfection
2.	Age group	Common in children/younger age; may be in adult/old in developed countries	Any age after 1° infection, later age than 1° infection
3.	Distribution	Lower part of upper lobe and upper part of lower lobe	Apex of one/both lobes due to high O_2 tension at apices
4.	Lesion	Ghon's complex	Simon focus
5.	Severity	Generally asymptomatic, less severe	May be symptomatic, more severe, fast to progress
6.	Involvement of lymphatics	Early involvement of lymphatics and LN	Due to pre-existing hypersensitivity, bacilli induce an immediate tisse response, which walls off the lesion and prevents early involvement of lymphatics and LN.

21. Classification of pneumoconiosis (1994, 99, 2001)

- Non-neoplastic lung reaction to inhaled mineral dusts, organic, inorganic particulates, chemical fumes and vapors.

Lung diseases caused by air pollutants

Mineral dust	
Coal dust	Anthracosis, macules, progressive massive fibrosis, Caplan's syndrome
Silica	Silicosis, Caplan's syndrome
Asbestos	Asbestosis, pleural plaques, Caplan's syndrome, mesothelioma, carcinoma of lung, larynx, stomach, colon
Beryllium	Acute berylliosis, beryllium granulomatosis, lung carcinoma
Iron oxide	Siderosis
Barium sulfate	Baritosis
Tin oxide	Stannosis
Organic dust that induces hypersensitivity pneumonitis	
Moldy hay	Farmer's lung
Bagasse	Bagassosis
Bird dropping	Bird-breeder's lung
Organic dust that induces asthma	
Cotton, flax, hemp	Byssinosis
Red cedar dust	Asthma
Chemical fumes and vapors	
Nitrous oxide, sulfur dioxide, ammonia, benzene, insecticide	Bronchitis, asthma, pulmonary edema, ARDS, mucosal injury, fulminant poisoning

22. Coal workers pneumoconiosis (CWP) (2001)

- Found in coal mine workers
- Forms:
  - Asymptomatic anthracosis
  - Simple CWP
  - Complicated or progressive massive fibrosis (PMF) CWP
- Carbon particles trigger immune-mediated reactions to produce damage to alveoli and its membrane; decreases local immunity (damage to PAM).

Simple anthracosis
- Present in almost all of coal miners; urban dwellers, tobacco smokers.
- Linear aggregates and streaks of carbon (anthracotic) pigment in pulmonary lymph nodes and lymphatic.

Simple CWP
- Upper lobes and upper part of lower lobe are mostly involved.

Presence of
- Coal macules [carbon particles in macrophages (1–2 mm in diameter)]
- Coal nodules (carbon macules having fine collagen fibers network)
- Centrilobular emphysema

Complicated CWP: In general, PMF is defined as confluent fibrotic reaction due to any pneumoconiosis, but mainly in CWP and silicosis.
- Intensely blackened scars > 2 cm; sometimes up to 10 cm.
- Multiple, bilateral, located more often in the upper parts of the lung.
- *Microscopic features:* Coal pigment, dense collagen fibers (intensive fibrosis), and

ischemic necrosis in central area of lesion, walls of respiratory bronchioles and pulmonary vessels are thickened scanty inflammatory infiltrate of lymphoid and plasma cells, alveoli are dilated.

Complications of PMF

– Pulmonary dysfunctions like dyspnea, chronic cough with black expectoration, decreased lung capacity, etc.
– Pulmonary hypertension
– Cor pulmonale
– Increased tuberculosis infection chances
– Increased risk of carcinoma of stomach, there is no increased risk of lung cancer due to PMF only.
– Right ventricular hypertrophy
– Chronic bronchitis
– Emphysema

Caplan's syndrome (viva): Coexistence of rheumatoid arthritis and pneumoconiosis.

23. Silicosis: Etiopathogenesis, pathology and complications (1994, 2003, 2011)

• "Knife grinders lung disease"
• Prolonged inhalation of silicon dioxide (silica)
• Most prevalent chronic occupational (pencil, slate, grinding, ceramic) lung disease in the world

Pathogenesis

• Silica has two forms: Crystalline and amorphous. The crystalline form (quartz, cristobalite and tridymite) are more fibrogenic and toxic than non-crystalline forms.
• Prolonged inhalation of silica particle leads to nodular fibrosing pneumoconiosis.

Morphology: (2000)

Gross

– Early stages: Tiny, discrete hardly palpable nodules in upper zone.
– Late stage: Larger nodule as hard collagenous scars, honeycomb pattern

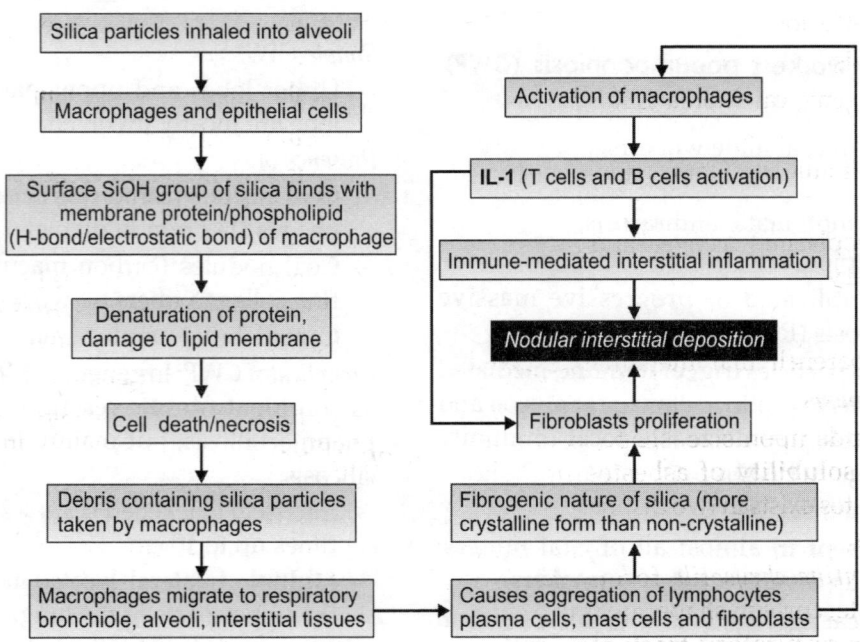

Fig. 15.5: Pathogenesis of silicosis

may be present in lung; fibrotic lesions are also seen in lymph nodes and pleura.

Microscopic features:

- *Silica nodule:* Concentric layers of hyalinized collagen surrounded by a dense capsule of more condensed collagen.
- Cavities may be present due to ischemia.
- *Polarized microscopy:* Nodule reveals birefringent silica particles.
- *Radiography:* Eggshell shadow—a central zone lacking calcification surrounded by concentration layer/zone of calcification.

- *Complications:* May develop PMF (see its complications in CWP), predisposes to pulmonary tuberculosis, lung cancer and cor pulmonale; Caplan's syndrome/rheumatoid arthritis.

24. Enumerate asbestos related diseases. Asbestosis (s/n) (1989, 95, 2011)

Asbestos related diseases due to prolonged exposure to asbestos dust:

1. Localized fibrosis; may cause diffuse pleural fibrosis
2. Pleural effusion
3. Asbestosis
4. Bronchogenic carcinoma (smoking co-risk factor)
5. Mesotheliomic carcinoma (smoking co-risk factor)
6. Other neoplasm: Laryngeal and some extra pulmonary

Asbestosis
- Diffuse parenchymal interstitial fibrosis
- *Pathogenesis*
  - Depends upon size, shape, concentration, solubility of asbestos particles. Asbestos exists in two distinct geometric forms.
  - *Serpentine chrysotile* forms are more flexible, curly in shape; are impacted in upper respiratory tract; removed by mucociliary action; and those reaches

lower part are digested, as they are soluble.

- Amphibole type asbestos are straight, stiff and brittle; easily reach deeper part of the lung, penetrate epithelial cells to reach *interstitium*.
- Initial injury occurs at bifurcation of small airways, where amphibole particles penetrate to interstitium.
- Alveolar and intersitial macrophages try to digest the fibers and are activated to release chemotactic factors and *fibrogenic* factors.
- Continuous release of mediators and inflammation in interstitial space; fibers deposition in the interstitium causes asbestosis.
- Asbestos is tumor initiator as well as tumor promotor.

- *Morphology*
Gross
  - Lungs are small, firm, with thickening of pleura.
  - Other features of interstitial lung diseases
  - First, lower lobe is involved; followed by middle and upper lobes or parts of lung.
  - Variable degree of subpleural fibrosis

- *Microscopic features*
  - Diffuse interstitial fibrosis
  - Asbestos bodies are golden-brown fusiform or beaded rods with a translucent center. It has asbestos fibers coated with an iron containing proteinaceous materials.
  - Enlarged airspaces; emphysema like condition—pleural plaque (dense collagen).

- *Clinical features*
  - Dyspnea
  - Cough
  - Sputum
  - Cor pulmonale
  - Progresses to heart failure
  - Death

25. Difference between TB and sarcoidosis

S. No.	Traits	TB	Sarcoidosis
1.	Cause	Infection of *Mycobacterium tuberculosis* complex	Unknown
2.	Granulomas:		
	a. Type	Caseating	Non-caseating
	b. Giant cells type	Langhans' giant cells	Foreign body giant cells
3.	Giant cell cytoplasmic inclusions		
	a. Schaumann's bodies	Absent	Present
	b. Asteroid bodies	Absent	Present
	c. Birefringent crystals	Absent	Present
4.	Steroid therapy	Worsen the problem in most cases	Dramatic improvement
5.	Diagnosis	Acid fast bacilli present	By exclusion methods

26. Classify bronchogenic tumors; its etiological factors (1993, 95, 97, 2004, 08, 10)

Classification

- Squamous cell carcinoma (epidermoid carcinoma)
- Adenocarcinoma (most common)
  - Acinar adenocarcinoma
  - Papillary adenocarcinoma
  - Bronchoalveolar carcinoma
  - Solid bronchioloalveolar carcinoma
- Small cell carcinoma
  - Oat cell carcinoma (lymphocyte like)
  - Intermediate cell carcinoma (polygonal)
  - Combined (with squamous cell carcinoma)
- Large cell carcinoma
  - Undifferentiated carcinoma
  - Clear cell carcinoma
  - Giant cell carcinoma
- Adenosquamous cell carcinoma
- Carcinoma with pleomorphic, sarcomatoid, or sarcomatous elements
- Carcinoid tumor: Typical and atypical tumors
- Carcinoma of salivary gland origin
- Unclassified carcinoma

Etiological factors: (2010)

- *Tobacco smoking*
  - Amount of daily smoking
  - Tendency to inhale
  - Duration of smoking
- *Industrial hazards*
  - All types of radiations; uranium
  - Coal
  - Iron
  - Asbestos
  - Mustard gas
  - Nickel
  - Chromates
- *Air pollution:* Indoor air pollution like radon
- *Molecular genetics:* Dominant oncogenes like *c-myc* (squamous cell carcinoma), *K-ras* (adenocarcinoma)

Tumor suppressor genes: Like p53 mutation, mutation and amplification of epidermal growth factor receptor (EGFR) gene.

- *Scarring:* Near the scar; mostly adenocarcinoma
- *Diet:* Vitamin A deficiency (increases risk)
- *Occupational:* Exposure to carcinogens

27. Squamous cell carcinoma of lung (1993, 95)

28. Difference between squamous cell and adenocarcinoma of lung

S. No.	Traits	Squamous cell carcinoma	Adenocarcinoma
1.	Sex	Male	Female
2.	Smoking history	Smokers	Non-smokers
3.	Location	Larger, more central bronchi	Tend to be peripherally located
4.	Growth rate	Highest of all bronchogenic carcinoma	Slower
5.	Local spread	Present (predominant)	Present, not so
6.	Distant metastasis	Later; low	Early
7.	Microscopy	Well-differentiated form—keratin and intercellular bridges; less differentiated form to poorly differentiated form may be present. Squamous metaplasia, epithelial dysplasia, carcinoma *in situ* present nearby	Two types: Bronchial-derived adenocarcinoma and bronchio-loalveolar. Vary from well glandular pattern (mucin secretion) to papillary to solid masses with occassional mucin producing glands
8.	Size	Larger	Smaller
9.	Scarring	Absent	May be present

29. Small cell (oat cell) carcinoma of lung (1986, 90, 91, 92, 2003)

- Highly malignat tumor; most aggressive of all lung tumors.
- *Site:* Hilum or central (bronchi) in location.
- Metastasizes widely, so incurable by surgery. Survival rate is only 15% at the end of one year.
- Most commonly associated with ectopic hormone production.
- Only in smokers; non-smokers only 1%.
- *Origin:* Neuroendocrine cells of the lining bronchial epithelium.
- *Morphology*

  Gross (all bronchogenic tumor)
  - Tumor is gray-white, firm to hard.
  - Foci of hemorrhage and necrosis in large tumors to produce yellow-white mottling appearance and soft to touch.
  - Cavity formation may follow necrosis.

  Microscopic features
  - *Oat cell:* Small epithelium cells, little cytoplasm, round to oval in shape, twice the size of lymphocyte, but like it, dark (hyperchromatic) nucleus and nucleoli not prominent.
  - *Variants:* Spindle small cell carcinoma, polygonal small cell carcinoma.
  - No glandular or squamous pattern.

  Electron microscopic features
  - Dense core neurosecretory granules.
  - Granules are similar to that found in neuro-endocrine *argentaffin/Kulchitsky* cells present along the bronchial epithelium.
  - Secrete polypeptide hormone.
  - Positive for neuron specific enolase (NSE), parathormone like hormones (PTHA) and polypeptide hormones.

30. Lab diagnosis of bronchogenic carcinoma (1997)

1. *Clinical features*
   - Cough
   - Dyspnea
   - Weight loss
   - ↓ed sputum production
   - Chest pain

2. Exfoliative cytology of sputum
3. Bronchial lavage
4. FNAC (radiologically guided)
5. Mediastinoscopy
6. Mediastinotomy
7. Thoracoscopy
8. Open lung biopsy
9. Chest drain
10. CT scan

31. Paraneoplastic syndromes associated with lung tumors (2000)

- *Hormone related syndrome*
  - ADH secretion (small cell carcinoma)—hyponatremia
  - ACTH secretion (small cell carcinoma)—Cushing's syndrome
  - Parathormone and parathyroid related peptides, prostaglandin E, and cytokines (squamous cell tumors)—hypercalcemia
  - Calcitonin—hypocalcemia
  - Gonadotropins—gynecomastia
  - Serotonin-associated with carcinoid syndrome
- *Other systemic manifestations*
  - Lambert-Eaton myasthenic syndrome—muscular weakness due to autoimmune antibody-mediated neuronal calcium channel damage.
  - Peripheral neuropathy—purely sensory (mostly).
  - Dermatological abnormalities including acanthosis nigricans.
  - Hematological abnormalities like leukamoid reactions.
  - Hypertrophic pulmonary osteoarthropathy.
  - Cardiovascular: Migratory thrombophlebitis, non-bacterial thrombotic endocarditis.

32. Bronchial carcinoids (1998)

- These are group of tumors earlier classified as adenoma (90%), but now known to be locally invasive, sometimes capable of metastasis.
- Remaining 10% includes adenoid cystic carcinoma and mucoepidermoid carcinoma.
- It comprises 1–5% of all lung tumors.
- *Age and sex:* Less than 40 yr, both sexes equally affected.
  - No association with cigarette smoking established.
- *Cell origin:* Neuroendocrine differentiation of the Kulchitsky cells of bronchial mucosa (compare with intestinal carcinoids).
- *Morphology*
  Gross
  - Growth pattern: Finger-like or spherical polypoid masses projecting into lumen of bronchus. Intact mucosa covers these growths.
  - *Size:* Usually less than 3–4 cm.
  Microscopic features
  - Pattern: Nests, cords and masses of cells separated by delicate fibrous stroma.
  - Tumor cells are regular with uniform round nuclei. Mitosis is infrequent.
  - Carcinoid adenoma may show cellular and nuclear pleomorphism, and are more aggressive.
  Electron microscopy: Cells have dense core granules (characteristics of neuroendocrine tumors).
  Immunocytochemistry: Cells showing serotonin, neutron specific enolase, bombesin and calcitonin.
- *Clinical features:*
  Due to intraluminal growth:
  - Persistent cough
  - Impairment of drainage of respiratory passage (2° infections)
  - Bronchiectasis
  - Atelectasis
  - Hemoptysis
  - Emphysema
  Metastasis and local invasion
  Production of vasoactive amine: Carcinoid syndrome.

33. Utility of bronchoalveolar lavage (1994)

Diagnosis of
- Pulmonary TB
- Chronic bronchitis
- Bronchogenic carcinoma
- Bronchiectasis
- Pneumonia

Treatment of
- Infective pathology
- Post-aspiration lavage (immediate)
- Surfactant therapy in ARDS (neonates)

34. Causes of hemoptysis

Inflammation
- Bronchiectasis
- Lung abscess

- Bronchitis
- Asbestosis
- Tuberculosis
- Pneumonia

Neoplasm
- Primary and metastatic lung cancer
- Bronchial adenoma

Others
- Pulmonary thromboembolism
- Primary pulmonary hypertension
- Trauma
- Foreign bodies
- Iatrogenic lung needle biopsy
- Pulmonary infarct
- Left ventricular failure
- Hemorrhagic diathesis
- Mitral stenosis

35. Difference between obstructive lung disease and restrictive lung diseases

S. No.	Traits	Obstructive lung disease	Restrictive lung disease
1.	Definition	A group of disorders associated with increased resistance to air flow owing to partial or complete obstruction at any level from trachea to terminal bronchioles.	A group of diseases associated with reduced lung compliance (expansion) either due to chest wall or skeletal abnormality or infiltrative parencymal disease
2.	Associated diseases	Chronic bronchitis, emphysema, acute bronchial asthmatic attack	Chest wall disorders (kyphoscoliosis), ARDS, ILD
3.	FVC	↓	↓↓
4.	FEV1	↓	↓
5.	FEV1/FVC (%)	N to ↓	N to ↑
6.	FEV1 (25–75%)	↓	N to ↓
7.	PEF	↓	N to ↓
8.	MVV	↓	N to ↓
9.	TLC	N to ↑	↓
10.	RV	↑	↓
11.	RV/TLC	↑	N

(FVC: Forced vital capacity, FEV1: Forced expiratory volume in one second, FEV1/FVC ratio—the percentage of the FVC expired in one second, $FEF_{25-75\%}$: forced expiratory flow over the middle one half of the FVC, PEF: Peak expiratory flow, MVV: Maximal voluntary ventilation, RV: Residual volume, TLC: Total lung capacity)

36. ARDS (Acute respiratory distress syndrome)

Severe, acute lung injury involving diffuse alveolar damage, increased microvascular permeability and non-cardiogenic pulmonary edema resulting in severe life threatening respiratory insufficiency and arterial hypoxemia.

Causes

Infection	Physical injury	Inhaled irritants
• Sepsis • Diffuse pulmonary infections: Viral, mycoplasma, miliary tuberculosis, pneumocystis pneumoniae • Gastric aspiration	• Mechanical trauma, head injury • Pulmonary contusions • Near drowing • Fractures with fat embolism • Burn • Ionizing radiation	• Oxygen toxicity • Smoke • Irritant gases and chemicals

Chemical injury	Hematologic conditions	
• Heroin or methadone overdose • Barbiturate overdose • Acetylsalicylic acid	• Multiple blood transfusions • DIC	Pancreatitis

Uremia	Cardiopulmonary bypass	Hypersensitivity reactions

Pathogenesis

- Activation of inflammatory mediators and cellular components resulting in damage to capillary endothelial and alveolar epithelial cells
- Increased permeability of alveolar capillary membrane
- Influx of protein-rich edema fluid and inflammatory cells into airspaces
- Dysfunction of surfactant
- Inflammatory mediators in ARDS: IL-1, IL-6, IL-8, MIP-1α, endothelin 1, VWF, endo-toxin, Fas ligand

Phases of ARDS

i. *Exudative phase* (1st week)
   - Alveolar and interstitial edema
   - Capillary congestion
   - Destruction of Type I alveolar cells
   - Early hyaline membrane formation
ii. *Proliferative phase* (2nd to 4th wk)
   - Increased type II alveolar cells
   - Cellular infiltration of alveolar septum
   - Organization of hyaline membranes
iii. *Fibrosis phase* (>3 to 4 wk)
   - Fibrosis of hyaline membranes and alveolar septum
   - Alveolar duct fibrosis

16

Gastrointestinal Tract

1. Pleomorphic adenoma/mixed parotid tumors (1990, 94, 95, 97, 98, 2002, 03)

- Benign tumors of salivary glands that arise from epithelium, but show both epithelial and mesenchymal differentiation. They were also called *mixed tumors* because it was thought to arise from ectoderm and mesoderm.
- *Site:* Parotid (60%), less common in submandibular; rare in minor salivary glands.
- *Origin:* Epithelial/myoepithelial/ductal reserve cell origin so called pleomorphic adenoma.
- Radiation exposure is thought be risk factor.
- *Morphology*
  Gross
  - Well demarcated
  - Round, may be multilobulated
  - Small, rarely more than 6 cm; average 2.5 cm in diameter
  - Firm in texture
  - Surface may be bosselated
  - Mostly encapsulated, but may be expansile growth
  - Cut surface: Variegated appearance (gray-white myxoid and blue translucent chondroid).

  Microscopic features
  - Heterogenicity in the histologic findings: Epithelial components dispersed in a matrix of varying degree of myxoid, hyaline, chondroid matrix.
  - Epithelial components: Ductal cells or myoepithelial cells forming various pattern like duct, acini, tubules, strands, sheets. Cuboidal cells lining ducts are common; well-differentiated squamous cells in sheets may also be present.
  - Mesenchyme elements: Loose connective tissue having myxoid, chondroid, mucoid or even bony matrix.

- *Clinical features*
  - Painless
  - Mobile discrete masses
  - Mostly present in superficial lobe of parotid
  - Slow growing tumor
  - Carcinoma conversion rare, but present.

2. Warthin tumors (Papillary cystadenoma lymphomatosum)

- Benign tumors of salivary gland that are restricted to parotid gland only.
- *Age:* 5th to 7th decade of life.
- *Sex:* Males are more affected than females.
- Mostly unilateral and solitary; may be multifocal and bilateral.
- *Smoking* is the most common risk factor associated with this tumor.
- *Histogenesis* is disputed, thought to arise from parotid ductal epithelium cells present

in the lymph nodes adjacent to or within parotid gland.

- *Morphology*

  Gross
  - Present in superficial parotid gland
  - Round to oval
  - Encapsulated
  - Small in size
  - Cut surface: Pale-gray surface, mucin or serous secretion containing narrow cyst or cleft (slit) like space showing papillary projections.

  Microscopic features: Epithelial components
  - It forms glandular or cystic structure.
  - The space is lined by double layer epithelium.
  - The inner (surface palisade) cell layer is columnar cells with abundant, finely granular, eosinophilic cytoplasm (*oncocytic* appearance, mitochondria in cytoplasm so granular).
  - The outer cell layer is cuboidal to polygonal.
  - Secretary cells are dispersed in the inner layer of columnar cells.

  Lymphoid stroma is present under the epithelium in form of prominent lymphoid tissue, often with germinal centers.

3. Achalasia cardia

It is a motor disorder of esophageal smooth muscle, characterized by
  i. Aperistalsis
  ii. Failure of relaxation of the LES with swallowing
  iii. Increased resting tone of LES

Pathogenesis
- It is due to dysfunction of inhibitory neurons containing nitric oxide and vasoactive intestinal polypeptide in the distal intestine. The cholinergic innervation of LES is intact or affected in advanced stage.
- There is neurogenic degeneration, either intrinsic (degeneration of ganglion of Aurebach's myentric plexus) or extrinsic (extraesophageal vagus nerve).
- As a result of abnormality, LES fails to relax and there is progressive dilatation of esophagus above the level of LES.

Clinical features
- 20–40 years of male and females are equally affected
- Presents with progressive dysphagia for both solid and liquids. The dysphagia is worsened by emotional stress and hurried eating.
- Regurgitation and pulmonary aspiration occurs because of retention of large volume of food in esophagus.
- Esophagitis with ulceration may occur.
- Pain is not commom.

Secondary achalasia may occur in chagas disease, polio, diabetes autonomic neuropathy, infiltrative disorders, e.g. malignancy, amyloidosis and sarcoidosis.

4. Barret esophagus (1996, 2004, 07, 08, 10)

- A condition of GERD (gastro-esophageal reflux disease) in which distal stratified squamous epithelium of esophagus is replaced by columnar cells (metaplasia).
- Males are more affected than females, seen in 40–60 years of age.
- A complication of long-standing and severe form of GERD.
- *Conditions associated that predispose to Barret esophagus*
  - Decreased LES tone in any diseased condition
  - Sliding hiatus hernia
  - Chronic gastric and duodenal ulcer
  - Nasogastric intubation
  - Neuropathy in alcoholics and diabetes milletus
  - Surgical vagotomy
  - Delayed gastric emptying, etc.

Pathogenesis
Due to chronic exposure to high acidity; inflammation and ulceration are common in lower part of the esophagus. In adaptive changes, there is in-growth of pleuripotent stem cells, which differentiate into columnar cells than are more resistant to acidity. In the environment of sustained low pH, these cells become dysplastic. Dysplasia may be low grade or high grade.

Morphology
Endoscopy: Red velvety mucosa present in-between smooth, pale, esophageal squamous mucosa above and light brown-pink gastric mucosa below.

Microscopic features
Three types of columnar epithelium have been described:
1. Intestinal type: The most common
2. Junctional type, and
3. Gastric fundic type
Metaplasia of squamous cells by columnar cells having:
• Goblet cells-intestinal type (Hallmark)
• Fundic gastric glands
• Cardiac mucosal glands
• Dysplasia-high or low grade

Clinical features
• Dysphasia
• Heartburn
• Hematemesis
• Melena
• Local ulceration
• Bleeding
• Stricture formation
• Development of adenocarcinoma (30–40 fold increased risk)

5. Carcinoma esophagus

It affects more commonly males than females of age more than 50 years.

It originates most commonly in the lower 1/3rd (55%) followed by middle 1/3rd (35%) and least common in upper 1/3rd (10%).

Esophageal carcinoma is of two common histological types:

Squamous cell carcinoma
Most common type worldwide and most common in India.

Occurs in upper and middle 1/3rd of esophagus.

Predisposing factors
• Alcohol
• Cigarette
• Achalasia
• Plummer-Vinson syndrome
• Celiac sprue
• Mucosal damage from physical agents—hot tea, lye ingestion, radiation
• Dietary deficiency of molybdenum, zinc, vitamic A

Adenocarcinoma
Most common type in the USA
Located in lower 1/3rd of esophagus

Predisposing factor:
Chronic gastric reflux (Barrett's esophagus)

6. Chronic gastritis: Pathogenesis, morphological changes and complications

7. Chronic gastritis: Etiopathogenesis (2002)

• Chronic inflammation of gastric mucosa and submucosa resulting in mucosal atrophy, epithelial metaplasia, dysplasia and predisposing to carcinoma development. There is usually no erosion of mucosa.

• *Etiology*
  – Infection: *H. pylori* (antral predominant);
  – Autoimmune (body-fundic predominant);
  – Toxic substance: Alcohol intake and tobacco smoking;

- Iatrogenic: Post-surgical like antrectomy, gastroenterostomy;
- Radiations;
- Other: Granulomatous conditions, amyloidosis, graft versus host reactions and chronic NSAIDs use.

*All environmental factors affect antral mucosa or both antral and body-fundic mucosa.

- **Morphology**

  Gross: Mucosa reddened, coarser texture, thick rugal folds, boggy appearance in early or thinned and flattened mucosa in long standing disease.

  Microscopic features
  - Chronic inflammatory infiltrate by lymphocytes, plasma cells in lamina propria.
  - Active inflammatory cells like neutrophils within surface and glandular epithelium are present.
  - Regenerative changes: Proliferation of mucosal cells.
  - *Metaplasia:* Intestinal metaplasia common.
  - Atrophy: In long-standing disease, there is loss of glandular structures, perietal cells, cystic dialatation of glands.
  - *Hyperplasia* of gastrin (inhibitors of acid secretion) producing G cells in the antral mucosa in autoimmune type of gastritis.
  - *Dysplasia:* Present in long standing disease.
  - *H. pylori* if present lie in the superficial mucosal layer and among the microvilli of epithelial cells. It is absent from areas having metaplasia.

- **Clinical features:**
  - Nausea
  - Vomiting
  - Upper abdominal discomfort
  - Mild form: Hypochlorhydric (not achlorhydria), pernicious anemia absent, serum gastrin level—normal or slightly increased.

- Severe form: Achlorhydria, pernicious anemia and hypergastrenemia.
- **Complications**
  - Peptic ulcer
  - Gastric carcinoma

8. Role of *Helicobacter pylori* in chronic gastritis (1998, 2002, 2011) or in gastric carcinoma (1998).

- Gram-negative non- invasive, non-sporing rod shaped bacteria.
- In chronic gastritis and peptic ulcer disease it has *strong causal association*; in gastric carcinoma and gastric lymphoma its role is *postulated* as etiological agent.
- **Virulence factors**
  - Motility
  - Urease
  - Protease
  - Phospholipase
  - Adhesin
  - Catalase
  - Mucinase
  - Hemolysin
  - Cytotoxins (pro-inflammatory substance): Cag A gene product: Duodenal ulcer, Vac A gene products: Vacoulating cytotoxin, lipopolysaccharide (endotoxin).

- **Role of H. pylori in peptic ulcer disease:**
  - It secretes urease, protease and phospholipase. Urease generates free ammonia that binds with H^+ and decrease acidity, thus colonization and survival of the organism is favored. Protease damages glycoprotein of gastric mucus. Phospholipases damage surface epithelial cells and these also release leukotrienes and eicosanoids. Increased production of proinflammatory cytokines (IL-1, IL-6, TNF-α).
  - Neutrophilic infiltrate and release of myeloperoxidase (hypochlorus, monochloramine) destroy cells.

- Colonization of *H. pylori* causes mucosal and lamina propria cells damage. There may be thrombotic occlusion causing ischemia.
- Other enzymes and products released by *H. pylori* are chemotactic to inflammatory cells.
- Through damaged mucosa, nutrients leak to surface microenvironment so bacilli are sustained.

9. Peptic ulcer: Etiopathogenesis, pathology and complications (1993, 2009)

10. Benign gastric ulcer/peptic ulcer (1991)

- Are chronic, most often solitary and less than 4 cm in size lesion present in any part of GIT that are exposed to acid and peptic juices.
- *Sites* (*in decreasing order*)
  1. First portion of duodenum
  2. Stomach, antrum
  3. Gastroesophageal junction in GERD
  4. Margins of gastrojejunostomy
  5. ZE syndrome—duodenum, stomach, jejunum
  6. Mecked diverticulum and its adjacent areas

  Pathogenesis: "Peptic ulcer results whenever defense mechanisms of stomach are impaired and/or damaging factors are more predominant."

- *Defense mechanism*
  - Mucus layer on surface
  - Bicarbonate secretion into mucosa
  - Mucosal blood flow
  - Apical surface membrane transport
  - Epithelial regenerative capacity
  - Prostaglandins secretion
  - Control of acid secretions

- *Damaging forces:* Gastric acid and peptic enzymes secretion aggravated by:
  - *H. pylori* infection

  - Alcohol
  - Personality
  - Ischemia
  - NSAIDs like aspirin
  - Gastric hyperacidity
  - Psychological stress
  - Shock
  - Cigarette
  - Duodenal-gastric reflux
  - Hypercalcemia
  - Delayed gastric emptying

- *Morphology*

  Gross
  - Size: Small, generally less than 2 cm
  - Shape: Round to oval
  - Sharply punched out lesion
  - Straight wall, mucosa may overhang the base
  - Base-clean up, smooth (peptic digestion)
  - Scarring

  Microscopic features: Varies according to stage of disease. In active ulcer undergoing necrosis, four distinct zones (from lumen to outward) are:
  - Zone of necrotic debris: Base and margins, thin layer necrotic fibrinoid debris.
  - Zone of nonspecific inflammatory infiltrate by neutrophils (predominant).
  - Zone of granulation tissue: Mononuclear WBC infiltrate.
  - Zone of fibrosis: Collagenous scar of fibrous scar.

- *Complications:* (1991, 92)
  - *Bleeding:* Most frequent complication (15–20% patients), life threatening (1/4th of ulcer death), and sometimes first indication of peptic ulcer. It is more commonly seen in posterior duodenal ulcers because of erosion of gastroduodenal artery.
  - *Perforation:* Emergency condition, life threatening (2/3rd of ulcer death), late presentation. It may result in acute

peritonitis, subphrenic abscess; may involve adjacent organs. Perforation occurs commonly in the ulcers located in the anterior part of duodenum. Deodenal ulcers tend to penetrate into pancreas causing pancreatitis. Gastric ulcers tend to penetrate into left hepatic lobe.

- *Obstruction:* Due to edema or scarring. It causes incapacitating, crampy abdominal pain. Mostly in case of pyloric channel ulcer. Present only in 2% cases.
- *Severe pain.*
- Tea pot stomach is caused due to longitudinal shortening of the gastric ulcer at the lesser curvature of the stomach and causes stomach to look like tea pot.

Hour glass stomach is caused due to cicatracia contraction of a saddle shaped ulcer at the lesser curvature.

11. Zollinger-Ellison (ZE) syndrome (1989)

- Also called gastrinomas (gastrin producing tumor).
- *Site:* Duodenum and parapancreatic soft tissues.
- *Origin:* Endocrine cells of both gut and pancreas undergo dedifferentiation and express a number of gene products.
- Hypergastrinemia induces hypersecretion of gastric acid. It causes ulcer in usual sites and also in unusual sites like jejunum.
- When total resection of the tumor is possible, then syndrome is eliminated.

12. Difference between duodenal and gastric peptic ulcer

S. No.	Traits	Duodenal ulcer	Gastric ulcer
1.	Age	25–50 yr (young)	Beyond 60 yr (old)
2.	Sex M: F	3:1	1.5–2:1
3.	Etiology	Most commonly associated with *H. pylori* infection	Disruption of mucosal barrier
4.	Site	1st part of duodenum (anterior wall)	Along lesser curvature
5.	Acid level	High	Mostly normal; increased only if gastrin level ↑ed
6.	Clinical features		
	Pain	Relieved after food intake	Aggravated after food intake
	Night pain	Common	No night pain
	Vomiting and hemetemesis	Less common	More common
	Melena	More common	Less common
	Weight loss	No weight loss	Marked weight loss
7.	Incidence	More common	Less common

13. Difference between gross features of benign and malignant peptic ulcer (2003)

14. Difference between benign and malignant peptic ulcer (1994, 95, 99, 2000, 01, 02, 08, 09, 11)

S. No.	Traits	Benign ulcer	Malignant ulcer
1.	Age	Comparatively younger age	Older age
2.	Sex	Male predominance very high	Equal or slightly more in male

(Contd.)

Difference between benign and malignant peptic ulcer (*Contd.*)

S. No.	Traits	Benign ulcer	Malignant ulcer
3.	Site	Along lesser curvature of pylorus and antrum	Along greater curvature of pylorus and antrum
4.	Ulcer base	Clear, may be hemorrhagic	Necrotic debris present
5.	Mucosal folds	Radiating from ulcer crater	Interrupted, flattening of the rugae around the ulcer due to infiltration by malignant cells.
6.	Shape/Barium meal	Sharply punched out lesion	Irregular
7.	Margins	Heaping up: rare and slight	Common and to greater degree
8.	Therapy	Good response	Poor response

*Size is no criteria for the differentiation into benign and malignant ulcers. Benign ulcers are generally less than 4 cm.

15. Classify tumors of stomach (1993)

Based on malignant potential

- *Benign*
  - Adenoma/adenomatous or neoplastic polyps
  - Spindle cell (stromal) tumors including leiomyoma
  - Lipoma
- *Malignant*
  - Gastric carcinoma
  - Leiomyosarcoma
  - Leiomyoblastoma (epitheloid leiomyoma)
  - Carcinoid tumor
  - Lymphoma

Based on origin

- *Non-epithelial/mesenchymal tumors*
  - Gastrointestinal stromal tumors (GIST)
  - Leiomyoma and leiosarcoma
  - Lipoma
  - Schwannoma
  - Granular cell tumor
  - Lymphoma
- *Epithelial tumors*
  - Intraepithelial gastric neoplasia (adenoma)
  - Adenocarcinoma
  - Small cell carcinoma
  - Carcinoid tumor

16. Gastric carcinoma: etiopathogenesis (1997), gross and microscopic features (1993)

17. Linitus plastica (1995)

Etiological factors:

- *Environmental factors*
  Diet:
  - Foods containing active nitrites or its precursor nitrates
  - Smoked and salted foods, pickles items
  - Less fresh fruits and vegetables
  - Cigarette smoking

- *Host factors*
  - Chronic gastritis (multifocal mucosal atrophy and intestinal metaplasia)
  - *H. pylori* infection
  - Partial gastrectomy—reflux of irritant biliary contents and chronic gastritis
  - Gastric adenoma
  - Barret esophagus—increased risk at junction (dysplasia)
- Genetic factors:
  - More in blood group A person
  - Family history
- *Racial factors:* More in blacks, American Indians

- *Geographical influence:* More in Japan, Finland and Iceland

Features/classifications
- According to *depth of invasion*
  - Early gastric carcinoma: Confined to mucosa and submucosa: Muscularis propria not infiltrated; may or may not involve peri-gastric lymph nodes.
  - Advanced gastric carcinoma: Extended to muscular wall (muscularis propria).
- According to *macroscopic features* (present in both early and advanced lesions):
  - Exophytic growth pattern: Tumor mass protruding into lumen.
  - Flat depressed: Usually not distinguished from mucosa. In advanced tumor, it has appearance of *"linitus plastica"*—infiltration of a part or entire stomach by tumor mass giving 'leather bottle' appearance.
  - Excavated: In early lesion, shallow crater is formed in contrast to large malignant ulcer in advanced lesion.
- *Histologic type:* (Lauren classification): *Intestinal type:*
  - Tumor cells form intestinal gland resembling colonic adenocarcinoma.
  - They permeates the wall.
  - They grows in expanding growth pattern as cohesive mass along broad fronts.
  - Cells have apical mucin vacuoles.
  - Mucin is present in the lumen of glands.

Diffuse/gastric type
- No gland formation.
- Scattered cells or small cell nests permeate mucosa and the gastric wall (infiltration).
- Arise from middle layer of mucosa.
- No intestinal metaplasia to develop carcinoma.
- Cells show *signet ring* appearance due to pushing of nucleus to periphery due to mucin formation.

Clinical features
- Abdominal pain
- Vomiting
- Anorexia
- Altered bowel habit
- Anemia
- Dysphasia
- Weight loss
- All gastric carcinomas eventually penetrate the serosa to spread to local and distant lymph nodes.
- May frequently metastasize to supraclavicular lymph nodes as a first clinical sign (virchow lymph nodes) or to periumbilical region to form a subcutaneous nodule (sister Mary Joseph nodule) or to bilateral ovaries (Krukenberg tumor).

18. Amoebic colitis: gross and microscopic features; its complications (1994, 98, 2001)

19. Amoebic ulcers

20. Difference between amoebic colitis and ulcerative colitis (1995, 96, 2003, 2011)

S. No.	Traits	Amoebic colitis	Ulcerative colitis
1.	Cause	*Entamoeba histolytica* (infective)	Unknown, idiopathic inflammatory bowel disease
2.	Transmission/risk	Fecal-oral route	Genetic predisposition, immunologic dysregulation
3.	Parts affected	Generalized, whole large intestine or localized to cecum, ascending colon, sigmoid, rectum, appendix in ↓ing order	Involves rectum and extends proximally to involve whole colon in severe cases

(Contd.)

Difference between amoebic colitis and ulcerative colitis (Contd.)

S. No.	Traits	Amoebic colitis	Ulcerative colitis
4.	Growth	Not such pattern	Retrograde
5.	Ulcers	Flask shaped (narrow neck and broad base) discrete ulcer with intervening normal mucosa. Size: Pin head to > 2.5 cm in diameter	Broad base ulcer with no narrow neck, continuous lesion no normal mucosa in between, size vary from small to very large
6.	Ulcer extension	Deep (base up to muscularis propria) or superficial	Usually superficial, limited to mucosa and submucosa
7.	Pseudopolyps	Absent	Present
8.	Risk of cancer	No	Increases
9.	Age	Any age, more in children	Peak 20–25 yr
10.	Morphology	Liquefactive necrosis few inflammating cells-neutrophils	Diffuse mononuclear infiltrates, crypt abscess

21. Difference between TB ulcer and typhoid ulcer of intestine (1993, 94, 95, 97, 98, 2002, 06)

S. No.	Traits	TB ulcers	Typhoid ulcer
1.	Causative organism	Mycobacterium tuberculosis	Salmonella typhi
2.	Site	Anywhere in small intestine; most common in terminal ileum and cecum, rarely colon	Most common in terminal ileum (Payer's patch); may occur in jejunum and colon
3.	Lymphocytic involvement	Mainly in lymphoid follicle, may involve Payer's patch	Mainly in Payer's patch, may also involve lymphoid follicle
4.	Orientation	Transverse to long axis of bowel due to spread by lymphatics	Longitudinal to long axis of bowel due to involvement of Payer's patch
5.	Size	Larger ulcer	Small ulcer
6.	Margins	Irregular, ulcer may encircle the gut	Regular
7.	Base of ulcers	Caseous materials present (white)	Caseous material absent, base is black due to sloughing of mucosa
8.	Microscopic features	Typical caseous granuloma, AFB, epithelioid cells, giant cell, etc.	Erythrophagocytosis, bacteria in macrophage
9.	Fibrosis and stricture	May be present on healing	Absent
10.	Perforation	Absent, less common	Present, more common
11.	Bleeding	Absent	Present

22. Difference between TB ulcer and amoebic ulcer (2007)

S. No.	Traits	TB ulcer	Amoebic ulcer
1.	Causative organism	*Mycobacterium tuberculosis*	*Entamoeba histolytica*
2.	Site	Most common in terminal ileum and cecum, rarely colon	Whole large intestine or localized to some part of large intestine
3.	Transmission	Hematogenous spread, ingestion of infected sputum, or direct spread from infected contiguous lymph nodes and fallopian tubes.	Feco-oral route
4.	Orientation of ulcer	Transverse to long axis of bowel	No such orientation
5.	Microscopic features	Epithelioid cell granuloma with or without granuloma	Liquefactive necrosis, few inflamma-tory cells-mainly neutrophils
6.	Perforation	Common	Uncommon
7.	Fibrosis and stricture	Common	Absent

23. Malabsorption syndrome (1990)

- Is defined as impaired absorption of nutrients like fat, fat-soluble and other vitamins, proteins, carbohydrates, electrolytes, minerals and water.

Classification of malabsorption syndrome:
- *Defective intramural digestion* of fat, proteins, and carbohydrates (enzyme deficiency). Defective bile secretion, bacterial overgrowth and modification, pancreatic insufficiency.
- *Primary mucosal cell abnormalities:* Defective terminal digestion and defective epithelial transport.
- *Reduced small intestinal surface area:* Crohn disease, Celiac sprue, etc.
- *Lymphatic obstruction.*
- *Infections* like tropical sprue, Whipple disease, parasitic infestation.
- Surgery/iatrogenic

Clinical features depend on type of malabsorption, nutrient specific deficiency or generalized symptoms.

- Passage of bulky, frothy greasy, yellow or gray stools, abdominal distension, and flatus.
- Weight loss and generalized muscle wasting.
- Anemia (Iron, pyridoxine, folate and vitamin B_{12} deficiency)
- Bleeding (vitamin K deficiency)
- Edema (protein deficiency)
- Dermatitis, mucositis, hyperkeratosis (vitamin A, zinc and essential fatty acid deficiency)
- Osteoporosis, osteomalacia (vitamin D and calcium deficiency)

24. Celiac sprue/non-tropical sprue (1995)

25. Difference between celiac sprue and tropical sprue

S. No.	Traits	Celiac sprue	Tropical sprue
1.	Synonyms	Gluten sensitive enteropathy, non-tropical sprue	Post-infectious sprue
2.	Race	A disease of whites	A disease of non-whites

(Contd.)

Difference between celiac sprue and tropical sprue (Contd.)

S. No.	Traits	Celiac sprue	Tropical sprue
3.	Cause	Idiopathic disease producing mucosal lesion in small intestine due to sensitivity to gluten and related proteins (water insoluble gliadin) of wheat and related grains. No organism is related	Infectious disease. But no specific causal agent is clearly demarcated. Enterotoxigenic bacterial overgrowth is found
4.	Role of immunity in pathogenesis	Cell mediated immunity plays important role	No role
5.	Site	Changes marked in proximal part (higher gluten exposure) of small intestine than distal part	Changes marked in all parts (marked in distal small bowel)
6.	Genetic predisposition	Present, HLA association	No
7.	Malignancy transformation	Intestinal lymphoma turns malignant	Intestinal lymphoma not hazardous
8.	Treatment	Stay away from gluten	Broad spectrum antibiotics

- Celiac sprue *microscopic* features:
  - Diffuse enteritis.
  - Atrophy or total loss of villi.
  - Surface epithelium: Vacuolar degeneration, loss of microvilli border, increased number of intraepithelial CD8+ T lymphocytes.
  - Crypt—increased mitotic figures, hyperplastic, elongated, tortuous to maintain mucosal thickness.
  - Plasma cell, lymphocytes, macrophages, eosinophils, mast cells infiltration in lamina propria.

26. Enumerate ulcero-inflammatory diseases of small and large intestine (1998, 1998)

- *Small intestine:*
  - Crohn's disease
  - *Campylobacter jejuni* ulcer
  - Typhoid ulcer
  - Drug induced ulcer
  - TB ulcer
- *Large intestine:*
  - Crohn's disease
  - Ulcerative colitis
  - *Shigella induced ulcer*
  - *Campylobacter jejuni ulcers*
  - *Amoebic ulcers*

27. Pathology and complications of TB intestine (1986)

Intestinal tuberculosis may have three forms: Primary, secondary and hyperplastic cecal tuberculosis.

- *Primary intestinal tuberculosis:*
  - It is caused by *Mycobacterium bavis* (ingestion of unpasteurized milk).
  - It involves mainly ileocecal region.
  - Lesions have predilection for mesenteric lymph; intestine is not involved significantly.
  - Gross: Lymph nodes are elnarged, caseous and matted (TB lymph node). Lymph nodes may heal by fibrosis and calcification.
  - Microscopically, lesions are seen in mucosa in early stage as Ghon's focus, later on mesenteric lymph nodes are

involved, which show tubercular granulomatous reaction.

- **Secondary intestinal tuberculosis**
  - Swallowing of sputum may result in 2° TB in intestine, if the patient has active pulmonary TB.
  - It involves mainly terminal ileum; colon in rare case.
  - Intestinal lesions are more prominent than lymph nodes lesion. Lesion starts in Payer's patches or lymphoid follicles in the form of small ulcers. It forms large ulcers (transverse to the long axis of the bowel), once it spread through lymphatics. It is microscopically similar to pulmonary TB.
- **Hyperplastic cecal tuberculosis:** A variant of secondary intestinal TB 2° to pulmonary TB involving cecum (sometimes ascending colon), which is palpable as lump.

Complications:
- Tuberculous peritonitis
- Transverse fibrous stricture
- Intestinal obstruction

28. Crohn's disease

- **Synonyms:** Terminal ileitis, skip lesion, regional enteritis, and granulomatous colitis.
- This is an idiopathic inflammatory bowel disease, characterized by
  - Sharply delimited and typically transmural involvement of bowel by an inflammatory process with mucosal damage;
  - Presence of non-caseating granulomas;
  - Fissuring with formation of fistulas.
- **Age:** Any age, but major peaks in teens and twenties, minor peak 50s and 60s.
- Smoking has strong correlation to the disease.
- **Morphology:**
  Gross:
  - Serosa: Granular and dull gray

- Creepy fat appearance
- Mesentery thickened, edematous and fibrotic
- Intestinal wall is rubbery and thick due to edema, inflammation, fibrosis and hypertrophy of muscularis propria
- Lumen is narrowed (string sign in X-ray)
- **Skip lesion (characteristics):** Sharp demarcation of the involved segment from uninvolved part
- Aphthous ulcer, linear ulcer (cobblestone appearance), fistula or sinus tract formation depending on the stage of the disease.

- **Histology:**
  - Mucosal hypertrophy
  - Chronic mucosal damage
  - Ulceration
  - Transmular inflammation affecting all layers
  - Non-caseating granuloma
  - Other changes like fibrosis
- **Clinical course:**
  - Presents with recurrent episodes of diarrhea, crampy abdominal pain, fever and melena.
  - Remission and relapses are common.
  - Patient may develop malabsorption fistula formation and intestinal stricture progressing into obstruction.
  - Extraintestinal manifestations include uveitis, sacroilitis, migratory polyarthritis, erythema nodosum, bile duct inflammatory disorder, obstructive uropathy and nephrolithiasis.

29. Ulcerative colitis (UC): etiopathogenesis (2001), morphology (1992, 2000) and its complications (1989, 90, 92, 99)

"UC is an ulcero-inflammatory disease limited to colon and affecting only the mucosa and submucosa except in very severe form".

- The lesion extends in a continuous fashion from rectum to proximal parts of colon (retrograde)

- There are no well-formed granulomas, no skip lesions are seen
- *Age:* 20–25 yr peak, more in female

- **Morphology**

  Gross

  - Mucosa may be slightly red, granular, friable and may bleed easily;
  - Broad based ulcers of mucosa are present; ulcers are aligned with the long axis of colon;
  - Pseudopolyps (due to regenerating mucosal bulging);
  - No mural thickening; normal serosa.

- **Histology**

  - Mucosal inflammation;
  - Chronic mucosal damage and ulceration (mostly limited to mucosa and submucosa);

- A diffuse, predominantly mononuclear inflammation in lamina propria is universal;
- Crypt abscess (due to neutrophilic infiltration of mucosal epithelium in crypt of lumen);
- Even after healing, submucosal fibrosis and mucosal architectural disarray of colonic gland atrophy may persist;
- Epithelial dysplasia is common.

- **Complications**
  - Toxic megacolon
  - Bleeding
  - Perianal fistula
  - Perforation
  - Development of colonic carcinoma

30. Difference between Crohn's disease and UC (1998, 2000, 04, 08, 10)

S. No.	Traits	Crohn's disease	UC
A.	Macroscopic features:		
	1. Location of lesions	Ileum, may be colon (may involve any part of GIT)	Only colon
	2. Pattern of distribution	Skip lesion	Diffuse, continuous
	3. Stricture formation	Early	Uncommon, late
	4. Wall appearance	Thickened	Thin
	5. Lumen dilation	Absent	Present
	6. Progression	Anterograde	Retrograde
B.	Microscopic features:		
	1. Pseudopolyps	Absent/slight	Marked
	2. Ulcers	Deep, linear	Superficial
	3. Lymphoid reaction	Marked	Mild
	4. Fibrosis	Marked	Mild
	5. Serositis	Marked	Absent or mild
	6. Granuloma	Present in 50%	Absent
	7. Fistula/sinus	Present	Absent
C.	Clinical features:		
	1. Fat/vitamin malabsorption	Present	Absent
	2. Malignant potential	Present, less	Present, more
	3. Response to surgery	Poor	Good

31. Precancerous lesion of GIT (1990)

- *Mouth*
  - Leukoplakia
  - Erythroplakia
  - Papillomas
- *Esophagus*
  - Long-standing esophagitis
  - Achalasia
  - Barret's esophagus
  - Plummer-Vinson syndrome
- *Stomach*
  - Chronic gastritis
  - Peptic ulcer (rare)
  - Chronic *H. pylori* infection
  - Pernicious anemia
- *Small and large intestine*
  - UC
  - Crohn disease
  - Juvenile polyps

32. Tubular adenoma of small intestine and colon (Neoplastic polyps)

33. Villous adenoma of small intestine and colon (1991, 94)

Adenomas of small and large intestines

- Age <40 yr (20–30% cases), >60 yr (40–50% cases).
- Male and female equally affected, familial predisposition present.
- All adenoma arise as the result of epithelial proliferative dysplasia, from mild to carcinoma *in situ*.
- Slow growth rate.
- The most worrisome lesions are villous adenomas greater than 4 cm in diameter.
- Malignant transformation depends upon polyp size, histologic architecture and severity of epithelial dysplasia.
- Adenomas are classified into four types based on epithelial architecture:
  1. Tubular adenoma
  2. Villous adenoma
  3. Tubular villous adenoma
  4. Sessile serrated adenoma

S. No.	Traits	Tubular adenoma	Villous adenoma
1.	Definition	>75% tubular architecture	>50% villous architecture
2.	Occurrence	90–95% most common	1% of total adenoma
3.	Location	90% cases in colon, mostly rectosigmoid	More in rectum and rectosigmoid
4.	Age	Comparatively earlier	Older age
5.	Gross	Small, pedunculated	Large, sessile-velvety or cauliflower like masses projecting 1–3 cm above normal mucosa
6.	Histology	Stalk has fibromuscular tissues and prominent blood vessels; covered by non-neoplastic mucosa. Tubule like structures lined by dysplastic cells (darkly stained) in colonic crypts, otherwise normal mucin secreting clear colonic mucosa	Frond like villiform of the mucosa covered by dysplastic, disordered columnar epithelium
7.	Risk of malignancy	Lesser	More malignant transformation, pre-malignant condition

34. Difference between familial polyposis (2002, 03) and UC (1992)

35. Difference between pseudopolyps of colon and polyposis coli (1998)

36. Peutz-Jegher's syndrome (1998)

37. Familial polyposis coli (2007)

38. Classify polyps of intestine

Non-neoplastic polyps

i. *Hyperplastic polyps*
   - Most common polyps of large intestine
   - Epithelial proliferations that are thought to result from delayed shedding of surface epithelial cells lead to piling of goblet and absorptive cells.
   - The crowding gives rise to serrated surface (histological hallmark)
   - May be single or multiple, classically less than 5 cm.
   - Has no malignant potential.

ii. *Inflammatory polyps*
   - It present with clinical triad of rectal bleeding, mucus discharge, and a lesion in the anterior rectal wall.
   - The abnormal anorectal sphincter leads to recurrent abrasion and ulceration of overlying rectal mucosa. The recurrent injury and healing causes some degree of mucosal prolapse and formation of inflammatory polyps.

iii. *Hamartomatous polyps:* It has following types of polyps-

iiia. *Juvenile polyps*
   - Focal malformation of mucosal epithelium and lamina propria.
   - Usually occurs in children of age less than 5 years
   - Lesions occur in rectum and presents with rectal bleeding or prolapse
   - It may be sporadic or syndromic. Sporadic polyps are usually solitary

(retention polyp) and no malignant potential
   - Individual with autosomal dominant inheritance have 3 to 100 or more polyps. Juvenile polyposis syndrome has higher risk of colonic adenocarcinoma.
   - Microscopically, cystically dialted glands filled with mucin and inflammatory cells are seen in a background of lamina propria with mixed inflammation.

iiib. *Peutz-Jegher's polyps*
   - It is seen in small intestine, colon and stomach
   - It is a part of Peutz-Jegher's syndrome, an autosomal dominant syndrome. It consists of polyp, melanotic mucoal and cutaneous pigmentation and increased risk of extraintestinal carcinoma (pancreas, breast, lung, ovary and uterus). Polyps are not pre-malignant.
   - The growth presents as large and pedunculated polyps with a lobulated appearance.
   - Histologically, there is extensive connective tissue and smooth muscle arborisation (intermixing) throughout polyp. The glands are lined by normal looking intestinal epithelium

iiic. *Cowden syndrome and Bannayan-Ruvalcaba-Riley syndrome*

iiid. *Cronkhite-Canada syndrome*

Neoplastic polyps

i. *Adenomatous polyps—Tubular and villous adenomas-has malignant potentials*

ii. *Familial polyposis (FAP) syndrome*
   - FAP is autosomal dominant disorder (mutation of adenomatous polyposis coli, APC gene on chr 5q21) developing numerous colorectal adenomas (may be in thousand, for diagnosis at least 100 adenomas should be present)

- FAP usually presents before 30 years of age, and conversion to colonic cancer is 100% by middle age unless prophylactic colectomy is done.
- It is associated with Gardner syndrome (polyps, multiple osteoma, epidermal cysts and fibromatosis) and Turcot syndrome (polyps, CNS tumor-medulloblastoma, glioblastoma)

iii. *Heredity nonpolyposis colorectal cancer (HNPCC) syndrome*

39. Colorectal carcinogenesis or Colorectal carcinoma: etiology and pathogenesis (2001, 06, 09, 11) or Difference between Right sided and Left sided colorectal carcinoma

Etiology
- *Dietary factors*
  - Excess energy intake relative to requirement.
  - Low contents of indigestible dietary fibers—increased transit time and altered intestinal bacterial flora.
  - High contents of refined carbohydrate (less vitamins A, C, E).
  - Intake of red meat (high cholesterol and hence high bile acid secretion, whose bacterial byproducts in the colon are irritant).
  - Decreased intake of protective micro-nutrients (lesser vitamins A, C, E).

(*Also see Neoplasia: cancer and diet*)

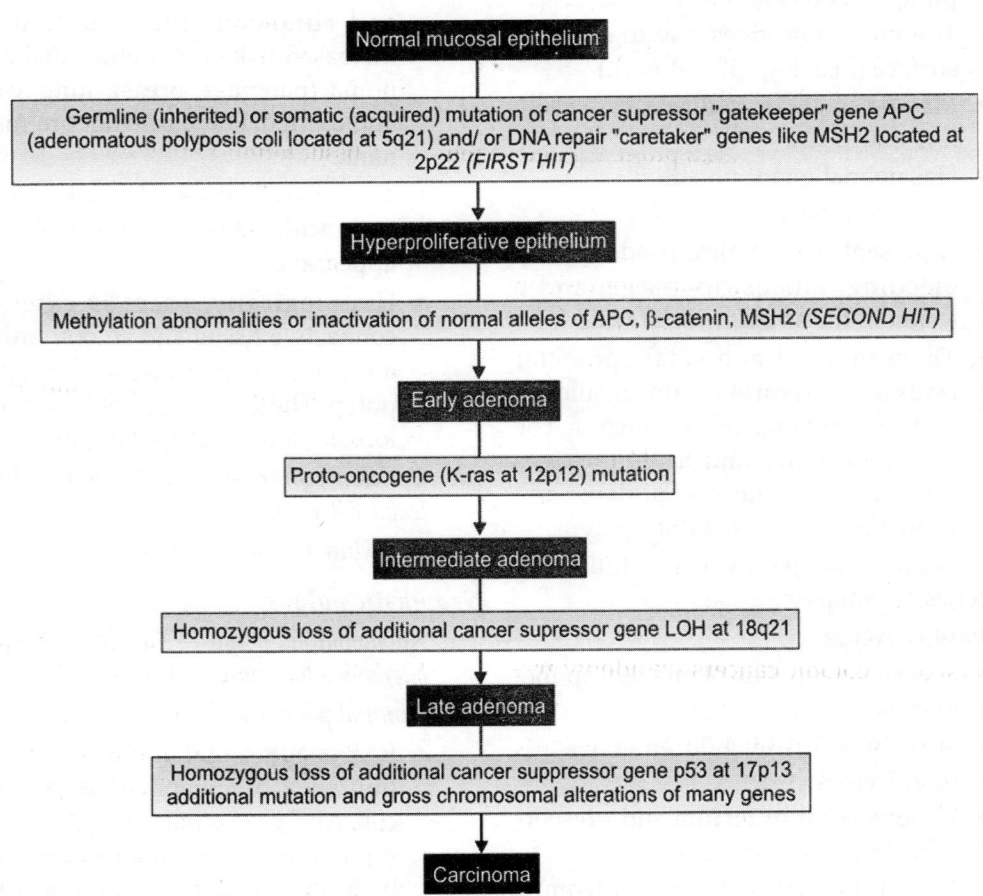

Fig. 16.1: Adenoma–carcinoma sequence

- Geographical variation
  - More common in North America and Northen Europe than South America, Africa and Asia.
  - *Familial history:* Only 1–3%; most are sporadic cases.
  - *Previous bowel diseases* like inflammatory bowel disease, adenoma and diverticular diseases.

Location
- Rectum (60%)
- Sigmoid and descending colon (25%)
- Cecum and ileocecal valve (10%)
- Ascending colon, hepatic and splenic flexures (5%)
- Transverse colon (rare)

- Mostly single

Two molecular pathways implicated in colonic cancer are:

i. *Adenoma-carcinoma sequence* (see Fig. 16.1)

ii. *Microsatellite instability pathway:* Sporadic gastrointestinal carcinomas, most commonly colorectal (hereditary non-polyposis colorectal cancer, HNPCC) and gastric carcinomas, may be associated with deficiencies of DNA mismatch repair (MMR) genes. Deficiency in cellular MMR leads to widespread mutagenesis and neoplastic development. The mutation is prominent in repetitive nucleotide regions, and these mutations are called microsatellite instability.

S. No.	Traits	Right sided proximal lesion of colorectal carcinoma	Left sided/distal lesion of colorectal carcinoma
1.	Location	Cecum and ascending colon	Descending colon and lower parts
2.	Gross appearance	Fungating polypoid carcinoma—Large cauliflower-like soft friable mass projecting into lumen	Carcinomatous ulcers—*Napkin ring* configuration, increased fibrous tissue forming annular ring and have central ulceration with slightly elevated margins
3.	Clinical features/presentation	Fatigue, weakness, iron deficiency anemia, bleed readily	Occult bleeding, change in bowel habits, crampy lower left quadrant discomfort, *melena, diarrhea* and *constipation*
4.	Diagnosis	Later, but not infiltrating	Early stage (theoretically) due to symptoms of *melena, diarrhea* and *constipation* but highly infiltrative at the time of diagnosis
5.	Prognosis	Good	Poor

- *Microscopic features* are common to both types of tumor:
  - 98% of all colonic cancers are adenocarcinomas.
  - Cell differentiation varies from tall-columnar cells invading mucosa and submucosa to undifferentiated anaplastic masses.
  - Stromal proliferation is high giving rise to firm, hard consistency to lesion.
  - Mucin production may be present, which have poorer prognosis.
  - *Variation:* Endocrine differentiation, signet ring appearance of tumor cells.

- *Spread of tumor*
  - Direct spread (circumferentially or transverse).
  - Lymphatic spread to local LN first, then regional and other LN group.

- Hematogenous spread to liver, lung, brain, ovary, etc.

40. Carcinoid tumor of GIT (1990, 97, 2000)

- Cells derived from epithelial stem cells in the mucosal crypts are present normally throughout the GIT mucosa.
- They coordinate the gut functions by releasing peptide and nonpeptide hormones.
- Due to their endocrine and paracrine functions they are called neuro-endocrine cells.
- Tumor arising from these cells is carcinoid tumor of GIT.
- *Age:* Any age; peak age: 50 yr.
- These cells may have argentaffin granules (stains positive with silver) or non-argentaffin granules.
- *Types* based on locations:

Midgut carcinoid:
- *Most common (60–70%)*
- *Argentaffin positive*
- *Terminal ileum:*
  - Later age—7th decade
  - Multiple
  - Female predominance
  - Metastasizes widely
- *Appendix:*
  - Most common gut carcinoid
  - Solitary
  - 3rd and 4th decade of life
  - Behave like locally malignant tumors; metastasis is rare
  - No sex predilection

Hindgut carcinoid:
- Occurrence (10–20%)
- Rectum and colon involved

Foregut carcinoid:
- Occurrence—10–20%
- Argentaffin negative
- Seen in stomach, duodenum and esophagus;

- *Morphology*
  Gross
  - Small button like submucosal elevations with intact or ulcerated mucosa;
  - Ileal and gastric carcinoids are multiple, whereas appendiceal carcinoids are solitary involving tip of the organ;
  - Cut surface is solid, yellow-tan.

  Microscopic features
  - Tumor cells are uniform in appearance (*monotonous* cell population) throughout the lesion forming discrete islands, strands, glands, trabeculae, or undifferentiated sheets;
  - Tumor cell has scant pink cytoplasm, round to oval stippled nucleus;
  - Mitoses infrequent;
  - Cellular atypia uncommon;
  - Other features: Well membrane bound secretory granules with osmophilic center (dense core granule), chromogranin A, synaptophysin, neuron-specific enolase may be present in cytoplasm.

41. Carcinoid syndrome (1993, 95, 97, 99, 2000, 01, 03, 07)

- It is present in 1% of all carcinoid tumor patients and 20% of patients when tumor has widely metastasized.
- Metastatic involvement of liver (loss of liver function) is prerequisite for the syndrome as liver converts active 5–HT into its inactive form 5–HIAA.
- *Secretory products* responsible for the syndrome: 5–HT (5-hydroxytyptamine, *serotonin*, most important), histamine, bradykinin, prostaglandins, etc.
- *Clinical features:* (*mnemonic: SHIVA*)
  - Cutaneous flushes and cyanosis present in most patients (*vasomotor disturbances*);
  - Diarrhea, cramps, nausea, vomiting in most patients (*intestinal hypermotility*);

– Cough, dyspnea, wheezing in 1/3rd patients (*asthmatic bronchoconstrictive attack*);

– Hepatic metastasis causing nodular liver (*hepatomegaly*) in some patients;

– *Systemic fibrosis* involving heart (right sided valves-stenosis and endocardial fibrosis), retroperitoneal and pelvic fibrosis, etc. in some patients.

42. Causes of melena (2000)

- Esophagitis (usually with hiatus hernia)
- Retching: Mallory—Weiss tear
- Peptic ulcer (acute and chronic): NSAIDs, *H. pylori*, stress induced
- Cancers of stomach and esophagus
- Vascular malformation of stomach
- Varices: Liver diseases and portal vein thrombosis
- Peptic ulcer in Meckel's diverticulum
- Crohn's disease of upper GIT
- Traumatic bleeding in upper GIT

43. Acute appendicitis (1993)

- Acute inflammation of appendix
- More common in older children and adult; rare in old aged person

Etiology

- *Obstruction*
  - Fecolith
  - Gallstone
  - Tumor
  - Foreign bodies
  - Ball of worms like *Oxyuriasis vermicularis*
  - Diffuse lymphoid hyperplasia
- *Others*
  - Inappropriate roughage intake
  - Hematogenous spread of infection to appendix
  - Vascular occlusion
- *Idiopathic reasons*

Pathogenesis

Obstruction or (and) infection causes secretion and accumulation of mucinous fluid in the lumen of appendix. Increased intraluminal pressure presses vein to cause collapse of venous drainage. Ischemic injury and bacterial proliferation result in further inflammation, edema, exudation and ischemic injury to appendix.

- "The *histological criteria* for the diagnosis of acute appendicitis in neutrophilic infiltration of the muscularis propria".

- *Stages of inflammation:*
  Normal appendix:
  - Serosa is glistening in color
  - No neutrophilic infiltrate

  Earliest stage:
  - Scant neutrophilic infiltration in mucosa, submucosa and muscularis propria
  - Subserosal vessels congested
  - Perivascular neutrophilic infiltration may be present

  Early acute appendicitis:
  - Organ swollen
  - Serosa hyperemic, dull, granular, red in color

  Acute suppurative appendicitis:
  - Serosa is coated with fibrinopurulent exudates
  - Ulceration and suppurative necrosis in mucosa may be visible

  Acute gangrenous appendicitis:
  - Hemorrhagic green ulceration in mucosa
  - Green black gangrenous necrosis
  - Followed by rupture and suppurative peritonitis

Clinical features

- Pain, first periumbilical; but after involvement of peritoneum it becomes localized to right lower quadrant
- Nausea, vomiting
- Abdomen tenderness in the affected area
- Increased WBC; mostly neutrophilia

Complications

- Perforation
- Adhesion
- Portal pylephlebitis
- Peritonitis
- Bacteremia

- Appendix abscess
- Hemorrhage
- Mucocele
- Liver abscess

44. Meckel's diverticulum (2000)

- This is the persistent proximal part of the vitello-intestinal duct which is present in the embryo, and which normally disappears during the 6th week of intrauterine life. It occurs in 2% subjects. Its lengths is 2 inches, and is situated about 2 feet proximal to ileocecal valve; attached to anti-mesentric border of the ileum. Its caliber is equal to that of ileum. Its apex may be free or may be attached to the umbilicus, to the mesentery, or to any other abdominal structures by fibrous hands.

- This is a true diverticulum having all three layers of bowel—mucosa, submucosa, and muscularis propria. It may have small region of gastric mucosa.

- *Significance*
  - It may cause intestinal obstruction.
  - Acute inflammation of diverticulum may produce symptoms that resemble those of appendicitis.

45. Difference between leukoplakia (2004) and erythroplakia

S. No.	Traits	Leukoplakia	Erythroplakia
1.	Definition	Is a white plaque on oral mucosa that can be removed by scrapping and can not be classified clinically or microscopically as another disease entity	Dysplastic leukoplakia—red, velvety, may be eroded area within oral cavity that may be slightly depressed or at the same level of surrounding
2.	Malignant transformation	5–6%	50%
3.	Histology	Orderly and regular hyperplasia of squamous epithelium with hyperkeratosis on the surface	Irregular stratification of epithelium Focal area of ↑ed and abnormal mitotic figure, hyperchromatism, loss of polarity, individual cell keratinization
4.	Occurrence	Common	Less

46. Define inflammatory bowel disease (IBD). Write briefly on its etiopathogenesis

(*Refer to textbook*)

17

Liver and Biliary Tract

1. Write briefly about bilirubin metabolism

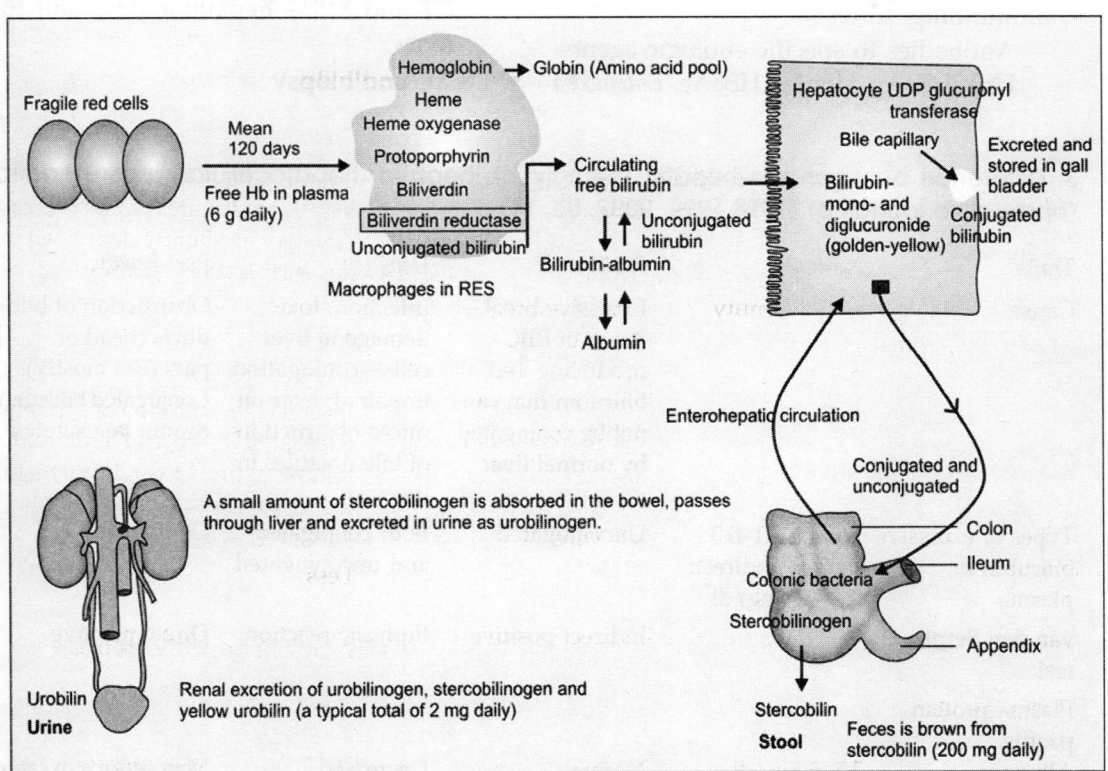

Fig. 17.1: Bilirubin metabolism

2. Enumerate liver function tests

- **Tests based on detoxification and excretory functions**
  - Serum bilirubin (total, direct and indirect)

- Urine bilirubin and urobilinogen
- Blood ammonia
- Serum enzymes
- Enzymes categories

- *Enzymes that reflect damage to hepatocytes:* Aspartate aminotransferase (AST or SGOT), Alanine aminotransferase (ALT or SGPT)
- *Enzymes that reflect cholestasis: LDH, 5' Nucleotidase, Gamma-glutamyl transferase (GGT), Bromosulphathein excretion test*
- **Tests for bio-synthetic function of the liver**
  - Estimation of plasma proteins: **Albumin and globulin**
  - Tests for reversal of A:G ratio: Thymol turbidity test
  - Tests for coagulability of blood: Factors I, II, V, VI, VII
- **Immunological tests**
  - Antibodies to specific etiologic agents- HBV-HBsAg, HBcAg, HBeAg, *Entamoeba*

histolytica, antibody to CMV, HCV, EBV, non-specific antibodies (anti-mitochondrial antibody-PBC, anti-smooth muscle antibody-auto immune hepatitis, pANCA-primary sclerosing cholangitis)
- Serum tumor markers (α-fetoprotein— ↑ in HCC)
- **Hepatobiliary imaging**
  - USG, CT scan—1st line investigation
  - ERCP, PTC—visualization of biliary tract
  - Doppler USG and MRI—hepatic vasculature and hemodynamics
  - CT and MRI—hepatic masses and tumors
- **FNAC and biopsy**

3. Difference between pre-hepatic (hemolytic), hepatic (hepatocellular), post-hepatic (obstructive jaundice) (1998, 1999, 2002, 03, 11)

Traits	Normal	Pre-hepatic	Hepatic	Post-hepatic
Cause	—	Excessive breakdown of RBC producing ↑ed bilirubin that cannot be conjugated by normal liver	Infection/toxic damage to liver cells—conjugation impaired; later on micro-obstruction of bile ductules in liver	Obstruction of bile ducts (head of pancreas mostly). Conjugated bilirubin cannot be excreted
Types of excessive bilirubin in plasma	Direct: 0.1–0.3 mg/dl; indirect: 0.2–0.7 mg/dl	Unconjugated	Both conjugated and unconjugated	Conjugated
van den Bergh test	—	Indirect positive	Biphasic reaction	Direct positive
Plasma protein profile:				
Albumin	3.5–5.5 g/dl	Normal	Decreased	May reduce in later stage
Globulin	2.0–3.5 g/dl	Normal	Increased	Normal
A:G ratio	1.7:1	Normal	Decreased	Usually normal
Serum enzymes level				
ALP/GGT	30–120 U/L	Normal	↑ed	↑↑ed
SGOP/AST	0–35 U/L	Normal	↑↑ed	↑ed/normal
SGPT/ALT	0–35 U/L	Normal	↑↑ed	↑ed/normal

(Contd.)

Difference between pre-hepatic (hemolytic), hepatic (hepatocellular), post-hepatic (obstructive jaundice) (Contd.)

Traits	Normal	Pre-hepatic	Hepatic	Post-hepatic
Urine bilirubin	Absent	Absent (acholuric jaundice)	Present (choluric jaundice)	Present (choluric jaundice)
Urobilinogen	0–4 mg/24 hr	↑	Decreased	Absent in complete obstruction
Fecal stercobilinogen	40–280 mg/24 hr	↑↑	Reduced	Absent, if complete obstruction
Fat	5–6% of total intake	Normal	Increased	↑↑
Thymol turbidity	—	Nil	Markedly ↑	Usually slight

4. Hereditary hyperbilirubinemia (1995, 98)

5. Gilbert syndrome (1994)

6. Dubin-Johnson syndrome (1994)

Disorder	Inheritance	Defect in bilirubin metabolism	Liver pathology	Clinical course
Unconjugated hyperbilirubinemia				
Crigler-Najjar syndrome type 1	AR	Absent UGT1A1 activity	Normal	Fatal in neonatal period
Crigler-Najjar syndrome type 2	AD	Decreased UGT1A1 activity	Normal	Generally mild course
Gilbert syndrome	AD (?)	Decreased UGT1A1 activity	Normal	Innocuous
Conjugated hyperbilirubinemia				
Dubin-Johnson syndrome	AR	Impaired biliary excretion of bil-glu due to mutation in canaliculi multidrug resistence protein (MRP2)	Pigmented cytoplasmic globules	Innocuous
Rotor syndrome	AR	Decreased hepatic uptake and storage. Decreased biliary excretion	Normal	Innocuous

7. Causes of portal hypertension (1990, 2003, 07) and its complications

It is characterized by prolonged elevation of portal venous pressure (≥ 12 mm Hg) due to increased resistance to portal blood flow.

- *Causes:* (see Table)

Complications

- *Ascites:* Transudate fluid (protein level <3 gm/dl, specific gravity 1.010, electrolyte concentration same as blood).

- *Varices* (porto-systemic shunts):
  - Esophageal varices (cardio-esophageal junction)
  - Hemorrhoids (veins around and in rectum)
  - Caput medusae (extending from umbilicus towards rib margin)
  - Retroperitoneal and falciform ligament anastomoses (periumbilical and abdominal wall collateral)
- Splenomegaly
- Hepatic encephalopathy
- Hematemesis and melena from variceal bleed

Pre-hepatic causes	Intra-hepatic	Post-hepatic
• Portal vein obstructive thrombosis • Narrowing of portal vein before ramification in liver • Tumor obstructing lumen • Congenital absence of portal vein	• Cirrhosis (*major cause*) • *Schistosomiasis* • Massive fatty change • Diffuse fibrosing granulomatous disease • Hepatic microvascular occlusive diseases • Metastatic tumor • Budd-Chiari syndrome	• Right sided heat failure • Constrictive pericarditis • Hepatic vein outflow obstruction

8. Mechanism of ascites in cirrhosis (1992)

- Ascites may be defined as the collection of excess of fluid in the peritoneal activity.
- Cirrhosis results in portal hypertension due to compression of central vein by perivenular fibrosis and expansile parenchymal nodule.
- Portal hypertension causes *increased resistance* in portal vein, abdominal capillaries (intestinal fluid leakage) which results in *transudation* of fluid into nearby peritoneal

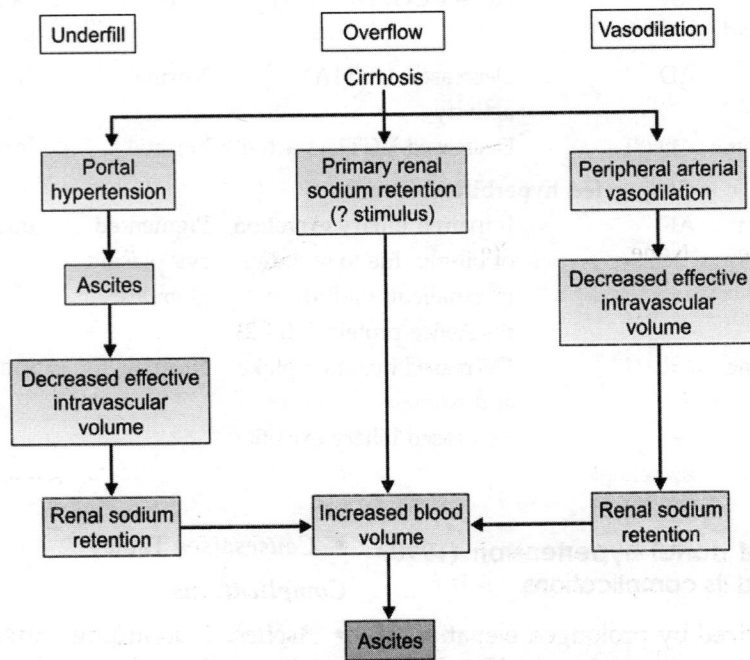

Fig. 17.2: Mechanism of ascites in cirrhosis

cavity and also helps in localization of fluid in peritoneal cavity.

- In cirrhosis, hepatic *lymphatic flow* increases (up to 20 L/day) but the capacity of thoracic duct lymph flow is fixed (800 ml/day); so protein rich and low triglycerides fluid accumulate as ascites.
- There is *decreased* synthesis of proteins including *albumin*, and also loss of albumin from blood/plasma into peritoneal cavity due to transudation (portal hyper-tension). This hypoalbuminemia results in reduced plasma osmotic pressure leading to loss of water into extravascular space.
- Due to decreased renal blood flow, impaired metabolism and excretion of *aldosterone*; there is increased serum level of aldosterone causing retention of salts and water.
- All these factors act together to cause ascites, which becomes clinically detectable when fluid is > 500 ml.

9. Brief outline of hepatitis viruses (summary)

Traits	Hepatitis A	Hepatitis B	Hepatitis C	Hepatitis D	Hepatitis E
Group: Genetic material	Picornavirus ssRNA	Hepadnavirus dsDNA	Flaviviridae ssRNA	ssRNA	Calciviridae ssRNA
Morphology	Icosahedral, non-enveloped	Double shelled, enveloped	Enveloped	Enveloped, replicative defect	Icosahedral, non-enveloped
Transmission	Fecal-oral	Parenteral, close contacts	Parenteral, close contacts	Parenteral, close contacts (endemic)	Water borne
Incubation period	2–6 wk	4–26 wk	2–26 wk	4–7 wk	2–8 wk
Age affected	Children	Any age	Adults	Any age	Young adults
Onset	Acute	Insidious	Insidious	Insidious	Acute
Illness	Mild	Occasionally severe	Moderate	Occasionally severe	Mild except pregnancy
Carrier state	None	Yes	Common	Yes	Unknown
Chronic hepatitis	None	5–10% of acute illness	>50%	5% (co-infection) 80% (superinfection)	None
Hepatocellular carcinoma	No	Yes	Yes	No	Unknown
Prognosis	Excellent	Depends on age	Moderate	Acute—good, chronic—poor	Good
Antigen	HAV	HbsAg, HbcAg, HbeAg	HCV, C100-3, C33c, NS-5	HbsAg, HDV	HEV
Antibodies	Anti-HAV	Anti-HBs, anti-HBc, anti-HBe	Anti-HCV	Anti-HBs, anti-HDV	Anti-HEV

(Contd.)

Brief outline of hepatitis viruses (summary) (Contd.)

Traits	Hepatitis A	Hepatitis B	Hepatitis C	Hepatitis D	Hepatitis E
Diagnosis	IgM Ab	HBs Ag or Anti-body HBc Ag	PCR for HCV RNA; 3rd generation ELISA for Ab detection	IgM and IgG Ab, HDV RNA in serum, HD Ag in liver	PCR for HEV RNA, IgM and IgG Ab
Prevalence	Worldwide	Worldwide	Probably worldwide	Endemic area	Only developing countries
Specific prophylaxis	Immunoglo-bulin and vaccine	Immunoglobulin and vaccine	Nil	HBV vaccine	Nil

10. Difference between hepatitis A and hepatitis B (1995)

(*Also see summary table*)

S. No.	Traits	Hepatitis A	Hepatitis B
1.	Mode of transmission	Infectious, fecal-oral route	Parenteral, close contact
2.	Carrier state	Absent	Present
3.	Chronic hepatitis	Absent	Present
4.	Age	Mostly childhood, <10 yr	All age group
5.	Viruses in:		
	Stool	Present: 2–3 wk before and 1 wk after onset of jaundice	Absent
	Body secretion	Not significant in saliva, semen, urine	Present in all physiologic and pathologic body fluids
6.	Viremia	Transient, so rarely transmitted by blood	Prolonged, remains in blood even during last stages of prolonged incubation period, also in active phage of acute and chronic hepatitis
7.	Vertical transmission	Absent	Present
8.	Fulminant hepatitis	Rare	More frequent
9.	Risk of hepatocellular carcinoma	Absent	Present
10.	Course of disease	Usually self-limiting	Variable, may be severe and fatal

11. Hepatitis B virus (1997, 2000, 01, 06)

(*Also see summary table, its sequelae, difference tables*)

Laboratory diagnosis

- HBsAg:
  - 1st marker to appear

- Present before transaminase appear
- Corresponds to onset of illness
- Present in circulation throughout the icteric/symptomatic course of the disease (up to 2 months, maximum 6 months): when absent from blood after appearing once, that means anti-HBs

antibodies have appeared in blood, which is protective in nature and remains for long time in blood.

- *Anti-HBc antibodies*
  - 1–2 wk after appearance of HBsAg;
  - No HBcAg in blood as it is enclosed within HBsAg coat;
  - *'Earliest antibody marker'* to be seen in blood: very long before anti-HBe or anti-HBs can be detected;
  - Life long: Prior infection can be detected even when all other viral markers become undetectable;
  - Initially IgM antibodies are predominant, after 6 months IgG type is dominant. Selective test positive for IgM type: recent infection, and IgG type: remote infection.
- *HBeAg*
  - Concurrently or soon after HbsAg;
    - Its presence in circulation: Denotes active intrahepatic viral replication;
    - Its disappearance coincides with fall of transminases level;
    - It is followed by appearance of anti-HBe antibodies.
- DNA polymerase, HBV DNA and virion (HBsAg): Its presence denotes high infectivity.
- HBV DNA: Denotes viral replication and infectivity.

  (*See textbook graph, also see microbiology table*)

12. Clinical feature and sequelae of hepatitis B (2008)

13. Sequelae/complications of HBV infection (2000, 04)

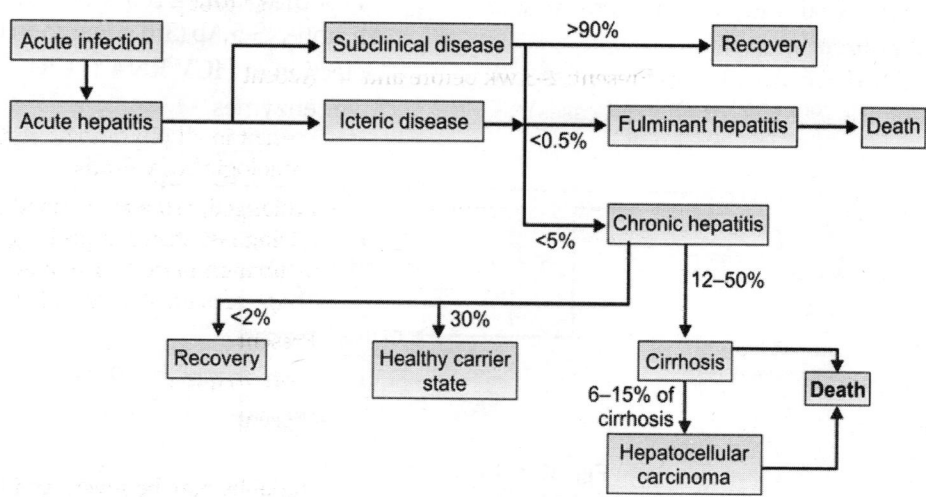

Fig. 17.3: Sequelae of HBV

14. Difference between chronic active and chronic persistent hepatitis (1994)

15. Chronic active hepatitis (1993, 2003)

Chronic active hepatitis: This is the form of chronic hepatitis where liver tissue destruction is continued; there is viral replication at pace. High titre of HbsAg, HbeAg, DNA polymerase, HBV, transaminases are present in circulation. Portal tracts show severe chronic inflammation with inflammatory cells extending into liver lobules disrupting the limiting plate of hepatocytes. Piecemeal necrosis, portal fibrosis, bridging necrosis and interface hepatitis are present.

Chronic persistent hepatitis: A form of chronic hepatitis where liver tissue destruction is minimal, viral replication is just sufficient to maintain constant viral population. HBsAg: Low, HBeAg: Absent, HBV: Absent, and DNA polymerase: Absent. Portal chronic inflammation is mild and restricted to portal triads, there is no disruption of the limiting plates. There is little or no necrosis and minimal fibrosis.

16. Non-A, non-B hepatitis (1991)

- Hepatitis caused by viruses other than HAV and HBV (e.g. HCV, HDV, HEV, HGV).

17. Serological diagnosis of HCV (2002)

18. Hepatitis C/Non-A non-B hepatitis (transfusion related) (1995, 98)

(*Also see summary table*)

- *Route* of transmission: Parenteral, close contacts; sexual and vertical transmission are infrequent.
- Most common cause of transfusion associated hepatitis (90–95% of all such cases).

- Carrier state and chronic hepatitis present.
- Chronic hepatitis is defined as symptomatic, biochemical or serological evidence of continuing or relapsing hepatic disease for more than 6 months. A carrier is an individual who harbors and can transmit an organism, but has no manifest symptoms.
- *Sequelae*
  - HCV is an unstable virus during its replication, giving rise to multiple types and subtypes of viral population. So, even elevated level of anti-HCV IgG does not offer much immunity during active infection.
  - Infection with HCV is persistent in nature causing more chronic disease (hepatitis) and thus cirrhosis (even more than HBV).
- *Laboratory diagnosis*
  - Detection of anti-HCV: Anti-HCV antibodies, anti-C100-3 Ab, anti-C33c Ab, anti-NS-5 Ab (3rd generation ELISA)
  - Detection of HCV RNA (PCR)
  - Liver enzymes

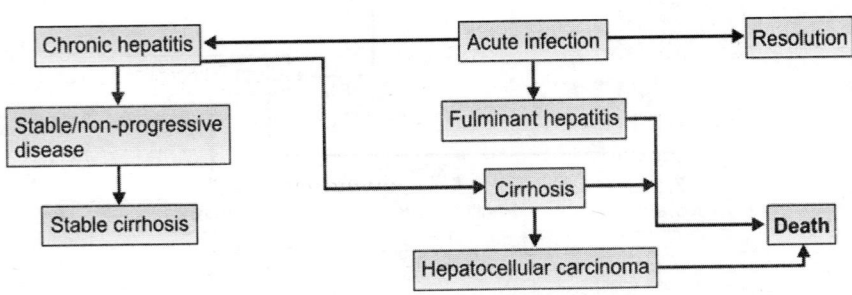

Fig. 17.4: Sequelae of HCV

19. Delta/D hepatitis (1996)

(*Also see summary table*)

- *Transmission:* Predominant transmission by nonparenteral router especially close personal contact (endemic areas).
  - Predominant transmission by parenteral route (same as HBV, non-endemic)
- HDV is an incomplete virus that is dependent on HBV for the outer coat layer HbsAg.

It causes hepatitis only in association with HBV. It may be confectious (HBV and HDV are introduced in patient simultaneously) or super-infectious a person having already HBV infection.

- *Sequelae*
  - Super-infection is more serious than co-infection. It may be due to preformed HbsAg particles availability in the former case.

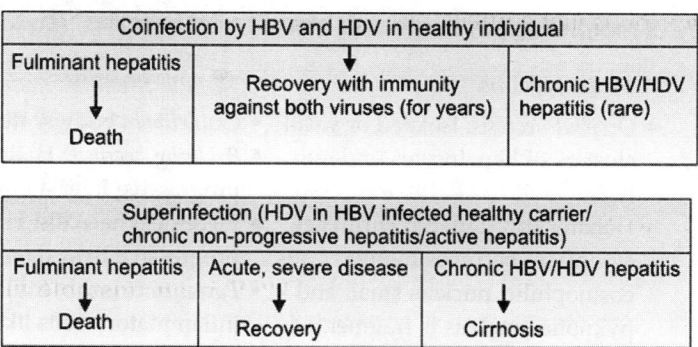

Fig. 17.5: Sequelae of HDV

- In coinfection, disease rarely progresses to chronic state; most of them recover (but less percentage of recovery and more fulminant hepatitis in comparison to HBV infection alone) in contrast to high degree of chronic progression and cirrhosis in superinfection.
- *Laboratory diagnosis:* (*See textbook graph*)
  - HDV RNA: Just before and early in the acute symptomatic phase, HDV RNA may be demonstrated in blood and liver cells by immunofluorescence technique.
  - Anti-HDV: IgM Ab: 2–3 wk after infection, most reliable indication of recent infection but short ilved. IgM is replaced by IgG in acute illness phage. In chronic illness IgM and IgG persists for months or longer.

20. HEV hepatitis/enterically transmitted/epidemic non-A and non-B hepatitis (1998, 2002)

(*Also see summary table*)

- *Transmission:* Drinking of fecal polluted water.
- Endemic outbreak.
- In India HEV is responsible for the majority of epidemic and sporadic hepatitis in adults.
- HEV is not associated with any carrier state or chronic liver disease or persistent viremia.
- A unique feature is the clinical severity and high case fatality rate of 20% in pregnant women, especially in the last trimester of *pregnancy*.

21. Comparative study of morphology in acute and chronic viral hepatitis* (1997, 2000)

	Acute hepatitis	*Chronic hepatitis*
Hepatocellular injury	• *Hepatocellular injury:* Marked in centrilobular zone. • *Ballooning degeneration:* Swollen hepatocytes are empty looking with granular cytoplasm having tendency to condense around nucleus. • Cholestasis: Canalicular bile plugs, not severe. • Fatty changes in hepatocyte in HCV infection.	• Throughout the lobule. Mild form around portal tract. • Lymphoid aggregates in portal tract, bile duct epithelial cell proliferation in HCV infection. • Cholestasis may be severe due to higher degree of fibrosis or secondary to cirrhosis. • Cases of chronic hepatitis B show scattered *ground-glass* hepatocytes (abundance of HBsAg in cytoplasm).

(Contd.)

Comparative study of morphology in acute and chronic viral hepatitis* (Contd.)

	Acute hepatitis	Chronic hepatitis
Hepatocellular necrosis	• *Dropout necrosis:* Isolated or small clusters of hepatocytes undergo lysis. • Hepatocytes undergo shrinkage, cytoplasm becomes highly eosinophilic, nucleus small and pyknotic, nucleus is fragmented and extruded from cell leaving a mass behind eosinophilic mass called *Councilman* body / acidophil body undergo apoptosis. • *Bridging necrosis:* In severe form, bands of necrosis linking portal tract to central hepatic vein, one central hepatic vein to another, one portal tract to another tract	• *Councilman* body scattered in lobule. • *Bridging necrosis:* Hallmark of progressive liver damage. • Piecemeal necrosis: Hallmark of progressive liver damage. • *Portal tract lesion:* Infiltration by inflammatory cells like lymphocytes, macrophage, plasma cells. Neutrophils, eosinophils rare. Bile duct proliferation.
Regeneration Sinusoidal cell reactive changes	Hepatocytes proliferation • *Kupffer cells* hypertrophy and hyperplasia – It contains phagocytosed cellular debris, bile pigment, lipofuscin granules • Panlobular infiltration of mono-nuclear cells (lymphocytes plasma cells, eosinophils) into sinusoids	Hepatocytes proliferation • *Kupffer cells* hypertrophy and hyper-plasia • Infiltration by chronic inflammatory cells
Portal tracts	• Inflammations predominantly mononuclear • *Piecemeal necrosis:* Hallmark of progressive liver damage	• *Inflammation: Confined to portal tract or interface hepatitis or bridging inflammatory necrosis* • *Fibrosis: Portal deposition or portal and periportal deposition or formation of bridging septa (Hall mark)*
Architecture	Liver architecture may be lost	Well preserved liver architecture in early stage, but may be lost once cirrhosis develop
Sequelae	Has varying sequelae depending on causative agent	*Post-necrotic cirrhosis* may develop
Causes	All hepatitis viruses—HAV, HBV, HCV, HDV, HEV	HBV, HCV, HDV (in association with HBV). Non-viral causes: Wilson disease, α1-antitrypsin deficiency, chronic alcoholism, drug induced and autoimmune diseases

*Chronic hepatitis is defined as symptomatic, biochemical, or serological evidence of continuing or relapsing hepatic disease for more than 6 months, with histologically documented inflammation and necrosis.

22. Piecemeal necrosis (2004)

- It may be present during *acute/chronic* hepatitis, inflammatory cells that are usually confined to portal tract area. If they are spilled to adjacent area (periportal area) resulting in necrosis of periportal hepatocytes: "interface hepatitis" is known as piecemeal necrosis.
- Hepatocytes are destroyed "piece by piece" away from portal area, and necrosed hepatocytes area present at the limiting plate in periportal zone. Infiltration by inflammatory cells is seen depending upon the type of inflammation (acute/chronic).
- Bile ducts undergo proliferation. Fibrosis in the area may be present.

23. Difference between macronodular and micronodular cirrhosis (1995)

24. Cirrhosis: Definition, causes, types and pathogenesis (1988, 92)

- **Definition:** Cirrhosis is the end stage of chronic liver disease defined by following:
  - Involve the entire liver;
  - Bridging fibrous septa either delicate bands or broad scars replacing multiple adjacent lobules;
  - Parenchymal nodule formation;
  - Disruption of the architecture of the entire liver.
- **Causes**
  - Alcoholic liver disease (60–70%)
  - Biliary cirrhosis (primary and secondary)
  - Viral hepatitis (post-necrotic cirrhosis) (10%)
  - Primary hemochromatosis
  - Nonalcoholic steatohepatitis (NASH)
  - Wilson disease
  - Indian childhood cirrhosis
  - Drug induced
  - α-1 antitrypsin deficiency
  - Cryptogenic (unknown cause) cirrhosis (10–15%)

- **Types**
  - *Micronodular (nodules less than 3 mm in size):* Early stage of alcoholic cirrhosis, nutritional cirrhosis, Laennec's cirrhosis, Indian childhood cirrhosis, hemochromatosis, Budd-Chiari syndrome, cirrhosis associated with biliary obstruction, jejuno-ileal bypass.
  - *Macronodular (more than 3 mm):* Postnecrotic cirrhosis, Wilson disease.
  - *Mixed:* Late stage of alcoholic cirrhosis.
- **Pathogenesis**
  1. "The central to pathogenesis in cirrhosis is *progressive fibrosis*."
  2. In the normal liver ECM consist of collagen type I, III, V and XI present around central veins in portal tract and in liver capsule.
  3. Liver does not have a true basement membrane instead, a delicate framework of type IV collagen and other proteins lie in the space between sinusoidal endothelium cells and hepatocytes (space of Disse)
  4. There is ↑ed deposition of type I and III collagen fibers in the space of Disse (*by Ito cells*); replacnig the delicate strands of type IV collagen.
  5. *Ito cells* (perisinusoidal hepatic stellate cells) are vitamin A fat storing cells, which under activation, lose retinyl ester stores to become myofibroblast like cells.
  6. These new fibers create delicate or broad *septal tracts*, which shunt the blood directly from portal triad to central hepatic venules bypassing blood flow and exchange to and from hepatocytes through sinusoids.
  7. *Continued fibrosis* in space of Disse also results in loss of fenestration (capillarisation of sinusoids) in sinusoidal endothelium and sinusoids become like capillaries impairing exchange of materials like nutrients, oxygen, protein formed by hepatocytes.

8. Liver damage and fibrosis stimulates remaining hepatocytes to *regenerate* and proliferate within the confines of fibrous septa. The net result is a fibrotic, nodular liver in which blood delivery to hepato- cytes is compromised: hepatocytes secretion of products decreases, stasis of bile, reduced net function of liver, increased resistance to blood flow through the liver.

25. Difference between morphological changes in alcoholic (1998) and post-necrotic cirrhosis (1999) (2001, 02, 03, 04)

or

Morphological features of alcoholic cirrhosis (2010, 11)

S. No.	Traits	Alcoholic cirrhosis	Post-necrotic cirrhosis
1.	Type	Initially micronodular, changes to mixed type (*hobnail appearance*) in long standing cases	Macronodular
2.	Gross	Initially liver is yellow-tan, fatty and enlarged, but later on in turns brown, shrunken, non-fatty organ. Cut section shows spheroidal or angular nodules of fibrous septa	Liver is small, shrunken, distorted shape with irregular and coarse scars and nodules. Cut section shows scars and varying size of macronodules
3.	Normal liver architecture	Hard to find	It is present in some areas
4.	Fibrous septa	They are initially delicate, later thick	Generally thick
5.	Inflammatory cells	Sparse infiltration of fibrous septa by mononuclear cells	Prominent mononuclear infiltration even forming follicles
6.	Mallory body	May be present, but rare	Absent
7.	Bile duct	Proliferation present, but not prominent	Extensive proliferation
8.	Fatty changes	Hepatocytes can be seen	Absent

26. Post necrotic cirrhosis: etiopathogenesis, morphological changes, complications

or

Difference between alcoholic cirrhosis and biliary cirrhosis (2008)

- *Pathogenesis and complications:* see pathogenesis of cirrhosis.
- *Morphological changes:* see difference table.

27. Fatty liver (2008)

Step 1. Starvation, toxins, DM, anorexia, alcohol abuse
Step 2 and 3. Anorexia, starvation

Step 4. Alcohol
Step 5. CCl$_4$

- Toxicity, protein energy malnutrition
- Defects in any of the six steps of uptake, catabolism or secretion result in accumulation of TGA in hepatocytes leading to fatty changes (Fig. 17.6).
- Chronic alcoholism (hepatotoxin altering mitochondrial and microsomal functions) produces fatty changes through multiple mechanisms like ↑ ed lipolysis, ↑ ed free fatty acid synthesis, ↓ ed triglyceride utilization, and ↓ ed fatty acid oxidation, also interfering with apoprotein synthesis.

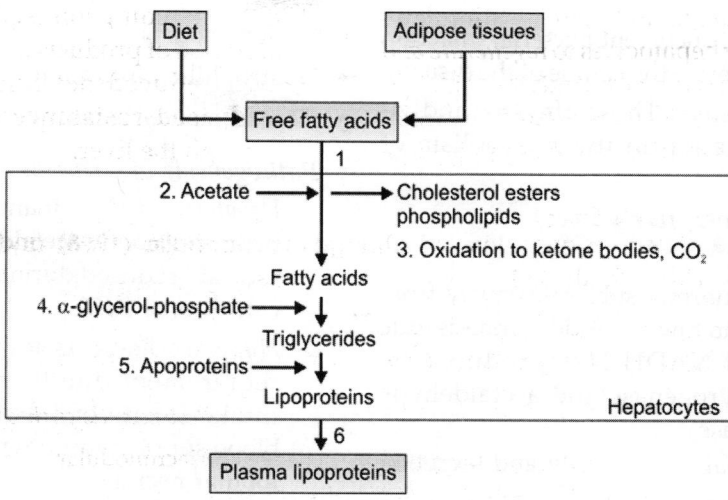

Fig. 17.6: Pathogenesis of fatty liver

Morphology

Gross

- Initially it is centrilobular but later on involve whole lobe
- Liver is large (4–6 kg)
- Yellow, greasy
- Soft organ
- Fragile
- No fibrosis at outset
- Fibrous tissue develop around the central vein and adjacent sinusoids

Microscopic features

- Hepatocytes show lipid vacuoles in its cytoplasm, which are initially small (microvesicular), but progressively coalesce to become macrovesicular; pushing nucleus to periphery.
- Such hepatocytes may rupture and lipoid vacuoles may coalesce to form fatty cysts.
- Stain for fat: frozen section; staining by Sudan dye IV, oil red-O and osmic acid.

28. Mallory bodies (1997, 2000, 03)

- These are eosinophilic cytoplasmic inclusions seen around nucleus in hepatocytes. These hepatocytes are degenerating and swollen (ballooning).
- This inclusion represents aggregates of cytokeratin intermediate filaments.
- Mallory bodies are characteristics, but not specific for alcoholic diseases.
- They are also present in primary biliary cirrhosis, Wilson disease, chronic cholestatic syndrome, Indian childhood cirrhosis, focal nodular hyperplasia, hepatocellular carcinoma and α_1-antitrypsin deficiency.

29. Pathogenesis of alcoholic liver disease (2006)

30. Etiopathogenesis and complications of alcoholic cirrhosis (1990, 94)

Alcoholic liver disease includes alcoholic steatosis, hepatitis and cirrhosis.

- *Etiology*
  - *Drinking pattern:* Even small amount for short period may be harmful, but large amount (50–60 g/d) for long period has been documented to have greater incidence of cirrhosis.
  - Gender: Women seen to be more susceptible to hepatic injury than men.
  - *Malnutrition:* Nutrients required for alcohol metabolism like vitamins and proteins deficiency that occur concurrently adds to the above cause.

- *Infection:* Concurrent bacterial infection may accelerate the course of the disease.
- *Genetic factors:* Those affecting individual variation in the metabolism of alcohol.

Alcoholic steatosis (fatty liver)
Pathogenesis

- Shunting of normal substrates away from catabolism and towards lipid synthesis (due to excess of NADH H + produced by alcohol dehyrogenase and acetaldehyde dehydrogenase)
- There is impaired assembly and secretion of lipoproteins
- Increased peripheral catabolism of fat

Gross: The liver is large, soft, yellow greasy.

Microscopic features: Even after moderate intake of alcohol, there is microvesicular lipid droplet accumulation in hepatocytes. With large and chronic alcohol intake, lipid accumulates creating large, clear macrovesicular globules that compress and displace the hepatocyte nucleus to the periphery of cell.

Alcohol hepatitis
Pathogenesis

- 15–20 years of excessive drinking can cause alcoholic hepatitis.
- Acetaldehyde, a major intermediate product of alcohol metabolism, induces lipid peroxidation and acetaldehyde—protein adduct formation, which disrupts cytoskeletal and membrane proteins.
- Alcohol directly affects microtubule organization, mitochondrial and membrane functions.
- Reactive oxygen species (ROS) generated during oxidation of ethanol can damage membrane and proteins. It in turn activates neutrophils, which again can cause inflammatory damage to hepatocytes.

Microscopic features

- Hepatocyte swelling and necrosis: hepatocyte swelling/ballooning (due to fat, proteins and water accumulation)

- Mallory bodies
- Neutrophilic infiltration
- Fibrosis: sinusoidal and perivenular fibrosis.

- **Pathogenesis of cirrhosis**
  - *Hepatotoxicity* by ethanol, its metabolic produce (mainly acetaldehyde) and free radical produced during metabolism by cytochrome P450.
  - *Hypoxia:* There is increased oxygen requirement due to chronic alcohol intake for its metabolism; impaired blood supply causes hypoxia and centrilobular necrosis.
  - Alcohol has inhibitory effect on the secretory action of hepatocytes resulting in accumulation of synthesized proteins within it.
  - Fat accumulation within hepatocytes takes place (*fatty changes*).
  - There is increased NADH: NAD (lactate: pyruvate) redox ratio causing *lactic acidosis.*
  - Immunologic mechanism is also proposed by which ethanol produces liver damage.
  - All these above factors result in common pathway (as explained in pathogenesis of cirrhosis) leading to alcoholic cirrhosis).

- **Complications**
  - Portal hypertension
  - Ascites
  - Hypoalbuminemia (edema)
  - Hepatocellular carcinoma
  - Variceal hemorrhages
  - Distended abdomen
  - Anemia
  - Increased clotting time / coagulation defects
  - Jaundice
  - Wasted extremities
  - Repeated infections

31. Biliary cirrhosis (2000, 2011)

Traits	Primary biliary cirrhosis	Secondary biliary cirrhosis	Primary sclerosing cholangitis
Cause	Autoimmune	Extrahepatic bile duct obstruction: Biliary atresia, gallstone, stricture, carcinome of head of pancreas	Unknown; May be auto-immune, 60% associated with inflammatory bowel disease
Male: Female ratio	1:6, 30–70 years	1:1	2:1, 30 years
Laboratory findings	Same as secondary, also ↑ed IgM auto-antibodies	Conjugated hyperbilirubi-nemia, ↑ed serum alkaline phosphatase, bile acids, cholesterol	Same as secondary, also ↑ed IgM, hypergammaglobuli-nemia
Clinical features	Same as secondary, also insidious onset	Pruritus, jaundice, malaise, dark urine, light stool, hepatosplenomegaly	Same as secondary, also insidious onset, 95% are AMA⊕, 20% ANA⊕, 60% ANCA⊕

Microscopic features

- *Primary biliary cirrhosis*
  - Chronic non-suppurative destructive cholangitis in small and medium intra-hepatic bile ducts.
  - Stage I: Bile duct lesion confined to portal tract.
  - Stage II: Widespread ductal proliferation with inflammatory infiltration beyond portal tract into surrounding hepatic parenchyma. Periportal mallory body may be present.
  - Stage III: Interconnecting portal tract fibrous scarring (florid duct lesion).
  - Stage IV: Micronodular type of cirrhosis.
- *Secondary biliary cirrhosis*
  - Bile stasis resulting in centrilobular necrosis of hepatocytes.
  - Proliferation, dilatation and rupture of bile ducts in portal areas resulting in 'bile lakes'.
  - Cholangitis and resultant inflammatory infiltrate.
  - Fibrosis starting from portal tract to adjoining areas with net result of micro-nodular cirrhosis.

- *Primary sclerosing cholangitis*
  - Obstruction of intrahepatic bile duct leads to proliferation of bile ductules, inflammation and necrosis of adjacent periportal hepatic parenchyma and cholestasis.
  - Large bile ducts shows periductal fibrosis that obliterates the lumen leaving a solid cord like scar with few inflammatory cells.
  - Fibrosing cholangitis.
  - Lymphocytic infiltrate around bile ducts: segmental involvement.
  - Obliteration of bile duct lumen due to periductal fibrosis.
  - Intervening bile ducts are inflamed, dilated and tortuous.
  - Cholestasis leading to biliary cirrhosis.
- ***Other features of primary sclerosis cholangitis***
  - Characteristic beading of contrast material seen in affected segment of biliary tree during retrograde cholangiogram (due to patchy involvement).
  - Associated with inflammatory bowel disease, pancreatitis and retroperitoneal fibrosis.

– Associated with antinuclear cytoplasmic antibodies (ANCA) with a perinuclear location is noted in 80% cases.
– Cholangiocarcinoma may develop in 10–15% cases.
– Median age is 30 years.

32. Hemochromatosis (1991)

- This is a condition characterized by excessive accumulation of iron in body, mainly in parenchymal organs like liver, pancreas.
- *Clinical features*
  – Micronodular cirrhosis
  – Skin pigmentation
  – Abdominal pain
  – Atypical arthritis
  – Risk of hepatocellular carcinoma
  – Deranged glucose homeostatis/diabetes mellitus
  – Hepatomegaly
  – Cardiac dysfunctions (arrhythmia, cardiomyopathy)
  – High level of serum iron and ferritin
- *Age:* 5th to 6th decade of life.
- *Sex:* Male predominance with slightly earlier presentation (in female menstrual and pregnancy loss of blood partially delays iron accumulation).
- *Pathogenesis*
  – *Genetic/hereditary hemochromatosis*: Homozygous recessive heritable disease. HLA-H linked.
    There is primary defect in *intestinal absorption* of dietary iron, leading to net iron accumulation of 0.5–1.0 gm/yr. There may be defect in plasma β_2 microglobulin.
  – *Secondary hemochromatosis*: Transfusion, iron dextran injection, ineffective erythropoiesis with ↑ ed erythroid activity, ↑ ed oral intake of iron, chronic liver disease, congenital atransferrinemia, etc.

Mechanism of iron toxicity
– Lipid peroxidation through iron catalyzed free radical reactions.
– Stimulation of collagen formation by stimulating Ito cells/hepatic stellate cells.
– Direct interaction of iron and reactive oxygen species with DNA resulting in cell injury.
– Iron is direct hepatotoxic.

- *Morphology*
  – Deposition of golden yellow pigment hemosiderin (which takes blue color with Prussian blue stain) in liver, pancreas, myocardium, pituitary, adrenal, parathyroid and thyroid glands.
  – Pancreas show diffuse interstitial fibrosis and parenchymal atrophy with hemosiderin deposits in the acinar and islet cells (causing diabetes).
  – Heart is enlarged with hemosiderin deposits in myocardial fiber (causing arrhythmias and cardiomyopathy).
  – Hemosiderin deposition in the synovium of joints leads to acute synovitis.
  – Testes are small and atrophied.
  – Inflammation is absent (characteristics).
  – Pigmentation of bile duct epithelium and Kupffer cell.
  – Liver is slightly larger than normal, dense, chocolate brown color.

33. α1-antitrypsin (1995)

- This is a plasma glycoprotein synthesized predominantly by hepatocytes, which acts as serum protease (like neutrophil elastase) inhibitor to prevent breakdown of elastin and collagen.
- Its deficiency causes pulmonary *emphysema* and cirrhosis.
- Neonates present with hepatitis and cholestatic jaundice.
- Adults present with hepatitis or cirrhosis.
- Increased risk of hepatocellular carcinoma.

- **Pathogenesis**
  - It is coded by *polymorphic gene* located on chromosome 14.
  - Most common genotype is *PiMM* (90% person): Normal phenotype.
  - Genotype PiZZ (homozygous) have abnormally low level of α-1 antitrypsin while *PiMZ* (heterozygous) have intermediate level.
  - These **defective variants** produce polypeptides that are abnormally folded, so blocking its movement/secretion from endoplasmic reticulum to Golgi apparatus. Thus, this abnormal polypeptide accumulates in hepatocytes.
  - In such group of people, there is decreased capacity to degrade abnormally folded or unassembled polypeptides.
  - α-1 antitrypsin deficiency is characterized by presence of round to oval cytoplasmic globular inclusions in hepatocytes. In routine H and E staining, these are acidophilic and poorly demarcated from surrounding.
  - They are strongly PAS positive and diastase resistance.

34. Indian childhood cirrhosis (1995, 96)

- This is an unusual and unexplained form of micronodular cirrhosis found in Indian subcontinent.
  - It is seen mainly in childhood between the age of 3 months and 3 yrs.
  - It has familial incidence thus showing genetic or common environmental origin (lately genetic origin has been ruled out).

- *Early stage* may show hepatomegaly and splenomegaly, which are insidious in onset.
- *Late stage:* It shows progressive liver damage. Histologically five groups of diseases are identified, of which type II is the most important. It is characterized by:
  - Ballooning degeneration of hepatocytes.
  - Liver cells showing mallory bodies and neutrophilic exudates surrounding hepatocytes.
  - Finally, micronodular cirrhosis results with aggressive fibrosis and scanty inflammatory cell response.
  - Focal necrosis, intracellular hyaline material may be present.
  - It may be confused with acute alcoholic hepatitis, but there is no *fatty changed* and almost *no regeneration* of parenchyma.
- Though mechanism of pathogenesis is not clear, but there is ↑↑ed Cu^{2+} and its binding proteins in liver in affected children as well as asymptomatic siblings. Also, level of non-toxic Zn has also been found to be increased. Genetic origin and causative role of Cu^{2+} has been dispelled. Instead, the possible hepatotoxic effects of post-puerperal domestic therapeutic remedies appear to be more plausible.
- *Clinical course:* In most of the children, non-specific symptoms like abdominal distension and enlargement of liver are followed by cirrhosis features like ascites, liver failure bleeding from portal hypertension leading to death.
- *Prognosis:* Bad, as there is no hepatocytes regeneration.

35. Difference between amoebic and pyogenic liver abscess (1993, 2010)

S. No.	Traits	Amoebic liver abscess	Pyogenic liver abscess
1.	Organism	E. histalytica	E. coli, Pseudomonas, Klebsiella, Enterobacter
2.	Area involved	Posterosuperior part of right lobe	Mainly right lobe, posterior part
3.	Lesion	Single, size vary greatly	Single or multiple, 1 cm or > 1 cm

(Contd.)

Difference between amoebic and pyogenic liver abscess (Contd.)

S. No.	Traits	Amoebic liver abscess	Pyogenic liver abscess
4.	Contents	The center of pus has large necrotic area containing reddish-brown, thick pus resembling anchovy or chocolate sauce. Abscess is surrounded by necrotic liver tissue	It has yellow colored typical pus. Large abscess may have thick fibrous capsule
5.	Microscopy	Single abscess having degenerated liver cells, leukocytes, RBC, connective tissues, debris, E. histolytica	Multiple small neutrophilic abscess (suppurative lesion)
6.	Stool	E. histolytica may be present	Absent
7.	Septicemia	Absent, less	Usually follow it due to spread
8.	Jaundice	Rare	Always present

36. Nutmeg liver/CVC liver (1993, 2001)

- **Cause:** Right sided heart failure, occlusion of inferior vena cava and hepatic vein.
- **Morphology**
  Gross features: The liver is enlarged, tense, and cyanotic with rounded edges. The central region (centrilobular) of lobule are red-brown and slightly depressed (due to loss of cells) and are accentuated against the surrounding zones of uncongested tan liver, so called *nutmeg liver*.
- **Microscopic features**
  - More marked hypoxia in centrilobular area, so centrilobular necrosis and hemorrhage.
  - Peripheral hepatocytes are less affected due to this chronic hypoxia and may show fatty changes.
  - Long standing CVC may show 'cardiac cirrhosis' leading to centrilobular fibrosis.

37. Hepatocellular carcinoma (HCC): Etio-pathogenesis (1993, 99, 2004, 08)

- HCC accounts for 80–90% of all liver cancers.
- Occurs more often in men than women, usually between 50 and 60 years of age.
- Predisposing factors:
  - Chronic hepatitis B and C
  - Alcoholic cirrhosis
  - Hematochromatosis
  - Wilson's disease
  - Alfatoxins
  - Primary biliary cirrhosis
  - α1-antitrypsin deficiency
- **Pathogenesis**
  - HBV infection: Repeated cell death and regeneration, mutation accumulation during rapid cell division (also in HCV infection); HBV DNA gets integrated with hepatocytes genome. It is proposed that HBV X-protein acts as transactivator of cellular and viral promoter helping in carcinogenesis.
  - Aflatoxin: Its metabolite binds to host DNA to form mutagenic adducts in genes like p53.
  - Alcoholic cirrhosis and primary hemochromatosis also play role in carcinogenesis.
  - Defect in DNA repair, point mutation or over expression of cellular gene.

Morphology
Gross
- Expanding type: More frequently, unifocal, large mass, yellow-brown, most often in right lobe, central necrosis, hemorrhage, occasional bile staining.
- Multifocal type: Less frequent, multifocal, multiple nodules of variable sizes, scattered throughout liver.
- Infiltrative type: Diffuse infiltrating.

Microscopy
- Histologic pattern:
  - Trabecular
  - Compact pattern
  - Pseudoglandular or acinar pattern
  - Cirrhous pattern
- Cell features: Cells resemble hepatocytes having vesicular nuclei with prominent nucleoli, cytoplasm is granular and eosinophilic. Cellular atypia and pleomorphism are present depending upon differentiation.

Investigations
- Markedly increased levels of α-fetoprotein and CEA
- USG and CT scan of abdomen
- FNAC or biopsy

38. Gallstones: Mechanism of formation, types, and complications (1997, 2000, 01, 07, 08, 10)

39. Etiopathogenesis of gallstone (2004)

40. Risk factors for gallstones (2009, 11)

Risk factors for gallstone include (five F): Fat, fertile (multiparous), flatulent female of forty (and more age)

Risk factors for cholesterol stones
- Demography: Northen Europeans, north and south Americans, native Americans, and Mexican Americans
- Advancing age
- Female gender and female hormones (oral contraceptive pills)
- Obesity and rapid weight reduction
- Gallbladder stasis and inborn disorders of bile acid metabolism
- Hyperlipidemia syndromes

Risk factors for pigmented stones
- Demography: Asian more than western
- Chronic hemolytic anemia syndromes
- Biliary infection
- Gastrointestinal disorders: ileal disease and cystic fibrosis with pancreatic insufficiency.

Cholesterol stones
"When the cholesterol concentration exceeds the solubilizing capacity of bile, i.e. supersaturated cholesterol can not remain in the dispersed form. Cholesterol nucleates into solid monohydrate crystals which further organize into cholesterol stone".

- *Four simultaneous defects*
  - Supersaturation of bile with cholesterol
  - Gallbladder hypomotility: Promoting nucleation
  - Cholesterol nucleation in bile is accelerated
  - Mucus hypersecretion: Trap crystal and fusion to form stone
- *Steps in cholesterol stone formation*

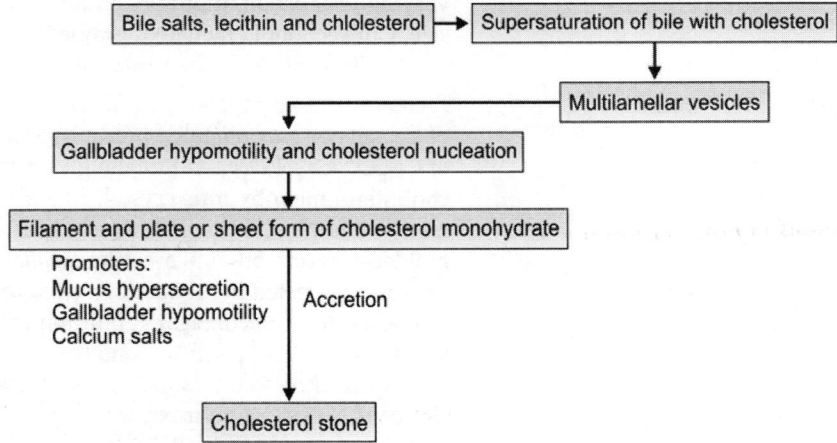

Fig. 17.7: Cholesterol stone formation

Pigment stones
- Mixture of insoluble calcium salts of unconjugated bilirubin along with inorganic calcium salts.
- *Cause:* Intravascular hemolysis and infection of biliary tract by *Escherichia coli*, round worm, opisphorchis sinensis (release of microbial glucuronidase), ↑↑ed unconjugated bilirubin.

Complications (2001, 10)
- When gallstones remain within gallbladder:
  - Cholecystitis
  - Biliary cirrhosis

- Cholecystitis may lead to perforation, generalized peritonitis, abscess formation
- Mucocele/hydrops
- Gallbladder cancer
- Biliary fistula
- Empyema
- When in the biliary tract:
  - Obstructive jaundice
  - Cholangitis
  - Cholecytocolic fistula
  - Pancreatitis
- When in GIT:
  - Gallstone ileus (intestinal obstruction)

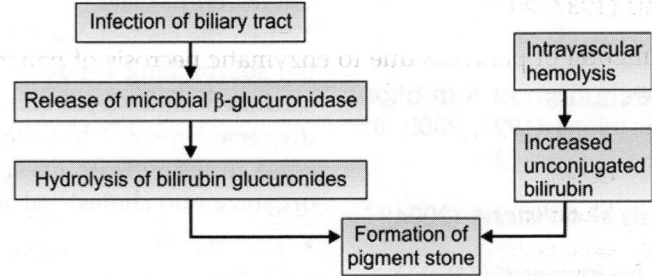

Fig. 17.8: Pathogenesis of pigment stone

Types of gallstones (viva) (1997)		
Cholesterol stone*	Pure cholesterol	Pale yellow, round to oval, finely granular, hard external surface, cut section reveals radiating glistering crystals, *radiolucent*
	Mixed	Cholesterol + $CaCO_3$, $Ca_3 (PO_4)_2$, and bilirubin in varying proportion, multiple, multifaceted, variable size, Cut section: Lamellated, gray-white to black, If > 10–20% of $CaCO_3$ then *radio-opaque*
Pigment stone	Black	Present in sterile gallbladder bile, oxidized polymers of Ca salts of unconjugated bilirubin; some amount of $CaCO_3$, $Ca_3 (PO_4)_2$, and mucin glycoprotein, cholesterol monohydrate crystal; Size: <1.5 cm, many in number, crumble to touch, speculated and molded contour, 50–70% are *ratio-opaque*
	Brown	Present in infected intrahepatic or extrahepatic ducts, pure Ca salts of unconjugated bilirubin, mucin glyco-protein, Ca salts of palmitate and stearate and greater amount of cholesterol; laminated, soft, greasy/soap like consistency, radiolucent

*Exclusively in gallbladder, cholesterol contents: 100–50%.

18

Pancreas

1. Acute pancreatitis (1987, 2003)

It is an acute inflammation of pancreas due to enzymatic necrosis of pancreas presenting as acute abdominal pain.

Causes

Metabolic	Genetic	Mechanical	Vascular
Alcoholism	Mutations in the	Gallstones	Shock
Hyperlipoproteinemia	cationic trypsinogen	Trauma	Atheroembolism
Hypercalcemia	and trypsin inhibitor	Iatrogenic injury	Vasculitis
Drugs (azathioprine)	genes	(operative injury, endoscopic procedure with dye injection)	
Infectious	Idiopathic pancreatitis		
Mumps			
CMV			
EBV			

Clinical features

- Acute, severe pain in abdomen, initially left upper quadrant followed by generalized pain in abdomen. Pain may radiate to back.
- Nausea and vomiting
- Cardiorespiratory symptoms (tachycardia, hypotension, tachypnea) followed by shock.

Laboratory diagnosis

- Leukocyte count: Increased, neutrophilia
- Serum amylase: It is a sensitive marker in the first 24 hours, if the value is more than four times of the normal value.
- Serum lipase: It is more specific than serum amylase, but appears later than amylase.
- Urinary amylase: Amylase is excreted in urine and level increases from 2nd day onwards and may remain elevated for 7– 10 days.
- Serum trypsin: This enzyme has the highest specificity and sensitivity for pancreatic injury, but its measurement requires use of radioimmunoassay.
- Hypocalcemia: Persistent hypocalcemia denotes poor prognosis. Hypocalcemia is due to precipitation in the areas of necrosis.

Pathogenesis

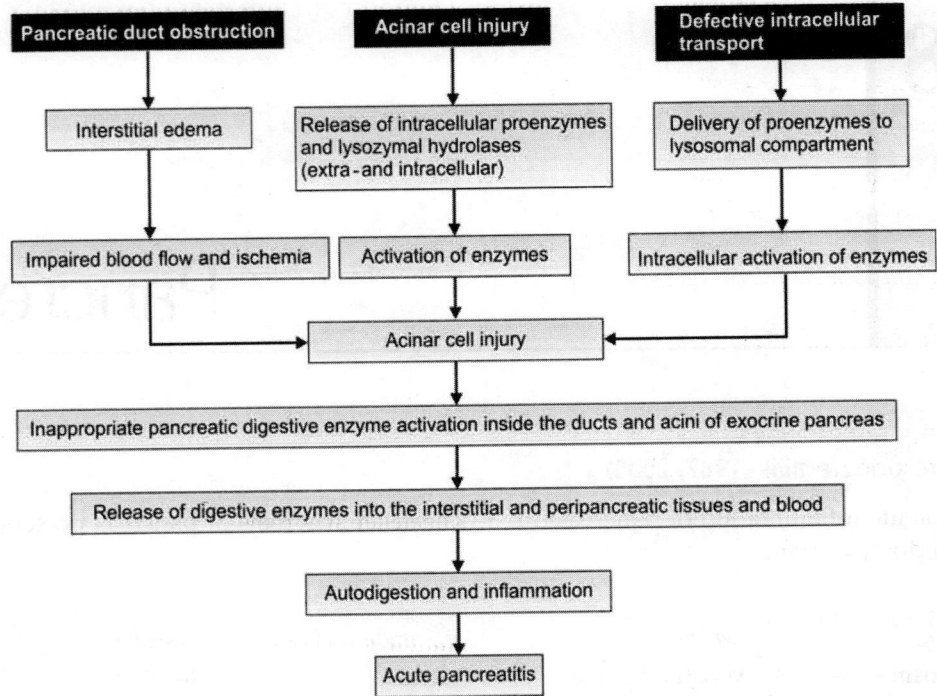

Fig. 18.1: Pathogenesis of acute pancreatitis

- Radiological: Ultrasonography and CT scan

Complications
- Systemic organ failure
- Shock
- Disseminated intravascular coagulopathy
- Acute respiratory distress syndrome
- Renal failure
- Pancreatic abscess
- Ileus (intestinal obstruction)
- Subcutaneous fat necrosis
- Pancreatic pseudocyst formation
- Chronic pancreatitis

2. Classify diabetes mellitus

Etiologic classification of diabetes mellitus (American Diabetes Association 2012)

Type 1 diabetes (β cell destruction, usually leading to absolute insulin deficiency)
- Immune-mediated
- Idiopathic

Genetic defects of β cell function
- Chromosome 12, HNF-1α (MODY₃)
- Chromosome 7, glucokinase (MODY₂)
- Chromosome 20, HNF-4α (MODY₁)
- Chromosome 13, insulin promoter factor-1 (IPF-1; MODY₄)

Type 2 diabetes (may range from predominantly insulin resistance with relative insulin deficiency to a predominantly secretory defect with insulin resistance)

Genetic defects in insulin action
- Type A insulin resistance
- Leprechaunism
- Rabson-Mendenhall syndrome
- Lipoatrophic diabetes
- Others

(Contd.)

Etiologic classification of diabetes mellitus (American Diabetes Association 2012) (*Contd.*)
- Chromosome 17, HNF-1β (MODY$_5$)
- Chromosome 2, Neuro D$_1$ (MODY$_6$)
- Mitochondrial DNA
- Others

Diseases of the exocrine pancreas
- Pancreatitis
- Trauma/pancreatectomy
- Neoplasia
- Cystic fibrosis
- Hemochromatosis
- Fibrocalculous pancreatopathy
- Others

Drug or chemical induced

Vacor
Pentamidine
Nicotinic acid
Glucocorticoids
Thyroid hormone
Diazoxide
β-adrenergic agonists
Thiazides
Dilantin
γ-interferon
Others

Uncommon forms of immune-mediated diabetes
"Stiff-man" syndrome
Anti-insulin receptor antibodies
Others

Gestational diabetes mellitus

Endocrinopathies
- Acromegaly
- Cushing's syndrome
- Glucagonoma
- Pheochromocytoma
- Hyperthyroidism
- Somatostatinoma
- Aldosteronoma
- Others

Other genetic syndromes sometimes associated with diabetes
Down syndrome
Klinefelter syndrome
Turner syndrome
Wolfram syndrome
Friedreich ataxia
Huntington chorea
Laurence-Moon-Biedl syndrome
Myotonic dystrophy
Porphyria
Prader-Willi syndrome
Others

Infections

Congenital rubella
Cytomegalovirus
Others

3. Laboratory diagnosis of diabetes mellitus (2003, 08)

American Diabetes Association 2012 diagnostic criteria of diabetes milletus

HbA1c ≥ 6.5% or

Fasting plasma glucose (FPG) ≥ 126 mg/dl (7.0 mmol/l). Fasting is defined as no caloric intake for at least 8 hours, or

Two hours plasma glucose ≥ 200 mg/dl (11.1 mmol/l) during an oral glucose tolerance test. The test should be performed as described by the World Health Organization, using a glucose load containing the equivalent of 75 g anhydrous glucose dissolved in water, or

In a patient with classic symptoms of hyperglycemia or hyperglycemic crisis, a random plasma glucose ≥ 200 mg/dl (11.1 mmol/l)

In the absence of unequivocal hyperglycemia or presence of acute metabolic decompensation, these criteria (1–3) should be confirmed by repeat test.

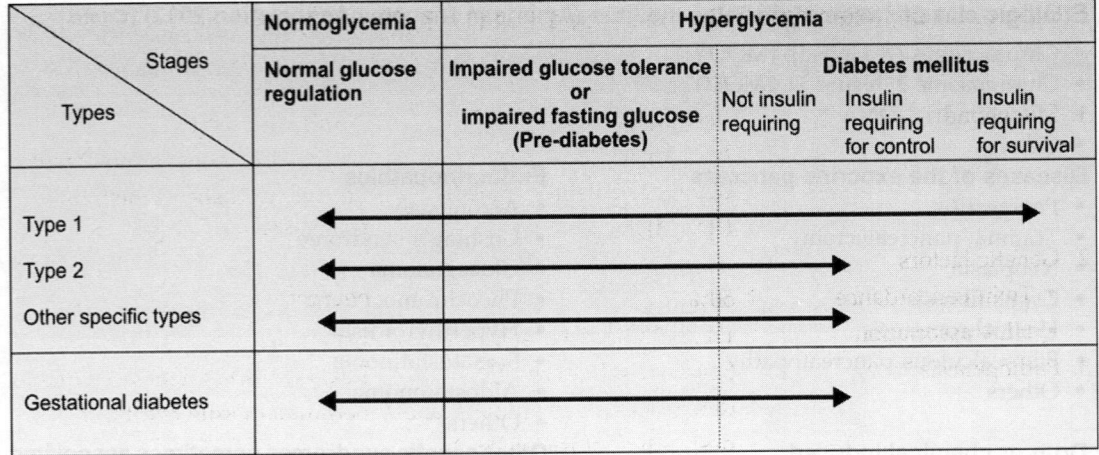

	Normoglycemia	Hyperglycemia			
	Normal glucose regulation	Impaired glucose tolerance or impaired fasting glucose (Pre-diabetes)	Diabetes mellitus		
Stages / Types			Not insulin requiring	Insulin requiring for control	Insulin requiring for survival
Type 1					
Type 2					
Other specific types					
Gestational diabetes					

Fig. 18.2

Impaired fasting glucose (IFG)
Fasting plasma glucose 110 to 125 mg/dl
Impaired glucose tolerance test (IGT)
Plasma glucose between 140 and 200 mg/dl, 2 hours after oral glucose load
A few other tests that aid to the diagnosis of diabetes mellitus are:
1. Urine glucose (Benedict's test) and ketone bodies (Rothera test)
2. Oral glucose tolerance test
3. Extended GTT
4. Blood lipid profile
5. Insulin and C-peptide assay.

4. Glucose tolerance test (GTT) (1991, 93, 99, 2004)

- This is designed to test the integrity and power of a person's metabolic mechanism for glucose utilization after a challenge dose to check pattern and extent of blood glucose level reduction after test dose.

- *Interpretation*

- *Procedure:*
  - Patient is advised to have high carbohydrate diet for at least 3 days prior to scheduled test.
  - Patient comes for test after overnight fasting (time varies according to different recommendations, should be approximately 8–12 hours).
  - Fasting blood sugar sample is taken.
  - 75 g of glucose dissolved in 300 ml of water is given. Some flavoring agents that do not interfere with glucose metabolism may be added to make it tasty.
  - Blood and urine specimens are collected at half an hour/smaller intervals for 2–3 hours.
- *Reading:*
  - Blood/plasma sugar level is determined by colorimetric/other techniques.
  - Urine sample is tested for glucosuria to predict rough value of renal threshold value for glucose.

Time	Over diabetes		Impaired glucose tolerance	
	Plasma*	Blood*	Plasma*	Blood*
Fasting (mg/dl)	≥126	>110	>200 (one value)	>180
After 2 hours of dose (mg/dl)	≥200	>180	140–200	120–180

*Venous blood taken. According to WHO 1999—DM diagnosis by oral GTT.

5. Difference between type 1 DM and type 2 DM (1998, 2000, 07, 11)

	Type 1 DM	Type 2 DM
1. Synonyms	Juvenile onset DM Earlier also known as insulin dependent diabetes mellitus (IDDM)	Adult onset DM Earlier also known as non-insulin dependent diabetes mellitus (NIDDM)
2. Genetic factors		
• Twin concordance	50%	90–100%
• HLA association	HLA-DR3 and HLA-DR4 linked	No
3. Pathogenesis	Severe absolute insulin deficiency due to autoimmune destruction of islet cells	Relative insulin deficiency due to peripheral tissue resistance
4. Islet cells	Early insulitis Marked atrophy and fibrosis β-cell depletion	No insulitis Focal amyloidosis and atrophy Mild β-cell depletion
5. Clinical features		
• Frequency	• 10–20%	• 80–90%
• Onset age	• < 20 yr	• > 30 yr
• Weight	• Normal	• Obese
• Ab against islet cells	• Present	• Absent
• Ketoacidosis	• Common	• Rare
• Symptoms onset	• Abrupt and severe	• Gradual and insidious
• Serum insulin level	• Decreased	• Normal to high
• Plasma glucagon	• High, suppressible	• High, resistant
• Treatment	• Insulin replacement	• Diet control, lifestyle modification, oral hypoglycemics, insulin

6. Complications of DM (1986, 96)

- Brain:
  - Cerebral vascular infarct
  - Hemorrhage
- Heart:
  - MI
- Eye:
  - Retinopathy
  - Cataract
  - Glaucoma

- Gangrene
- Delayed wound healing

- Atherosclerosis of aorta, large- and medium-sized arteries
- Peripheral neuropathy

- Diabetic nephropathy Nephrosclerosis:
  - Glomerulosclerosis
  - Arteriosclerosis
  - Pyelonephritis
- Hypertension
- Microangiopathy

- Peripheral vascular atherosclerosis (accelerated)

- Autonomic neuropathy

- Pancreas (Type 1 DM):
  - Insulitis—islet cells loss
  - Leukocyte infiltration—β cell degranulation
  - Amyloid deposition (Type 2)
- Infections (Defective immunity)
- Ketoacidosis, hyperosmolarity

7. Advanced glycosylation end products (AGEs) (2001, 09, 11)

- AGEs are formed as a result of nonenzymatic reactions between intracellular glucose-derived dicarbonyl precursors (glyoxal, methylglyoxal, and 3-deoxyglucasone) with the amino groups of both intracellular and extracellular proteins.
- The degree of glycosylation is proportional to the blood sugar level, and this process is accelerated in the presence of hyperglycemia.
- Some of *properties:*

Chemical properties	Biological properties

• Cross-linking polypeptides of same protein-like collagen
• Trap nonglycosylated proteins like LDL, Ig
• Induces resistance to proteolytic digestion of AGE
• Lipid oxidation
• Nucleic acid damage
• Nitric oxide inactivation
	• Binds to AGE receptors on monocytes and mesenchymal cells
	• Induce
	  – Monocytes emigration
	  – Cytokine and growth factor release
	  – ↑ed vascular permeability
	  – ↑ed cellular proliferation
	  – ↑ed ECM production

- These products bind to a specific receptor (RAGE) presents on the inflammatory cells (macrophages and T cells, endothelium, and vascular smooth muscle). The vascular response results in:
  - Release of pro-inflammatory cytokines and growth factors from intimal macrophages.
  - Generation of reactive oxygen species in endothelial cells.
  - Increased procoagulant activity on endothelial cells and macrophages.
  - Enhanced proliferation of vascular smooth muscle cells and synthesis of extracellular matrix.

In addition to this receptor-mediated changes, AGEs can directly cross-link extracellular matrix proteins. The net result is decreased in vascular lumen compromising blood supply and functions of organs.

8. Ketoacidosis (1993)

Ketoacidosis is a pathological metabolic state associated with high concentrations of ketone bodies formed by the breakdown of fatty acids and the deamination of amino acids due to severe insulin deficiency and relative or absolute increase in glucagon. Acetoacetic acid, β-hydroxybutyric acid and acetone are ketone bodies. Acetoacetic acid and β-hydroxybutyric acid produce metabolic acidosis in the patient. Ketoacidosis is most common in untreated type 1 DM (sometimes type 2 DM) when the liver breaks down fat and proteins in response to a perceived need for respiratory substrate.

Predominant signs and symptoms are nausea and vomiting, pronounced thirst, excessive urine production, increased respiratory rate and abdominal pain that may be severe, clinical evidence of dehydration such as dry mouth, tachycardia and low blood pressure.

Pathogenesis: (also see Fig. 18.3)

9. Cells forming the islets of Langerhans and their functions (viva)

   i. Alpha cells: Secrete glucagon (increases blood glucose)

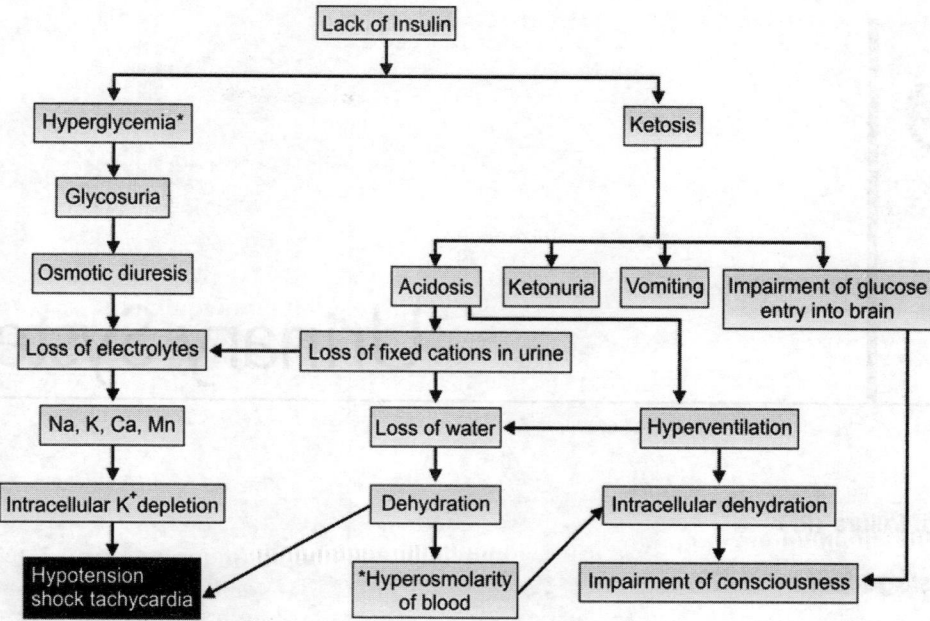

* Hyperglycemia also causes hyperosmolarity of blood directly.

Fig. 18.3: Pathogenesis of ketoacidosis

ii. Beta cells: Secrete insulin (decreases blood sugar level, anabolic hormone)
iii. Delta cells: Secrete somatostatin (inhibits the secretion of other islet hormones)
iv. Delta-1 cells: Secrete vasoactive intestinal peptide (VIP), which regulates and stimulates gut mobility.
v. PP cells: Secrete pancreatic polypeptide (stimulates gastric secretion and inhibits intestinal mobility).

10. Islets tumors of pancreas (1994)

(*Refer to textbook*)

19

Urinary System

1. Renal failure (RF)

2. End stage kidney (1992)

3. Laboratory findings of chronic renal failure (2001, 04)

4. Difference between acute and chronic renal failures—laboratory findings (1999)

S. No.	Traits	Acute RF	Chronic RF
1.	Definition and description	• Now renamed acute kidney injury (AKI) to incorporate the broad spectrum of kidney damage ranging from asymptomatic cases with transient changes of GFR to rapidly fatal derangement with severe oliguria, anuria and severe electrolyte imbalance and uremic encephalopathy. • Defined as an abrupt (within 48 hours), reduction of kidney function manifesting as increase in serum creatinine level or reduction in urine output or both.	• Now better termed chronic kidney disease (CKD). • It implies damage to the kidney, structurally or functionally, by some chronic processes. • Defined as either kidney damage or reduction in GFR to < 60 ml/min/1.73 m^2, or both, persisting for 3 months or more.
2.	Reversibility	Usually reversible, if managed timely	Leads to progressive and irreversible deterioration of renal function
3.	Causes	• Pre-renal – Caused due to decreased renal flow (hypovolemia, decreased cardiac output) – Functional integrity of kidney remains preserved	Caused by conditions leading to chronic insults to kidney Examples: Diabetes (DM nephropathy), hypertension (HTN nephropathy), chronic glomerulonephritis

(Contd.)

Difference between acute and chronic renal failures—laboratory findings (Contd.)

S.No.	Traits	Acute RF	Chronic RF

		• Renal
		  – Functional integrity of kidney is not preserved as actual site of injury in kidney itself
		  – Sites of injury: Vascular, glomerular and tubular
		• Post-renal
		  – Causes: Obstruction (ureter, bladder and urethra), functional (neurogenic bladder)
			Chronic pyelonephritis, reflux nephropathy, congenital defects in kidney (e.g. polycystic kidney disease)

	Clinicopathological profile		
	Urine output	Usually oliguria (a few are non-oliguric as in case of AKI due to nephrotoxic drugs)	Normal urine output is maintained till the last stage of disease.
	Azotemia	Not well-tolerated (patient develops symptoms even with modest rise in blood urea)	Well-tolerated (remain asymptomatic even with high levels of urea)
	Metabolic acidosis	Poorly tolerated	Well-tolerated
	Hypertension	May develop HTN, but being acute in nature and does not lead to organ damage	Develops chronic HTN leading to 2° damage to other organs as HTN retinopathy
	Growth retardation	No growth retardation	May lead to growth retardation, if disease occurs in childhood (due to anemia, ↓ appetite, growth hormone resistance and renal osteodystrophy)
	Anemia	Does not cause anemia	Causes anemia
	Skeletal damage	Does not produce damage to bone	Leads to renal osteodystrophy
	Glucose intolerance	Not present	Usually present due to insulin resistance

Laboratory diagnosis

Methods/sample	Traits	Acute RF	Chronic RF
Blood	Urea	Normal/↑ed	↑↑ed
	Creatinine	↑ed	↑↑ed
	Calcium	Normal/low	↓ed
	Phosphate	↑ed	↑↑ed
	Sodium	↑ed/↓ed	↑/↓ed
	Potassium	↑ed	↑↑ed
	Parathormone	Normal	↑ed
	Alkaline phosphatase	Normal	↑ed
	Erythropoietin	Normal	↓ed
Renal physiology	GFR	↓↓ed	↓↓ed

(Contd.)

Laboratory diagnosis (*Contd.*)

Methods/sample	Traits	Acute RF	Chronic RF
Urine	Urine output	↓↓ed	Initially normal, ↓ed later
Hematological	Hemoglobin	Normal (no anemia)	↓ed (anemia present)
examination	TLC	Usually normal	Normal
	Platelet count	Normal	Normal (but defective function, hence bleeding tendency)
	Reticulocyte count	Normal	N/↑/↓ed
	PBS	Normocytic normochromic RBCs, Burr cells may be present.	Normocytic normochromic RBCs, Not Burr cell
Radiological	USG	Normal kidney size	Small contracted kidney

5. Pathogenesis of chronic kidney diseases

Progressive and irreversible damage to kidney by some chronic process.

Its pathophysiology involves two steps:

I. Initation
- Various etiological factors like congenital defects, immune complex deposition, toxins, etc. may cause initial damage to kidney.
- This leads to loss of nephrons.

II. Progression
- Kidenys compensate for loss of nephrons by functional and structural changes in remaining nephrons.
- This includes:
  - Glomerular hyperfusion—increase in glomerular blood flow in the remaining nephrons, thus increasing "single nephron GFR".
  - Glomerular hyperfiltration—proportionate increase in tubular reabsorption.
  - Increase in volume of remaining glomeruli, i.e. increased capillary lumen volume and hypertrophy of cellular and extracellular constituents of glomeruli.

Thus kidneys compensate for loss of nephrons.

But once there is critical loss of nephron mass due to persistent chronic injury, the renal failure becomes progressive. The burden of progressively increasing hypoperfusion and hyperfiltration into the remaining nephrons ultimately cause pressure damage of the surviving glomeruli leading to distortion of glomerular architecture followed by sclerosis.

This constitutes the mechanism for progressive damage to kidney structure and function leading to chronic kidney disease.

6. Renal function tests

- *Urine examination*
  - Physical examination (color, specific gravity, pH, volume, osmolality)
  - Chemical analysis (protein, glucose, Hb, electrolytes—Na^+/K^+/Cl^-)
  - Microscopic examination (blood cells and casts)
  - Bacteriologic examination.
- *Blood examination*
  - Blood urea (BUN)
  - Serum protein
  - Serum creatinine
  - Serum cholesterol

- Serum electrolytes
- Serum uric acid
- *Renal clearance tests (CT)*
  Test for glomerular function:
  - Insulin CT
  - Creatinine CT
  Test for tubular function:
  - Urea CT
  - Para-amino hippuric (PAH) CT
- *Concentration and dilution tests*
  - Concentration test (fluid deprivation test)
  - Dilution test (excess fluid intake test)
- *Others*
  - Intravenous pyelography
  - Ultrasonography
  - Arteriography
  - FNAC
  - Renal biopsy

7. Difference between adult and childhood polycystic kidney disease

S. No.	Traits	Adult	Childhood
1.	Inheritance	Autosomal dominant	Autosomal recessive
2.	Pathologic features	Large, multicystic kidney associated with liver cyst and Berry aneurysm	Large cystic kidney at the time of birth
3.	Kidney cyst	Cortical and medullary cyst	Distal tubule and collecting duct cyst
4.	Clinical features	Hematuria, flank pain, hypertension	Bilateral abdominal mass
5.	Typical outcome	Chronic renal failure begins at the age of 40–60 yr	Death in infancy and childhood
6.	Complications	Subarachnoid hemorrhage, colonic diverticulum and mitral valve prolapse	Hepatic fibrosis, splenomegaly, esophageal varices

8. Pathogenesis of glomerular disease. Immune mechanism of glomerulonephritis.

Injury to glomeruli may be immune-mediated or nonimmune-mediated. Immune mechanism seems to underline most cases of primary GN and may cases of the secondary glomerular diseases.

Immune mechanism of glomerulonephritis

- Mostly antibody-mediated.
- Role of T cell-mediated injury has been found in certain glomerulonephritis.

Antibody-mediated GN

- *Circulating immune complex nephritis*
  - Antigens are not of glomerular origin. They may be endogenous (e.g. DNA in SLE) or exogenous (streptococcal, viral, malarial, spirochetal).
  - Antigen–antibody complexes are formed in circulation, and then trapped in glomeruli because of their physico-chemical properties and hemodynamic factors of glomeruli (Fig. 19.1).
- *In situ immune complex nephritis:* In situ antigens are already present in the glomeruli, either as an intrinsic part of glomeruli itself (fixed intrinsic tissue antigen) or non-glomerular exogenous antigen (planted antigen) already planted within the glomeruli.
- *Cytotoxic antibodies*
  - Antibodies against glomerular cell antigens may react with cellular components and cause injury by cytotoxic or other mechanisms. There is no immune deposition in this case.

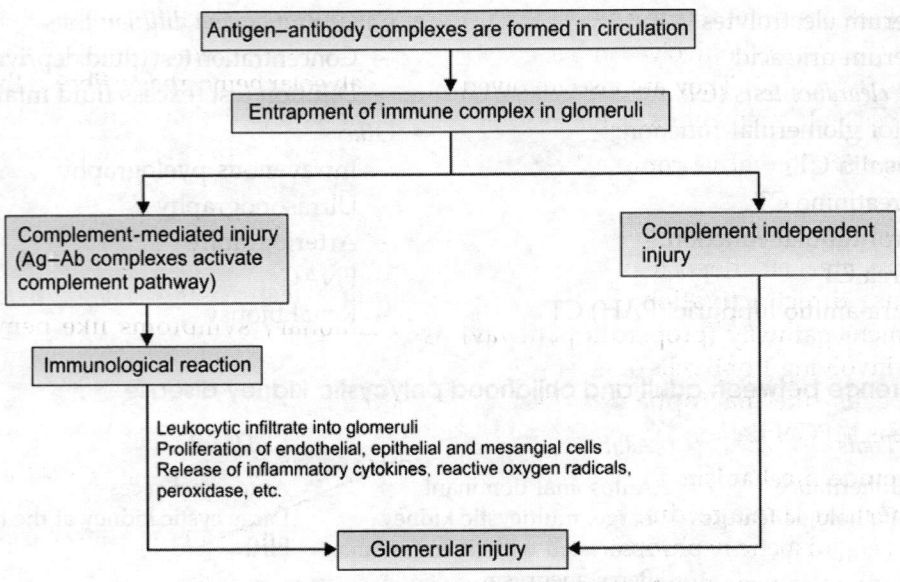

Fig. 19.1: Circulating immune complex nephritis

Fixed intrinsic tissue antigens

1. Goodpasture syndrome	• Ab is directed against fixed Ag that are normal components of GBM (a component of the *non-collagenous* domain of the α_3 chain of collagen type IV). • Homogeneous, diffuse linear pattern of deposits
2. Heymann nephritis	• Ab directed against 'Ag complex' located on the basal surface of visceral epithelial cells. This Ag complex is partially homologous to Heymann Ag found in rat. • Granular, interrupted deposits along the sub-epithelial aspect of the GBM
3. Others	Such as antibody directed against mesangial Ag

Planted Ag

These are non-glomerular Ags, which get planted in glomerulus by interacting with various intrinsic components in the glomerulus.

For example, cationic molecules can bind to glomerular capillary anionic sites; larger aggregated proteins like IgG can deposit in mesangium; DNA has affinity for GBM components.

Many exogenous (infectious agents, drugs), endogenous (DNA, Ig, immune complex) Ags can act as planted antigens

Cell-mediated glomerular injury

Sensitized T cells may be involved in some forms of glomerular injury. They are also involved in progression of many glomerulonephritis.

Activation of alternative complement pathway

Some bacterial endotoxins, polysaccharides, IgA aggregates, etc. deposited in glomeruli may cause direct activation of alternative complement pathway (properdin pathway) without involving T or B cells or other inflammatory cells like macrophages. Classical example is MPGN IIa.

Non-immune mechanism

- Glomerular damage due to metobolic insult, e.g. diabetic nephropathy.
- Glomerular damage due to hemodynamic alteration, e.g. hypertensive nephropathy.
- Injury associated with deposition diseases: Amyloidosis, cryoglobulinemias.
- Direct damage by infectious agents: Hepatitis, *E. coli*: Derived nephropathy.
- Inherited: Alport's syndrome.

9. Goodpasture syndrome (2002)

It is a syndrome characterized by clinical complex of anti-GBM nephritis and pulmonary hemorrhage.

- **Age:** 5–40 yr; M:F = 6:1
- **Pathogenesis:** It is an autoimmune disorder. Antibodies are formed against a component of NCI domain of α_3 chain of type IV collagen (α_3 chain being preferentially expressed in GBM and pulmonary alveolar BM).

- **Predisposing factors**
  - Viral infection
  - Genetic predisposition (HLA-DR2)
  - Exposure of hydrocarbon solvent
  - Smoking

- **Morphology:** Lung
  - Gross: Heavy with areas of red-brown consolidation

- Microscopic features: Focal necrosis of alveolar walls associated with intra-alveolar hemorrhage, fibrous thickening of septa and organization of blood in the alveolar space. Hemosiderin laden-macrophages (Heart failure cells, HF cells) are seen.
- **Kidney:** (*see in type I RPGN from table*).
  Clinical features: (*Renal syndrome from table*)
  Pulmonary symptoms like hemoptysis, dyspnea, and pulmonary embolism appear earlier.

10. Nephrotic syndrome: Definition, its causes (2003) and enumerate types of glomerular nephritis causing it (1993, 98, 2001)

11. Difference between urinary findings of nephritic and nephrotic syndromes (1997, 99, 2000, 02, 04)

Nephrotic syndrome is characterized by:
- Massive proteinuria (with daily loss of 3.5 gm or more of protein)
- Hypoalbuminemia, (with plasma albumin level < 3 gm/dl)
- Generalized edema
- Hyperlipidemia and lipiduria

Nephritic syndrome patients usually present with hematuria, red cell casts in urine, azotemia, oliguria and mild to moderate hypertension.

Causes of nephrotic syndrome

- Primary glomerular diseases
  - MGN
  - IgAN
  - FSGS
  - MPGN
  - MCD

- **Systemic disease**
  - Diabetes mellitus
  - Amyloidosis
  - SLE
  - Infections (malaria, syphilis, HIV, hepatitis)
  - Drugs (gold, penicillamine)
  - Miscellaneous (bee-sting allergy, hereditary nephritis)
  - Neoplasm (melanoma)

S. No.	Traits	Nephritic	Nephrotic syndrome
1.	Proteinuria	<1.0 g/day	>3.5 g/day
2.	Hematuria	+nt	−nt
3.	Oliguria	+nt	−nt
4.	Lipiduria	−nt	+nt
5.	Casts	Red cell casts	Lipid cell casts
6.	Urine	Coca-colored and smoky urine	Frothy urine
7.	Azotemia	+nt	−nt
8.	Hyperlipidemia	−nt	+nt
9.	Edema	Less	More marked

12. Post-streptococcal/acute proliferative/ post-infectious glomerulonephritis (PSGN): Etiopathogenesis (2003), clinical features, lab diagnosis (1997), urinary findings and morphological features (1998)

13. Membranous glomerulonephritis (MGN): Etiopathogenesis (2001) and pathology (1998)

14. What is the minimal changes disease (MCD)/lipoid nephrosis? Renal changes and lab diagnosis

15. Difference between type I and type II membranoproliferative glomerulonephritis (MPGN)

16. IgA nephropathy

Type	Etiology	Mechanism	LM	EM	IFM	Clinical
PSGN	Gr A β-hemolytic streptococci. *Other important lab diagnosis: 1. ↑anti-streptococci Ab titer (anti-DNAs B and anti-cationic proteinase) 2. ↓serum C3, 3. Presence of cryoglobulin in serum	Ab-mediated against circulating or planted Ag like endostreptosin, proteinase	Diffuse hyper-cellular glomeruli due to proliferation of endothelial and mesangial cells, and in-filtration of neutrophils and monocytes	Subepithelial humps	Granular deposits of IgM, IgG, and C3 in GBM and mesangium	Nephritic syndrome
MGN	Idiopathic, infection (malaria, syphilis, hepatitis), drugs (gold, peni-cillamine, NSAIDs), auto-immune (SLE), neoplasm (lung, colon), metabolic disorders (DM)	Ag–Ab mediated, in situ immune complex formation (similar mechanism as Heymann neph-ritis in rat)	Diffuse thicke-ning of GBM, paucity of neutrophils and macrophages in glomeruli	Subepithelial deposits, irregular silver stained spikes	Granular deposits of IgG and C3	Nephrotic syndrome, non-selective proteinuria
MCD	Idiopathic; asso-ciated with HIV, heroin, drugs,	Loss of glomerular polyanions defective charge barrier	Normal	Foot process effacement and lipid	No deposits	Nephrotic syndrome, selective

(Contd.)

Glomerulonephropathy (Contd.)

Type	Etiology	Mechanism	LM	EM	IFM	Clinical
	lymphoma, may follow respiratory tract infection or prophylactic immunization			laden cells in PCT		proteinuria
FSGS: (Focal segmental glomerulosclerosis)	Idiopathic, HIV; heroin; consequence of glomerular capillary hypertension like congenital oligonephropathy, acquired nephron loss, adaptive response (obesity, sickle cell anemia)	Ablation nephropathy	Focal and segmental sclerosis affecting 50% of glomeruli with entrapment of amorphous hyaline material	Foot process effacement, focal detachment of epithelial cells, denudation of underlying GBM	Focal deposit of IgM and C3	Nephrotic syndrome, subnephrotic proteinuria
MPGN type I	Idiopathic; associated with autoimmune (SLE), infection (HIV, hepatitis), liver disease (cirrhosis, hepatitis),	Immune-complex mediated	Diffuse, enlarged, hypercellular glomeruli; mesangial proliferation (↑ed matrix and macrophages infiltration),	Subendothelial deposits	Granular subendothelial deposits of IgG, C3, C1q and C4	Nephrotic syndrome
MPGN type II	lymphomas, heroin, thrombotic, microangiopathic	Autoantibody, alternative complement pathway (C3NeF)	BM thickening, reduplication, and splitting (double contour or tramtrack appearance)	Dense deposits in proper GBM	Granular deposits of C3 on either side of GBM	Hematuria, chronic renal failure
IgA N	Idiopathic, hereditary, infection (GIT, respiratory tract), gluten enteropathy, liver diseases	↑ mucosal and serum IgA synthesis, circulating IgA immune complex +nt	Mesangial widening and proliferation	Mesangial and paramesangial dense deposits	Mesangial deposition of IgA with IgG, IgM and C3	Recurrent hematuria and proteinuria
CGN	End stage of all above glomerular diseases	According to disease	Hyalinized glomeruli transforming them into a cellular eosinophilic mass	According to disease	No deposition	Chronic renal failure

*Write features/laboratory findings of any above diseases as general features of nephritic/nephrotic syndrome (given in difference table) in addition to features listed above.

*The histopathologic hallmark of nephritic syndrome is massive influx of inflammatory cell in glomerular tuft leading to extensive destruction of various glomerular components, while in nephrotic syndrome the characteristic injury is damage to GBM leading mainly to increased leakiness of GBM causing only proteinuria and its consequences.

17. Rapidly progressive glomerulonephritis (RPGN) (1989, 90)

- Not a discrete glomerulonephritis; rather, a specific clinicohistologic stage seen in various glomerulopathies.
- Characterized clinically by *rapid* and *progressive* loss of renal function.
- Characterized histologically by formation of *crescents*.
- The course of any glomerulonephritis may proceed to develop RPGN.
- Clinical features belong to those of nephritic syndrome (severe oliguria/uremia).

- If patient is not treated promptly, death occurs within weeks to month.
- Histologic picture dominated by the presence of crescent in most of glomeruli, hence also known as crescentic glomerulonephritis.
- Pathophysiology: Most cases are immunologically mediated.

Crescent formation is due to continued growth of parietal cells into Bowman's space. The Bowman's space gets filled with parietal cells, macrophages, other inflammatory cells and entangled fibrin strands leading to hard crescent-like structure.

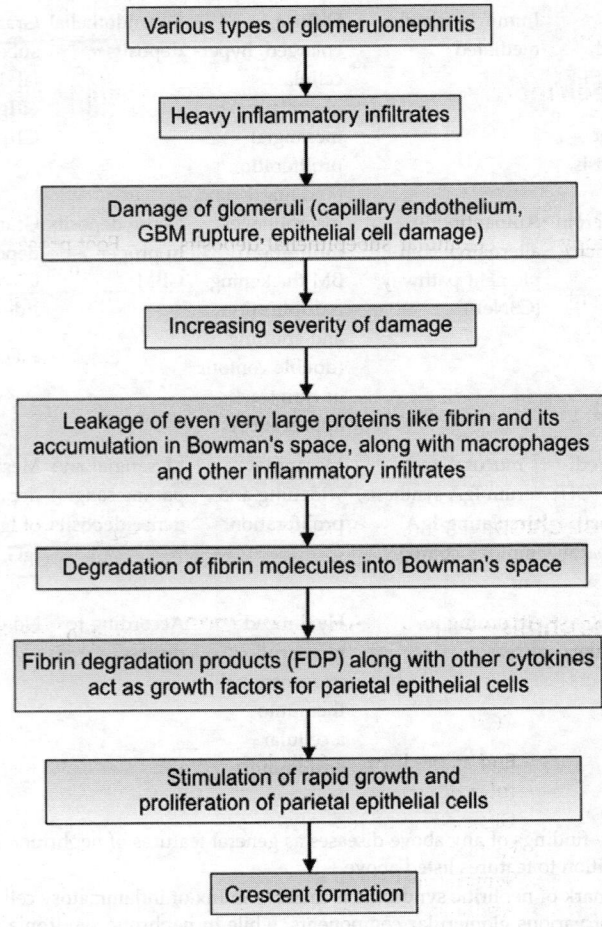

Fig. 19.2: Pathogenesis of RPGN

A practical classification divides RPGN into three groups on the basis of immunological findings:

Type	Etiology	Mechanism	LM	EM	IFM	Clinical
RPGN type I	Idiopathic, Goodpasture syndrome	Anti-GBM Ab	Enlarged and hypercellular glomeruli contains area of focal necrosis and crescents formed by proliferation of parietal cells and migration of monocytes and macrophages into Bowman capsule. Fibrin strands are prominent between cellular layers in crescents	No deposits; rupture of GBM +nt	Linear deposition of IgG and C3	Nephritic syndrome, progress into renal failure over weeks to months
RPGN type II	Idiopathic, post-infectious, SLE, Henoch-Schonlein purpura	Immune complex		Subepithelial deposits	Granular deposition of IgG and C3	
RPGN type III	Idiopathic, Wegener granulomatosis, microscopic polyarteritis nodosa	Pauci-immune (ANCA assoaciated)		No deposition	No or little deposition	

18. Difference between membranous nephropathy and minimal changes diseases (1994)

S. No.	Traits	Membranous nephropathy	Minimal changes
1.	Age	Adult	Children
2.	Light microscopy (LM)	Thickening of GBM	Normal GBM
3.	Electron microscopy (EM)	Granular subepithelial deposits	Foot process effacement and lipid laden cells in PCT
4.	Immunofluorescent microscopy (IMF)	Granular deposit of IgG and C3	Not such deposition
5.	Proteinuria	Non-selective	Highly selective
6.	Hypertension	+nt	−nt
7.	Hematuria	+nt	−nt
8.	Corticosteroid therapy	No response	Good response

19. Difference between chronic glomerulonephritis (CGN) and chronic pyelonephritis (CPN) (1993, 2000)

20. Chronic pyelonephritis—etiopathogenesis (2003), morphological changes and laboratory findings (1995)

S. No.	Traits	CGN	CPN
1.	Disease	End stage disease of all glomerular disorders	Chronic tubulointerstitial renal disorder
2.	Surface	Diffusely, granular, cortical surfaces	Depressed area on dilated and blunted calyx
3.	Scar	Symmetrical	Asymmetrical
4.	Glomeruli	Acellular, ↓ in number, show hyaline obliteration	Normal, may show periglomerular fibrosis

(Contd.)

Chronic pyelonephritis—etiopathogenesis (2003), morphological changes and laboratory findings (Contd.)

S. No.	Traits	CGN	CPN
5.	Tubules	Atrophied	Atrophy in some area and hypertrophy in other and dilatation (thyroidization)
6.	Renal pelvis and calyx	Normal	Dilated
7.	Arteriolar changes	Arteriolar sclerosis	Hyaline arteriosclerosis
8.	Clinical presentation/ lab diagnosis	Proteinuria, azotemia, hypertension	Polyuria, nocturia, pyuria, bacteriuria, mild proteinuria and gradual onset of hypertension and renal insufficiency

Etiopathogenesis of CPN: Two forms:
1. Chronic obstructive pyelonephritis: Can be bilateral as with obstructive anomalies of urinary tract (posterior urethral valves) or unilateral (calculi and unilateral obstructive anomalies of the ureter).
2. Reflux nephropathy: (a) Superimposition of a urinary infection on congenital vesicoureteral reflux and intrarenal reflux and (b) Occasionally causes renal damage in the absence of infection in case of severe obstruction (sterile reflux).

21. Uremic complications of chronic glomerulonephritis (2009)/chronic renal failure

These comprise pathological changes outside kidney in patients with chronic uremia. These are:
- Uremic pericarditis
- Uremic gastroenteritis
- Uremic encephalopathy
- Secondary hyperparathyroidism leading to nephrocalcinosis and renal osteodystrophy
- Hypertension (may lead to left ventricular hypertrophy)
- Uremic pneumonitis (diffuse alveolar damage, pleural effusion and lung damage)

22. Difference between acute pyelonephritis and chronic pyelonephritis

S. No.	Traits	Acute pyelonephritis	Chronic pyelonephritis
1.	Definition	Acute suppurative inflammation of kidney caused by bacterial infection.	Chronic tubulointerstitial renal disorders having chronic tubular inflammation and renal scarring with pathologic involvement of calyces and pelvis
2.	Etiology	Urinary obstruction, instrumentation, catheterization, pregnancy, DM, pre-existing renal lesions	Chronic obsturctive pyelonephritis, reflux nephropathy
3.	Pathology	Bacterial infection and renal lesion associated with UTI	Bacterial infection plays a dominant role, but vesicoureteal reflux and obstruction are also involved.

(Contd.)

Difference between acute pyelonephritis and chronic pyelonephritis (Contd.)

S. No.	Traits	Acute pyelonephritis	Chronic pyelonephritis
4.	Gross	Patchy interstitial suppurative inflammation and tubular necrosis (hallmarks)	Coarse discrete corticomedullary scar overlying blunted or dilated calyx
5.	Microscopic	Tubules showing coagulative necrosis with outline preserved	Tubules show atrophy in some areas and dilatation in other. Dilated tubules filled with colloid (thyroidization).
6.	Clinical	Sudden onset with back pain, fever, malaise	Onset is insidious (silent onset).

23. Diabetic nephropathy/renal changes in DM (1990, 93,95, 98, 2001, 02, 04)

- Four types of lesions are seen in diabetic nephropathy.

1. Morphological changes in glomeruli

Three changes are seen:

i. *Capillary basement membrane thickening:* Widespread thickening of GBM with mesangial widening.

ii. *Diffuse glomerulosclerosis:* Involvement of all parts of glomeruli. It consists of:
- Overall thickening of GBM
- Diffuse increase in mesangial matrix with proliferation
- Exudative lesions: Capsular hyaline drops (an eosinophilic hyaline thickening of the parietal layer of Bowman's capsule which bulges into glomerular space), and fibrin caps (a homogeneous, brightly eosinophilic material appearing on the wall of a peripheral capillary of a lobule).

iii. *Nodular glomerulosclerosis (**Kimmelstiel-Wilson lesion**/intercapillary glomerulosclerosis):* These lesions are specific for juvenile onset diabetes or islets-cells antibodies positive DM. The pathological changes are:
- One or more nodules are seen in glomeruli (ovoid/spherical, laminated, hyaline, acellular mass which are PAS +ve and contains lipid and fibrin)

- Surrounding capillaries are thickening.
- Nodules compress capillaries and obliterate glomerular tufts leading to tubular atrophy and interstitial fibrosis.
- With effects of these changes, small and contracted kidney is outcome.

2. Vascular lesions
- Atheroma of renal arteries
- Hyaline arteriosclerosis of afferent and efferent arterioles
- These vascular lesions are responsible for renal ischemia which results in tubular atrophy and interstitial fibrosis.

3. Diabetic pyelonephritis: Poorly controlled diabetics are susceptible to bacterial infection. *Papillary necrosis* is an important complication which may result in acute pyelonephritis.

4. Tubular lesions (Armani-Ebstein lesions): In untreated diabetics, who have high blood sugar level, the epithelial cells of PCT develop extensive glycogen deposits appearing as vacuoles.

- **Pathogenesis of glomerulosclerosis**
  - Metabolic defects: Insulin deficiency and recurrent hyperglycemia.
  - Biochemical changes in GBM: ↑ collagen and fibronectin, ↓ proteoglycan heparin sulfate.
  - Non-enzymatic glycosylation of Hb and other proteins (collagen and BM materials) resulting in thickening of GBM.

- Hemodynamic changes ($\uparrow$ GFR, $\uparrow$ glomerular filtration area) associated with glometer hypertrophy.
- **Clinical features:** Patients present with three glomerular syndromes including non-nephrotic proteinuria, nephrotic syndrome, and chronic renal failure.

24. Difference between nephrotoxic ATN and ischemic ATN (1998, 2004)

25. Acute tubular necrosis (ATN) (1990, 93)

- ATN is a disorder characterized morphologically by destruction of tubular epithelial cells and clinically by acute suppression of renal function.
- **Caused by:**
  - Organic vascular obstruction

- Acute tubulointerstitial nephritis
- DIC
- Severe glomerular disease (RPGN)
- Massive infection
- Urinary obstruction
- *Clinical course*
Three stages:
  - Initial: Lasting for about 36 hours; slight $\downarrow$ in urine output and $\uparrow$ BUN.
  - Maintenance: Sustained $\downarrow$ in urine output, salt and water overload (hyperkalemia) and rise in BUN concentrations.
  - Recovery: $\uparrow$ urine output and hypokalemia.
- *Prognosis*
  - Depends on clinical setting
  - Up to 50% of patients with ATN may not have oliguria and may in fact have $\uparrow$ urine output.

S. No.	Traits	Ischemic ATN	Nephrotoxic ATN
1.	Definition	ATN which is caused by renal ischemia	ATN which is caused by toxic agents
2.	Etiology	Hypotension, shock, $\downarrow$ ed renal perfusion	Drugs like gentamycin, other antibiotics, radiographic contrast agents, poisons, heavy metals and organic solvents
3.	Pathogenesis	• Tubular injury • Persistent and severe disturbances in blood flow	Tubular injury plays a dominant role
4.	Morphology	Focal tubular epithelial necrosis and apoptosis at multiple points along the nephron, rupture of BM (tubulorrhexis) and occlusion of tubular lumens by casts	Acute tubular injury which is non-specific according to agent, like in case of mercuric chloride poisoning injured cells not yet dead may contain large acidophilic inclusions.
5.	Tubular necrosis	Patchy, relative short lengths are affected, with large skip areas in between	Extensive necrosis is present with no skip areas
6.	Parts of tubules affected	Straight segments of proximal tubules and ascending limbs of loop of Henle	PCT with many toxins (like Hg), but DCT and ascending loop of Henle may be affected.
7.	Casts	Eosinophilic hyaline and pigmented granular casts consists of Tamm-Horsfall protein with Hb, myoglobin and other plasma proteins	Non-specific according to agent like lipid casts in case of CCl_4 poisoning

26. Difference between benign and malignant nephrosclerosis (1997, 98, 2000, 01, 04)

27. Malignant nephrosclerosis

28. Kidney in hypertension (HTN) (1990)

29. Renal change in malignant HTN (1993)

S. No.	Traits	Benign nephrosclerosis	Malignant nephrosclerosis
1.	Seen in	Benign hypertension, DM, ↑ age	Malignant hypertension
2.	Gross	Leather grain appearance	*Flea bitten* appearance due to tiny petechial hemorrhage
3.	Microscopy	• Narrowing of the lumens of arterioles caused by thickening and hyalinization of the walls (hyaline arteriosclerosis) • Fibroelastic hyperplasia of arteries and arterioles	• Hyperplastic arteriolitis (onion-skinning) due to proliferation and elongation of smooth muscle cells • Necrotizing glomerulitis (neutrophils infiltration and thrombosed capillaries) • Fibrinoid necrosis of arterioles • Necrotizing arteriolitis
4.	Renin	Normal	↑ed
5.	Aldosterone	Normal	↑ed
6.	Proteinuria	Mild	Marked
7.	Sign of malignant hypertension	Absent	Present such as retinopathy, encephalopathy
8.	Renal failure	Rare	More common

30. Types of renal calculi/stones or urinary calculi. Pathogenesis, gross-appearance and complication of renal calculi. Urolithiasis (short note) (1992, 93, 95, 96)

Types	Incidence (M:F)	Causes	Pathogenesis	Gross
Calcium stone	75% (2–3:1)	Idiopathic hypercalcemia, hyperoxalouria, hyper-uricosuria, hypocitraturia, distal renal tubule acidosis	Supersaturation of ions in urine, alkaline pH of urine	Small, smooth contour, or irregular jagged mass of spicules
Structive stone [MgNH₄ (PO)₃] Triple stone/ Stag-horn stone	10–15% (1:5)	UTI by urease containing organisms like *Proteus*	Alkaline urinary pH due to ammonia from urea (by urease)	Large, solitary, branching structure due to progressive accretion of salts
Uric acid stone	6% (3–4:1)	Gout, dehydration, idiopathic, malignant tumors	Acidic urine, ↓ solubility of uric acid	Smooth, yellow brownish, hard, multiple
Cystine stone	1–2% (1:1)	Hereditary	Least soluble cystine precipitate as crystals	Small, smooth yellow, multiple, round
Others	Up to 10% (1:1)	Inherited abnormality of amino acid metabolism	Xanthinuria	—

- *Clinical features*
  - Ureteral colic pain
  - Hematuria
- *Complications*
  - Urethral obstruction and stricture formation
  - Local trauma, which causes ulcer and bleeding
  - UTI
  - Hydronephrosis
  - Pyonephrosis

31. Short note on urinary casts (1986, 88, 91, 93)

- Casts are proteinaceous plugs (made up of Tamm-Horsfall protein) formed within the nephron and washed out by the flow of tubular fluid.

- *Two types*
1. Cellular
   - Leukocyte casts: Seen in pyelonephritis
   - Fatty or lipid casts: In nephrotic syndrome
   - Red cell casts: In nephritic syndrome
   - Epithelial casts
2. Non-cellular
   - *Hyaline casts* are structureless, transparent proteinaceous plugs, made up of Tamm-Horsfall proteins (a specific urinary glycoprotein normally secreted by the cells ascending thick limb and distal tubules). They are increased in ATN and proteinuria.
   - *Granular casts* are similar to hyaline casts except that granular aggregates of proteins are embedded in them. For example, Bence-Jones tubular cast.
   - *Broad waxy casts* (renal failure casts): Seen in CRF in the dilated nephron.

32. RCC—classify renal tumors (2000) or morphological changes in RCC (1997, 2003, 04)

Cell type	Benign	Malignant
Epithelial tumors of renal parenchyma	Adenoma, oncocytoma	RCC (hypernephroma)
Epithelial tumors of renal pelvis	Transition cell papilloma	TCC
		Squamous cell carcinoma
		Adenocarcinoma of renal pelvis
Embryonal tumors	Mesoblastic nephroma, Multicystic nephroma	Wilms' tumor
Non-epithelial tumors	Angiomyolipoma, fibroma	Sarcoma
Miscellaneous	Reninoma	—
Metastatic tumors	—	—

Age: More than 60 yr

Sex: M:F = 2–3:1

Epidemiology: Tobacco, obesity, hypertension, unopposed estrogen therapy, exposure to asbestos, petroleum products and heavy metals.

Majority of cases of RCC are sporadic, but about 5% are inherited which are associated with:

1. von Hippel-Lindau (VHL) syndrome
2. Hereditary clear cell RCC
3. Hereditary papillary RCC

- *Clinical features*
  - Three classic diagnostic features are painless intermittent hematuria, palpable abdominal mass and costovertebral pain.
  - RCC also produces a number of paraneoplastic syndromes (hyperkalcemia, hypertension, Cushing syndrome, etc.).
- *Metastasis*
  - Tendency to metastasize widely before giving rise to any local signs and symptoms.

Types and features of RCC

Traits	Clear cell RCC	Papillary RCC	Chromophobe RCC	Collecting duct (Bellini duct) carcinoma
Incidence	70–80%	10–15%	5–8%	1%
Genetics	3p deletion in VHL gene	Trisomy of 7, 16, 17, and loss of Y	Multiple chromosome loss and hyperdiploidy	Several chromosomal abnormality, no definite pattern
Gross	Solitary, unilateral, bright yellow to gray-white which distorts the renal outline	Multifocal, bilateral, golden yellow papillae may be seen, hemorrhagic and cystic area present	Same as clear cell RCC	Seen in medullary region
Microscopy	Solid to tubular growth pattern, round cells with clear and granular cytoplasm (glycogen and lipid) may show nuclear atypia and giant cells.	Papillary growth pattern, cuboidal to low columnar cells, psammoma bodies present	Solid sheets of cells around the blood vessels, pale eosinophilic cells with perinuclear halo	Irregular channels lined by highly atypical epithelium, in a hobnail pattern

- Most common sites are lung and bones
- It also invades renal vein and grows as a solid column of mass even up to inferior vena cava and right side of heart.
- **Prognosis:** Average 5 yr survival is about 45–70% in the absence of distant metastasis and 15–20% in case of renal vein invasion.

33. Wilms' tumor/nephroblastoma: Pathogenesis (1998, 2000, 03)

Most common primary renal tumor of childhood.
- **Age:** Childhood; 2–5 yr
- **Sex ratio:** 1:1
- **Associated with three syndromes**
1. *WAGR syndrome*
   - Aniridia
   - Genital anomalies
   - Mental retardation
WT-1 gene nonsense or frame shifts mutation
WT-1 gene presents at 11p13—its protein product is a transcriptional factor

2. *Denys-Drash syndrome*
   - Gonadal dysgenesis (male pseudohermaphroditism)
   - Nephropathy (renal failure)
WT-1 gene missense mutation affecting DNA binding properties

3. *Beckwith-Wiedemann syndrome*
   - Enlargement of body organs
   - Hemihypertrophy
   - Renal medullary cyst
   - Abnormally large cells in adrenal cortex (adrenocytomegaly)
WT-2 gene presents on 11p15.5, function is unknown
WT-2 mutation increases Wilms' tumor chances.

- *Morphology*
   - Gross: Tumor mass is large solitary well-circumscribed
     Cut section: Soft, homogeneous, tan to gray color, foci of hemorrhage and necrosis may be present.

– Microscopic feature: Mixture of primitive epithelial cells (in the form of abortive tubules or glomeruli) and stromal cells (fibrocystic or myxoid in nature)

Small, spindled, anaplastic, sarcomatoid tumor cells are present.

- **Clinical features:** Palpable abdominal mass, hematuria, pain and hypertension.

Metastasis: Through blood to lung and liver.

Renal hilar, para-aortic lymp nodes are involved.

Prognosis: 5 yr survival rate is above 75%.

34. Difference between nephroblastoma/Wilms' tumor and RCC (1994, 95)

S. No.	Traits	RCC	Wilms' tumor
1.	Age	Adult	Children
2.	Genes associated	VHL, MET	WT-1 and WT-2
3.	Psammoma bodies	+nt	−nt
4.	Gross	See clear cell RCC	See Wilms' tumor
5.	Microscopy	See clear cell RCC	See Wilms' tumor
6.	Paraneoplastic syndrome	Very common	Not common
7.	Tendency to invade renal vein	Invade renal vein	Do not invade
8.	Prognosis	Comparatively poor	Better

35. Causes of hematuria, polyuria, enlarged kidney, contracted kidney, proteinuria and glycosuria

Hematuria
Lesion of the urinary tract
Kidney
Polycystic kidney, ruptured kidney, TB, *acute nephritic syndrome,*
Renal tumor (RCC and Wilms' tumor), infarction, IgA nephropathy
Ureter
Stones, papilloma or carcinoma of urothelium
Urinary Bladder:
Rupture, cystitis, TB, TCC, stones
Prostate-BHP, carcinoma
Urethra
Rupture, urethritis, TCC and stones
Diseases of the adjacent viscera
Acute appendicitis, salpingitis and pelvic abscess
General disorders
Blood disorders, infarction, congestion (RHF) and collagen diseases
Drugs
Like salicylates and anticoagulant drugs

Contracted kidney
CGN, CPN, diabetic nephropathy, benign nephrosclerosis, amyloidosis, senile nephrotic syndrome, end stage of MGN and polyarteritis nodosa
Enlarged kidney
RPGN, PSGN, ATN, polycystic kidney, acute drug induced interstitial nephritis, initial stage of MGN and sometimes amyloidosis
Polyuria
>2.5 l in 24 hours
Excessive fluid intake, diuretic therapy, chronic kidney disease, diabetes insipidus, mental disorder, DM and primary aldosteronism
Glycosuria
DM, renal glycosuria, pregnancy, alimentary glycosuria, IV infusion of glucose and ↑ intracranial tension
Proteinuria
Kidney diseases (like nephrotic syndrome, acute glomerulonephritis, TB of kidney, RCC and renal vein thrombosis), muscular exertion, high fever, heavy metal poisoning and orthostatic albuminuria (only when the person is active on his feet)

36. Tumors of urinary bladder

Urothelial (transitional) tumors: 90% of all urinary bladder tumors
    Exophytic papilloma
    Inverted papilloma
    Papillary urothelial neoplasm of low malignant potential
    Low grade and high grade papillary urothelial cancers
    Flat non-invasive urothelial carcinoma (carcinoma *in situ*)
Mixed carcinoma
Adenocarcinoma
Small cell carcinoma
Sarcomas

37. Transitional cell carcinoma (TCC) urothelial tumor: Pathogenesis (2000, 02, 03), and its grading

WHO grading of TCC (1973)

Papilloma
TCC Grade I
TCC Grade II
TCC Grade III

ISUP (International Society of Urological Pathology) classification 1998 adopted by WHO in 2004:

Urothelial papilloma
Urothelial neoplasm of low malignant potential
Urothelial carcinoma, low grade
Urothelial carcinoma, high grade

Age: 50–80 yr
Sex: M:F = 3:1
Epidemiology
- Cigarette smoking
- *Schistosoma hematobium* infections
- Heavy long-term exposure to cyclophosphamide
- Industrial exposure to arylamines
- Long-term use of analgesics

Pathology
Chromosome 9 monosomy or deletion of 9p and 9q as well as deletions of 17p, 13q, 11p and 14q. 9p deletions (9p21) involve the tumor-suppressor gene p16 (MTS 1, INK 4a), which encodes an inhibitor of a cyclin-dependent kinase and also the related p15.

Two models
1. *Two pathway model:* Initiated by deletions of tumor-suppressor gene (9p and 9q) a few of which may acquire p53 mutation and progress to invasion.

2. *Linear model of progression:* Initiated by p53 mutations, directly results in induction of potentially invasive tumors.

Clinical features: Painless hematuria, frequency, urgency and dysuria.

Complications: Stricture formation, hydronephrosis and pyonephrosis.

Prognosis: Depends on tumor grade or blood group Ag (tumor cells expressing A, B and H Ag have a better prognosis).

38. Bence-Jones proteinuria (1994, 2000)

- Bence-Jones, proteins are light chains secreted in multiple myeloma and amyloidosis.
- Its presence and amount indicate stage of renal failure.
- Bence-Jones proteinuria results in renal failure by *two mechanisms:*
  - Direct toxic to epithelial cells
  - It combines with the Tamm-Horsfall protein under acidic condition to form large histologically distinct tubular casts which obstruct the lumen and also induce peritubular inflammatory reaction (casts nephropahty).
- *Detection*
  - **Heat coagulation test:** At 45 °C, it starts precipitating and remains at top till 58 °C; beyond this temperature it dissolves in the urine and again reappears on cooling at 60 °C.
  - **Immunoelectrophoresis:** More sensitive method, it detects even minute quantity of the protein.

20

Male Genital Tract

1. Testicular atrophy (1999)

Testicular atrophy is a progressive degenerative change in testes resulting in decreased male fertility.

Causes

1. Progressive atherosclerotic narrowing of testicular blood vessels as in old age
2. End stage of all inflammatory conditions (orchitis)
3. Cryptorchidism
4. Hypopituitarism
5. Obstruction of flow to semen
6. Malnutrition and cachexia
7. Prolonged administration of female sex hormone
8. Exhaustion atrophy due to high level of pituitary follicle stimulating hormone
9. Klinefelter's syndrome (primary genetic disorder)
10. Irradiation
11. Prolonged administration of antiandrogens (for treatment of carcinoma prostate)

Morphology

- *Gross:* Testes are small in size and firm in consistency due to fibrotic changes.
- *Microscopic examination*
  - Initially spermatic tubules show hyalinization and thickening of basement membrane; later on, these appear as dense cords of hyaline connective tissues

which are outlined by prominent and thickened basement membrane.
- Increased interstitial stroma, Leydig cells are not affected and they appear prominent.
- Sertoli cells are present, but there is no spermatogenesis.

2. Classify common testicular tumors

Germ cell tumors (95%)
- Seminomatous tumors
  - Seminoma
  - Spermatocytic seminoma
- Non-seminomatous tumors
  - Embryonal carcinoma
  - Yolk sac (endodermal sinus) tumor
  - Choriocarcinoma
  - Teratoma

Sex cord-stroma tumors
- Leydig cell tumor
- Sertoli cell tumor

Note: Most germ cell tumors are aggressive cancers capable of rapid, wide dissemination, although with current therapy most can be cured. Sex cord-stromal tumors are generally benign.

3. Etiology of germ cell tumors of testes

For unexplained reasons, there is a worldwide increase in the incidence of germ cell tumors.

In the 15–34 yr age group, they constitute the most common tumor of men and cause approximately 10% of all cancer deaths.

1. Environmental factors are explained by population migration studies.
2. Race: These tumors are more common in whites than blacks (5:1 ratio, USA).
3. Testicular dysgenesis syndrome (TDS): cryptorchidism, hypospadias and poor sperm quality.
4. Klinefelter's syndrome
5. Family history: The relative risk of developing germ cell tumor of fathers and sons of patients with testicular germ cell tumors is four times higher than normal, and is 8–10 times higher between brothers (genetic polymorphism at Xq27).
6. Excess 12p copy number either in the term of i(12p) or increased 12p an aberrantly banded marker chromosome.

4. Clinical features of germ cell tumors

- It presents with painless enlargement of the testes.
- All testicular tumors are derived from totipotent germ cells, so "forward" and "backward" differentiation can be seen; so metastatic tumor may sometimes show a different histology as compared to the primary lesion.
- Most testicular tumors are derived from intratubular germ cell neoplasia (IT GCN) which is also seen commonly in the nearby tissue.
- Biopsy of a testicular mass is associated with a risk of tumor spillage and metastasis; therefore, any testicular mass is considered neoplastic unless proven otherwise, and radical orchidectomy is performed based on this assumption.

Spread

Lymphatic spread: It is common to involve retroperitoneal para-aortic nodes followed by mediastinal and supraclavicular nodes.

Hematogenous spread: Primarily to lungs, but may involve liver, brain and bones.

Clinical stages of testicular tumors

Stage I: Tumor confined to the testes, epididymis or spermatic cord.

Stage II: Distant spread confined to retroperitoneal nodes below diaphragm.

Stage III: Metastasis outside the retroperitoneal nodes or above the diaphragm.

Tumor markers in germ cell tumors (male)

Testicular tumors	Tumor markers
Embryonal carcinoma	HCG, AFP
Yolk sac tumor	AFP, α_1-antitrypsin
Choriocarcinoma	HCG
Mass of tumor cells/ burden	Lactate dehydrogenase

Role of serum markers

- In evaluation of testicular mass
- In staging of testicular germ tumors
- In assessing tumor burden
- In monitoring response to therapy

5. Seminoma (1990, 93, 97, 2000, 01, 07)

- Most common type of germ cell tumor (50%)

Age: In thirties, never in infants

Note: Seminomas contain an isochromosome 12p and express OCT 3/4 and NANOG. Approximately 25% of these tumors have c-KIT activating mutations.

Morphology: Three histological variants:

1. *Typical (classical) seminoma (85%)*
   Gross
   - Testis is bulky, sometimes ten times of normal testis.
   - Cut surface—homogeneous, gray-white, fleshy lobulated and well-circumscribed surface
   - Hemorrhage and necrosis are absent.
   - Tunica albuginea are generally intact, but sometimes extension to epididymis, spermatic cord and scrotal sac may be present
   - Usually replaces the entire testes

Microscopic examination

- Tumor has sheets of uniform seminoma cells which are divided into poorly demarcated lobule by delicate fibrous septa.
- *Seminoma cell* is large and round to polyhedral and has a distinct cell membrane; a clear or watery appearing cytoplasm (glycogen or lipid contents). It has a large central nucleus with one or two prominent nucleoli.
- Mitoses vary in frequency
- Stroma varies
- Infiltration of T lymphocytes in septa is seen and may form granulomas.

Immunocytochemical tests

- Seminoma cells are diffusely positive for c-KIT, OCT 4
- α-fetoprotein is absent.
- HCG (except 15% cases where syncytial giant cells resembling syncytiotrophoblasts of placenta are present) is also absent.
- Tumor cells contain placental alkaline phosphatase (PLAP).
- Sometimes, scattered keratin positive cells are also present.

2. *Anaplastic (5–10%)*

Tumors with greater cellularity, more nuclear irregularity, more number of tumor giant cells, three or more mitoses per high power field are classified as anaplastic seminoma: Prognosis of both classical and anaplastic seminomas are similar.

3. *Spermatocytic seminoma (4–6%):* Classified separately.

Clinial features: Large testicular swelling, may be associated with diffuse pain.

6. Spermatocytic seminoma

- Clinically and histologically distinct from typical seminoma.
- *Age:* More than 65 years
- Slow-growing tumor that rarely metastasizes. Very good prognosis.

Morphology

Gross: Larger than typical seminoma; cut surface is pale-gray, soft and friable, sometimes reveals mucoid cyst.

Microscopic examination

- Spermatocytic seminoma contains three intermixed cell population (small cells, medium-sized cells and giant cells)
- Medium-sized cells are the most numerous and have round nucleus and eosinophilic cytoplasm.
- Small cells have narrow rim of eosinophilic cytoplasm resembling secondary spermatocytes.
- Giant cells are scattered and are either uninucleate or multinucleate.

Electron microscopy: Tumor cells showing cytoplasmic and nuclear features of spermatic maturation.

7. Metastasis of testicular tumors (2004)

- All testicular tumors are derived from totipotent germ cells, so "forward" and "backward" differentiation can be seen, though most of the tumors metastasize "true". For example, embryonal carcinoma may present as teratoma picture in secondary depots. Conversely, teratoma may present as choriocarcinoma in lymph nodes.
- Lymphatic spread is common to all forms of testicular tumors. Retroperitoneal para-aortic nodes are first involved, followed by mediastinal and supraclavicular nodes.
- Hematogenous spread is primarily to lung; may also involve liver, brain and bones.
- Seminoma metastasizes primarily through lymphatic; hematogenous spread occurs later.
- Non-seminomatous germ cell tumors (NSGCT) metastasize early and hematogenous route is more frequently involved.

8. Non-seminomatous germ cell tumor (2008)

or

Difference between seminoma and non-seminomatous testicular tumors

S. No.	Traits	Seminoma	Non-seminoma
1.	Definition	Only one histologic type	Umbrella designation that includes one histologic type (embryonal cell carcinoma) as well as more than one histologic type or mixed
2.	Stage	70% patients present in stage I	60% in stages II and III
3.	Localization	Localized to testes for long	Metastasize early
4.	Metastasis	Mainly lymph node; hematogenous spread later	Hematogenous spread more frequent
5.	Gross	Area of necrosis and hemorrhage is rare, shape of testes maintained	Common, shape of testes distorted
6.	Microscopic	Less tendency to infiltrate tunica, epididymis, spermatic cord	Greater tendency to infiltrate tunica, epididymis, spermatic cord
7.	Hormone	15% tumors secrete HCG	Secrete HCG, AFP, LDH, PLAP, etc.
8.	Radiation	Radiosensitive	Radio-resistant
9.	Behavior	Less aggressive	More aggressive
10.	Prognosis	Good	Bad

9. Embryonal carcinoma

- These occur mostly in 20–30 yr of age group.
- These tumors are more aggressive than seminomas.

Morphology

Gross: Cut surface of tumor is variegated, has poorly demarcated margins. There are foci of necrosis and hemorrhage. Extension through the tunica albuginea into the epididymis and cord is seen frequently.

Microscopic examination

- Tumor cells grow in alveolar or tubular patterns sometimes with papillary convolutions.
- They lack well-formed glands.
- More undifferentiated lesions display sheets of cells.
- The tumor cells have epithelial appearance, they are large and anaplastic. They have hyperchromatic nuclei with prominent nucleoli. Cellular and nuclear pleomorphism is present. Mitotic figures and giant cells are seen frequently.

- They are positive for markers OCT 3/4 and PLAP (similar to seminoma) as well as distinguishing markers cytokeratin and CD30; they are negative for c-KIT.

10. Yolk sac tumor of male (2004)

- Also called endodermal sinus tumor, orchioblastoma, and infantile embryonal carinoma.
- Most common testicular tumor of infants and young children up to age of 3, and has good prognosis in this age group.
- In adults, pure form is rare; but combination with embryonal carcinoma is frequent.
- AFP level is elevated in all cases of yolk sac tumor.

Morphology

Gross

- Tumor is nonencapsulated.
- Cut surface shows homogeneous, yellow-white, mucoid appearance. Area of necrosis and hemorrhage may also be seen.

Microscopic examination

- Tumor cells form a variety of patterns— loose reticular network, papillary, tubular and solid arrangement.
- The characteristic pattern is a lace-like (reticular) network of medium-sized cuboidal or flattened cells.
- In approximately 50% of tumors, structures resembling endodermal sinuses (Schiller–Duval bodies) are seen. Schiller–Duval bodies consist of a mesodermal core with a central capillary and a visceral and parietal layer of cells resembling primitive glomeruli. Eosinophilic and hyaline-like globules are present within and outside the cytoplasm. These globules are positive for α-fetoprotein (AFP) and α₁-antitrypsin. The presence of AFP is highly characteristic.
- Intracellular and extracellular PAS positive hyaline granules may be present.

11. Teratoma of testes (1990, 98, 2001)

- Complex tumor composed of tissue organoid components derived from more than one germ layer (endoderm, mesoderm and ectoderm).
- More common in infants and children (40% of infant testicular tumors), but they may occur at any age up to adult life.
- Pure form is present mostly in infants and children; in adults pure form is rare.
- In adults, pure teratoma comprises 2–3% of all germ cell tumors.
- The frequency of teratomas mixed with other germ cell tumors is proximately 45%.
- Elevated HCG or AFP is found in 50% cases.

Morphology

- *Gross:* Large (5–10 cm in diameter) may involve whole testes, gray-white. Cut surface has variegated (heterogeneous) appearance: Gray-white solid area, cyst and honeycombed area, and foci of cartilages and bones.
- Hemorrhage and necrosis indicate mixture with embryonal carcinoma, choriocarcinoma or both.

Microscopic examination: Three types:

- *Mature (differentiated) teratoma*
  - Benign tumors; more in infants and children.
  - Composed of disorderly mixture of a variety of well-differentiated structures like cartilage, smooth muscle, intestinal and respiratory epithelium, mucous gland, cyst lined by squamous and transitional epithelium, neural tissues, bones and fat, all embedded in a fibrous or myxoid stroma.
  - Pure matured form is present mostly in infants and children and has very good prognosis.
  - In adult, pure mature form is rare; there is always hidden malignant teratoma. *So all testicular teratomas in adult are thought to be malignant.*
  - Dermoid cyst is rare in testes.
- *Immature teratoma:* Malignant; more in adults.
  - Intermediate between mature teratoma and embryonal carcinoma.
  - Incompletely differentiated structures; organoid fashion is absent. Some areas of well-formed structures lie in the dominant poorly formed structures.
- *Teratomas with malignant transformation:* This term is used when a malignant, non-germ cell tumor arises in teratoma.
  - Clear evidence of malignancy in the derivatives of one or more germ cell layers.
  - There may be a focus of squamous cell carcinoma or a sarcoma, mucin-secreting adenocarcinoma.
  - These non-germ cell tumors do not respond to chemotherapy, so surgery is the only option.

12. Choriocarcinoma (1987, 89)

- Highly malignant form of testicular / ovarian tumor.

- May arise in placental tissue or other totipotent cells of mediastium and abdomen.
- Pure form of choriocarcinoma is rare; mostly mixed pattern.
- *Age:* 2nd decade of life
- The serum and urinary level of HCG are greatly elevated in all cases.
- *Morphology*
  Gross
  1. Very small (rarely more than 5 cm in diameter) lesion
  2. Generally do not cause testicular enlargement, detected only as small palpable nodule
  3. Sometimes due to ischemic necrosis, tumor lesion is replaced by fibrous scar and is not detected by palpation
  4. Areas of hemorrhage and necrosis are extremely common.

  Microscopic examination: Two types of cells are seen without forming placental type villi:
  1. Syncytiotrophoblast: They are large and have many irregular or lobular hyperchromatic nuclei, abundant eosinophilic cytoplasm. HCG is present in cytoplasm.
  2. Cytotrophoblast: These are regular, polygonal cells with distinct cell borders, clear cytoplasm and single uniform nucleus. They grow in cords and masses.
- Metastasizes early through bloodstream to lungs, liver, bone and other viscera.
- These tumors of ovary are unresponsive to chemotherapy in contrast to that of placental origin.

13. Nodular hyperplasia (benign hypertrophy or hyperplasia) of prostate (1988, 90, 2008)

- Hyperplasia of prostatic stromal and epithelial cells, resulting in the formation of large and discrete nodule in *transition and periurethral zones.*
- *Age:* BPH is extremely common in men over 50 years of age. Its incidence increases with age.

- Histologic evidence of BPH can be seen in approximately 20% of men over 40 years, 70% by age 60 and 90% by age 80 years.

Pathogenesis
- The basic pathology behind BPH is an increased number of epithelial cells and stromal components in the periurethral area of the prostate. This increase in number of cells is due to increase in cellular proliferation as well as reduction of the rate of cell death (hence accumulation of senescent cells in the prostate).
- The main hormone responsible for these effects is dihydrotestosterone (DHT).
- DHT is formed from testosterone in the stromal cells of prostate by the enzymes type 2 5α-reductase.
- DHT acts in autocrine and paracrine fashions on stromal cells as well as epithelial cells to produce different growth factors.
- These growth factors stimulate epithelial and fibroblast proliferation as well as decrease the death of epithelial cells. The net result is increased epithelial and stromal cells resulting in enlarged prostate.
- Testosterone has the same effect, but is very less potent than DHT.

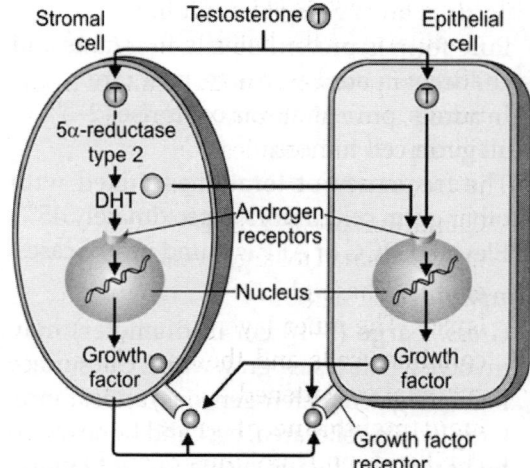

Fig. 20.1: Simplified diagram of pathogenesis of BPH. Growth factors: Fibroblast growth factors (FGF-7, FGF-1 and 2)

- Estrogen increases the level of androgen receptors, thus providing DHT more sites for action. Estrogen level increases with age, so its role might be significant.

Morphology

- *Gross*
  - The weight of prostate may vary from 60 to 100 g or more (normal weight of prostate is 7–16 g).
  - The early nodules are composed almost entirely of stromal cells, and later predominantly epithelial cells.
  - In nodule with primary glandular proliferation, the cut surface of prostate is yellow-pink with a soft consistency and a milky-white prostatic fluid oozes out of these areas.
  - In nodules with primarily stromal (fibromuscular) proliferation, surface is pale-gray, tough looking, does not exude fluid; and is less clearly demarcated from the surrounding uninvolved prostatic tissue.
  - The nodules do not have true capsule, but a plane of cleavage (formed by compression of surrounding prostatic tissue) is present.

- *Microscopic examination*
  - Nodularity is the hallmark of BPH.
  - The composition of nodule ranges from purely stromal fibromuscular nodule to fibroepithelial nodules with a glandular predominance.
  - Glandular proliferation shows aggregation of small to large cystically dilated glands. These glands are lined by two layers. The inner layer is composed of columnar cells and the outer layer by cuboidal or flattened epithelium. Basement membrane of gland is intact. Papillation and infoldings of epithelium are present.
  - The stromal component shows fibrous and muscular proliferation.

  - Sometimes squamous metaplasia and foci of infarction may be present.

Clinical features: Clinical presentation depends on weight of prostate as well as on many unknown factors. Patient may be asymptomatic despite presence of mild enlarged prostate or may present with mild sign and symptoms of increased frequency and urgency to frank renal failure due to hydronephrosis.

- *Early complains:* Due to compression of urethra: Increased frequency, nocturia (urgency), problem in starting and stopping the stream of urine, overflow dribbling, painful micturition.
- *Late complains:* Secondary to retention of urine in the bladder: Infection (UTI), cystitis, hypertrophy, urine retention or trabeculation in urinary bladder, *hydronephrosis* may occur.

14. Lab diagnosis of carcinoma prostate

1. *Digital rectal examination:* Most of the prostatic tumors are located in posterior lobe, so per rectal examination makes it easy to palpate any prostatic tumor mass.
2. *Transrectal ultrasonography:* For early detection of tumor and its local spread, US-guided biopsy is also done.
3. *Biopsy:* To confirm diagnosis. Normal prostatic glands have two cell lining (layers), but cancer cells lack basal cells. This change can be detected by using immunohistologic markers.
4. *Computed tomography scan:* Lymph node involvement.
5. *Magnetic resonance imaging:* Lymph node involvement.
6. *Pelvic lymphadenectomy:* For microscopic metastasis.
7. Osteoblastic metastasis (detected by skeleton survey or radio nuclide scanning) in bone is diagnostic of prostatic cancer.

8. *Tumor markers:* Prostatic acid phosphatase and PSA.

9. α-methylacyl-coenzyme A-racemase (AMACR) is up-regulated in cancer cells and can be detected by using immunohistochemistry. Its sensitivity varies from 82–100%.

10. PCA3: A gene on chromosome 9q that possibly encodes a regulatory RNA for tissue growth.

11. EZH2 (enhancer of zeste 2): Loss of E catherin (adhesion protein) from prostatic cancer cells is associated with high levels of EZH2 and may contribute to prostatic cancer progression.

Prostatic acid phosphatase (PAP): Secreted by prostatic epithelium (normal as well as cancerous). Serum level is highly raised in prostatic cancer extending beyond the capsule or in metastatic cases. Normal values 1–3 ng/ml units. If level is 3–5 ng/ml prostatic cancer is suspected, but more than 5 ng/ml unit is diagnostic of the cancer.

15. Carcinoma prostate (1993, 2007)

- 1st most common form (2nd common: Lung cancer) of cancer and 2nd leading cause of cancer death in males.
- *Age:* Men over 50 yr.

Etiopathogenesis of carcinoma prostate
Etiology of carcinoma prostate is multifactorial, but none has been clearly established.

1. *Age:* More than 50 yr
2. *Race:* Most common in blacks and least common in Asians.
3. *Family history:* Increased incidence, if there is family history of carcinoma prostate.
4. *Hormone:* Androgen plays an important role in prostatic cancer. The growth and survival of prostate cancer cells depend on androgens which bind to androgen receptors and induce the expression of pro-growth and pro-survival genes.

5. Environmental factors and dietary factors like increased fat consumption.
6. Genetic factors like inherited polymorphism and chromosomal rearrangements.
- In approximately 70% of cases, carcinoma of prostate arises in the peripheral zone of the gland, classically in a posterior location, where it may be palpable on rectal examination.

Morphology
- *Gross*
  - Size of prostate: Enlarged, normal or smaller.
  - Location of tumor: Peripheral zone, most commonly in posterior lobe.
  - Malignant part is firm and fibrous.
  - Cut section is homogeneous and may show yellowish irregular areas.

Microscopic features: Four histologic types: Adenocarcinoma, transitional cell carcinoma, squamous cell carcinoma and undifferentiated carcinoma.

Adenocarcinoma is the most common (96%)
  - Most adenocarcinomas produce well-defined gland pattern.
  - Groups of acini are either closely packed in back-to-back arrangement without intervening stroma or haphazardly distributed.
  - Glands lack branching and papillary infoldings (differentiate from normal gland)
  - These glands are typically smaller than benign glands and are lined by a single uniform layer of cuboidal or low columnar epithelium. The outer basal cell layer (typical of normal gland) is absent.
  - Nuclei are large and often contain one or more large nucleoli. Nuclear pleomorphism (size/shape) is marked.
  - Mitotic figures are infrequent.
  - There is little or no stroma between acini.
  - Glands may be well-differentiated to almost undifferentiated.

- Tumor cells may be clear cells (foamy cytoplasm), dark cells (homogeneous basophilic cytoplasm) or eosinophilic cells (granular cytoplasm).
- There is invasion of intraprostatic *perineural* spaces.

- **Metastasis of carcinoma prostate**

Local extension: Involves periprostatic tissue, seminal vesicles, and the base of urinary bladder.

Lymphatic spread: Spread of prostatic cancer occurs through lymphatics early to obturator nodes and eventually to para-aortic nodes.

Hematogenous spread: Occurs chiefly to bones and viscera.

The bony metastasis is typically osteoblastic. The bones most commonly involved (in descending order of frequency) are lumbar spine, proximal femur, pelvis, thoracic spine and ribs.

Grading of carcinoma prostate

Gleason system

In this system, prostate cancers are classified into five grades on the basis of glandular pattern of differentiation.

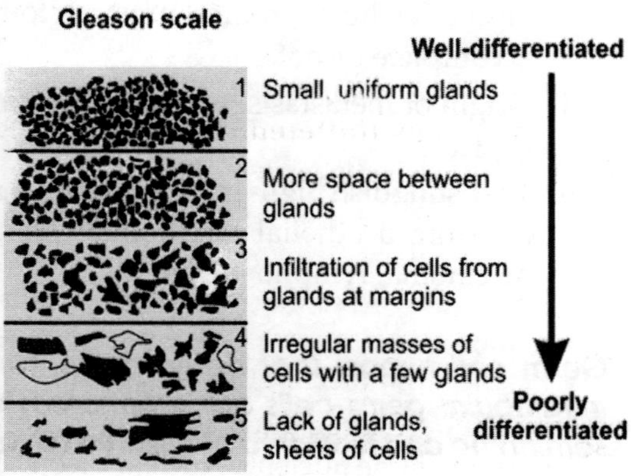

Gleason scale

Well-differentiated

1 Small uniform glands

2 More space between glands

3 Infiltration of cells from glands at margins

4 Irregular masses of cells with a few glands

5 Lack of glands, sheets of cells

Poorly differentiated

Fig. 20.2: Gleason score for carcinoma prostate

Grade 1 represents the most well-differentiated tumors, in which the neoplastic glands are uniform and round in appearance and are packed into well-circumscribed nodules.

By contrast, grade 5 tumors show no glandular differentiations and the tumor cells can infiltrate the stroma in the form of cords, sheets and nests.

The other grades fall inbetween.

Each tumor is assigned by a primary grade (1–5) according to the most frequent pattern and a secondary grade (1–5) according to the second most frequent pattern or the highest grade.

The two grades are added to obtain a combined Gleason grade or score (2–10).

Gleason score	Severity
2–4	Incidental finding on TURP samples for BPH; good prognosis
5–7	Most of the treatable carcinoma prostate; good prognosis
8–10	Advanced carcinoma prostate; poor prognosis

Staging of prostatic adenocarcinoma using TNM system

TNM designation extent of primary tumor (T)	Anatomic findings
T_1	Clinically inapparent lesion (by palpation/imaging studies)
T_{1a}	Involvement of $\leq 5\%$ of resected tissue
T_{1b}	Involvement of $\geq 5\%$ of resected tissue
T_{1c}	Carcinoma present on needle biopsy (following elevated PSA)
T_2	Palpable or visible cancer confined to prostate
T_{2a}	Involvement of $\leq 5\%$ of one lobe
T_{2b}	Involvement of $\geq 5\%$ of one lobe
T_{2c}	Involvement of both lobes
T_3	Local extraprostatic extension
T_{3a}	Extracapsular extension
T_{3b}	Seminal vesical invasion

(Contd.)

Staging of prostatic adenocarcinoma using TNM system (Contd.)

TNM designation extent of primary tumor (T)	Anatomic findings
T_4	Invasion of contiguous organs and/or supporting structures including bladder neck, rectum, external sphincter, levator muscular or pelvic floor.
Status of regional lymph nodes (N)	
N_0	No regional nodal metastasis
N_1	Metastasis in regional lymph nodes
Distant metastases (M)	
M_0	No distant metastasis
M_1	Distant metastasis present
M_{1a}	Metastasis to distant lymph node
M_{1b}	Bone metastasis
M_{1c}	Other distant sites

16. Prostate specific antigen (PSA)

- Normally produced by prostatic epithelial and secreted in the serum.
- It cleaves and liquefies seminal coagulum after ejaculation by its enzymatic activity (protease function).
- Its serum level increases in prostatic cancer, nodular hyperplasia of prostate, prostatitis and other diseased conditions of prostate.
- PSA is organ specific and not tumor/disease specific.
- It may be presumed to have very high serum level of PSA in cancer as compared to nodular hyperplasia, but their values may coincide. So *criteria* other than its serum level to be looked for.

1. *PSA density:* Ratio between serum PSA value and volume of prostate gland.
2. *PSA velocity:* Rate of change of serum PSA level with time.
3. Use of reference value according to age, race or other local criteria.
4. Percentage of free PSA: Ratio of free PSA (minor component) and total PSA in serum multiplied by 100. Major portion is bound to α_1-antichymotrypsin protein. *Percentage of free PSA is lower in patients with prostatic cancer than other non-neoplastic diseases.*

- Percentage of free PSA is useful in differentiating between prostatic cancer and other non-neoplastic diseases in two extreme values, but in the range of 4–10 ng/ml it is most useful in combination with rectal examination and transrectal ultrasonography (normal cut off value—less than 4 ng/ml).

Uses of PSA:

1. Diagnosis of prostatic diseases.
2. Response to chemotherapy in cancer.
3. To check whether radical prostatectomy is complete or not.
4. Origin of metastasis, whether it is from prostate.
5. To distinguish high-grade prostatic cancer from urothelial carcinoma, colonic carcinoma, lymphoma, etc.

Germ cell tumors that do not arise from intratubular germ cells are spermatocytic seminoma and teratoma of children (viva).

21

Female Genital Tract

1. Cervical intraepithelial neoplasm (CIN) (1988, 92, 93, 97, 99, 2000, 03, 04, 08)

CINs are precancerous lesions that give rise to carcinoma cervix (squamous cell carcinoma of cervix).

Human papillomavirus has been implicated in CIN. Harald zur Hausen was awarded the Nobel prize in 2008 for discovery of HPV as a cause of cervical cancer.

LSIL: Low grade squamous intraepithelial lesion.

HSIL: High grade squamous intraepithelial lesion.

CIN I
- Indistinguishable histologically from condylomata
- Dysplasia is present in lower 1/3rd layer of stratified squamous cells.

Appearance
- Lesion may be raised (acuminatum) or macular (flat condyloma)
- Koilocytic atypia (viral cytopathic effect) are seen. Nuclear alteration (enlarged nucleus, hyperchromasia, coarse chromatin granules, variation of nuclear sizes and shapes) and cytoplasmic halos (disruption of cytoskeleton).

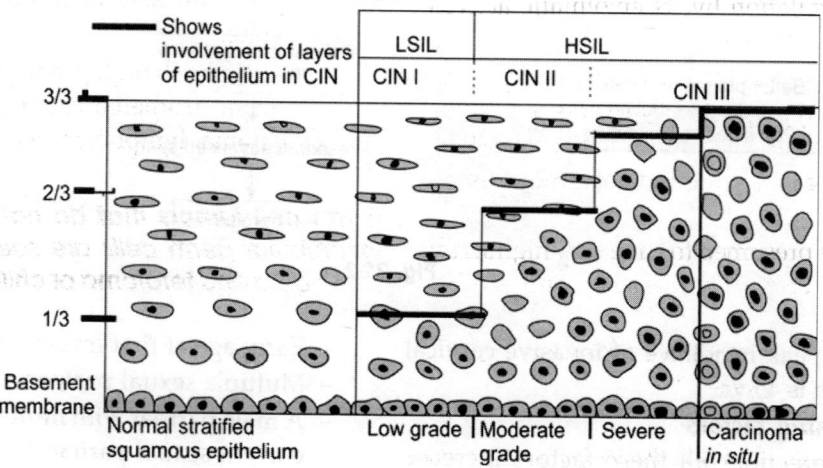

Fig. 21.1: Diagram depicting varying degree of involvement of stratified squamous epithelium in CIN

CIN II

- Dysplasia is limited to basal 2/3rd layer of stratified squamous cells.
- Atypical cells in lower layer are seen.
- *Atypical cells have:*
  - N/C ratio increased
  - Loss of polarity
  - Abnormal mitoses
  - Anisokaryosis
  - Mitotic figures
  - Hyperchromasia
  - Loss of maturation
  - Expansion of the immature basal cells above the lower third of the epithelial thickness
- Upper layer cells differentiated though abnormal
- Aneuploid cell population
- High risk HPV type

CIN III/carcinoma *in situ*

- Dysplasia spread to whole layer
- Complete loss of polarity
- Atypical cells throughout all layers
- A stage prior to malignancy (pre-malignant)

A low grade lesion does not always progress to a high grade lesion. Likelihood of regression in CIN I is 50–60%, persistence is 30% and progression to CIN III is 20% with CIN III likelihood of regression is only 30% and of progression is 60–70%.

2. Role of viruses in uterine cervix cancer (1998)

3. Grading and staging of carcinoma cervix (1998, 2004)

4. Carcinoma cervix: Predisposing factors, etiology, morphology and diagnosis (1995, 2009, 10)

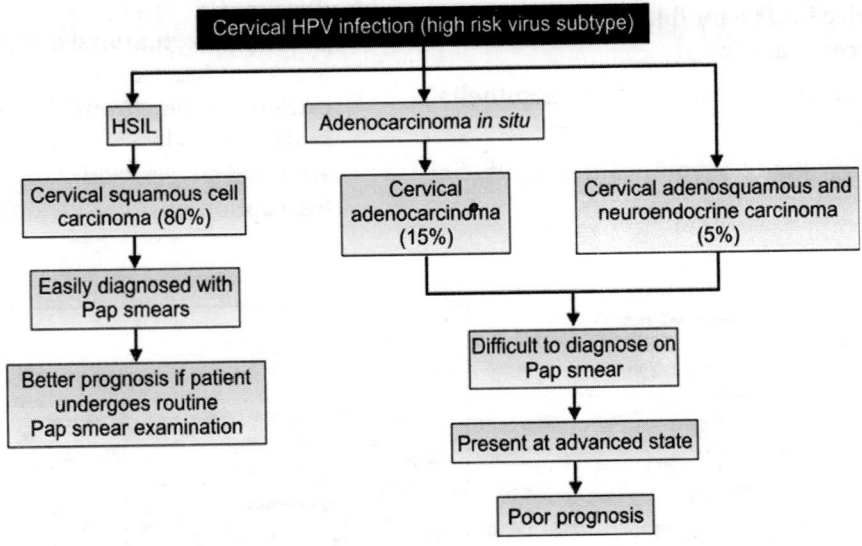

Fig. 21.2

Age: The peak incidence of invasive cervical carcinoma is 45 yr.

Predisposing factors

- HPV infection (all these factors increase transmission of HPV):
  - Early age at first intercourse
  - Multiple sexual partners
  - A male partner with multiple previous/current sexual partners.
  - Lack of circumcision in male sexual partners.

- Use of oral contraceptives
- Cigarette smoking and use of nicotine
- High parity
- Family history of cervical cancers
- Associated other genital infections
- Immune suppression
- Certain HLA subtypes
- Persistent infection with a high oncogenic risk HPV (HPVs 16 and 18)

Morphology
- *Gross*
  - Invasive cervical carcinoma may be either fungating (exophytic growth, most common) or infiltrative.
  - The cancer can grow to involve all contiguous structures.
- *Microscopic examination*
  - Squamous cell carcinoma: Tumor consists of nests and tongues of malignant squamous cells (either keratinized, i.e. well-differentiated or non-keratinized, i.e. moderately to undifferentiated). Cancer cells invade the underlying stroma.
  - Adenocarcinoma: Cancer shows proliferation of glandular epithelium composed of malignant endocervical cells with large, hyperchromatic nuclei and relatively mucin depleted cytoplasm. The glands appear dark as compared to normal gland.
  - Adenosquamous subtype is composed of intermixed malignant glandular and malignant squamous epithelium.
  - Neuroendocrine cervical carcinoma is histologically similar to small cell (oat cell) carcinoma of lung.

Staging
  i. *Stage 0:* Carcinoma *in situ* (CIN III, HSIL)
  ii. *Stage I:* Carcinoma confined to the cervix
    - Ia: Diagnosed only by microscopy (pre-clinical carcinoma), but have:
      - Ia1: Stromal invasion no deeper than 3 mm and no wider than 7 mm (microinvasive carcinoma)
      - Ia2: Maximum depth of invasion of stroma deeper than 3 mm and no deeper than 5 mm taken from base of epithelium; horizontal invasion not more than 7 mm.
    - Ib: Histologically invasive carcinoma confined to cervix, but greater than stage Ia2.
  iii. *Stage II:* Carcinoma extends beyond the cervix, but pelvic wall not involved. Carcinoma also involves vagina, but without the involvement of lower third.
  iv. *Stage III:* Pelvic wall and lower one-third of vagina are also involved by carcinoma. On PR examination, there is no cancer free space between the tumor and pelvic wall.
  v. *Stage IV:* Extension of carcinoma beyond true pelvic wall, or may involve mucosa of bladder or rectum, or have systemic/local metastasis.

Diagnosis: Biopsy
Screening: Pap smear, HPV DNA testing
5 yr survival rate with appropriate treatment
Stage 0: 100%
Stage I: 90%
Stage II: 82%
Stage III: 35%
Stage IV: 10%

5. Endometriosis

- Presence of endometrial glands or stroma in abnormal location outside the uterus is known as endometriosis.
- *Age:* Third and fourth decades.
- *Sites* in decreasing order of frequency (*remember for viva*):
  a. Ovaries
  b. Uterine ligaments
  c. Rectovaginal septum
  d. Culde sac
  e. Pelvic peritoneum
  f. Large and small bowel and appendix
  g. Mucosa of the cervix, vagina and fallopian tubes.
  h. Laparotomy scars

- *Theories* that are proposed to explain it:
  - *Metastatic theory (regurgitation/transplanted)*: Due to regurgitation of menstrual blood through fallopian tubes, endometrial tissue is transplanted from uterus to peritoneal cavities. This is the most widely accepted theory.
  - *Metaplastic theory*: Coelomic epithelium gives rise to endometrial tissues *in situ*, so endometriosis develops.
  - *Vascular or lymphatic dissemination theory*: It explains the presence of endometrial tissues at extra pelvic sites like lung or lymph nodes.
- Genetic, hormonal and immune factors are attributed to the increased risk of endometriosis in certain women.
  - There is profound activation of inflammatory cascade in endometriosis leading to high level of PGE2, IL-1β, TNF and IL-6.
  - Estrogen production by endometriotic stromal cells is markedly upregulated due to high level of steroidogenic enzyme aromatase.

Morphology
- *Gross*
  - Red-blue or yellow-brown nodule present on or just beneath serosal surface.
  - Extensive hemorrhage, may cause fibrotic adhesion of different layers.
  - Large cystic space filled with brown blood debris, may distort ovaries (often bilateral) and change its appearance to *chocolate cyst*.
- *Histologic diagnosis* of endometriosis is made, if two of three features are found:
  - Endometrial glands
  - Endometrial stroma
  - Hemosiderin laden macrophages are identified
- *Clinical features*
  - Dysmenorrhea
  - Dyspareunia
  - Infertility
  - Pelvic pain due to intrapelvic bleeding and periuterine adhesion

6. Adenomyosis

Adenomyosis is defined as the presence of endometrial tissue within the uterine wall (myometrium). The endometrial tissue grows downward in continuity with endometrium into myometrium.
- Histologically adenomyosis consists of irregular nests of endometrial stroma, with or without glands in between muscle bundle. The cells are separated from basalis by at least 2 to 3 mm.
- Adenomyosis presents with irregular and heavy menses (menometrorrhagia), colicky dysmenorrhea, dyspareunia, and premenstrual pelvic pain.

7. Endometrial hyperplasia (1998, 2002)

There is increased proliferation of endometrial glands relative to stroma resulting in increased gland to stromal ratio and associated with prolonged, profuse and irregular uterine bleeding in menopausal or postmenopausal women. These hyperplasia may progress to carcinoma.
- Risk factors of endometrial hyperplasia:
  - Prolonged stimulation of endometrium
    - Anovulation
    - ↑ estrogen production from endogenous or exogenous source (hormone replacement)
  - Obesity
  - Menopause
  - Polycystic ovarian disease
  - Excessive cortical function
  - Inactivation of PTEN (tumor suppressor gene)

Based on histopathology, International Society for Gynecological Pathology has classified endometrial hyperplasia into four classes:

1. Simple hyperplasia without atypia (cystic or mild hyperplasia)

- Glands vary in size and shape and have cystic dilatation.
- Mild increase in gland to stroma ratio
- Epithelial growth patterns are similar to normal proliferative phase, but mitoses are not that frequent.
- They rarely progress to adenocarcinoma (1%)
- They may turn into cystic atrophy once estrogen stimulation is withdrawn.

2. Simple hyperplasia with atypia

- This pattern is uncommon
- Architecturally tissue pattern seems simple hyperplasia, but glandular epithelial cells show cytologic as well as some nuclear atypia, i.e. loss of polarity, prominent nucleoli and open chromatin pattern.
- Approximately 8% of these lesions progress to carcinoma

3. Complex hyperplasia without atypia

- There is increased number and size of endometrial glands, marked crowding as well as branching of glands.
- There is a little stroma
- Mitotic figures are frequent
- Glands remain distinct and nonconfluent
- Epithelial cells are cytologically normal
- Only 3% of these hyperplasia progress to carcinoma

4. Complex hyperplasia with atypia

- These have complex hyperplasia with epithelial cellular atypia and resemble well-differentiated adenocarcinoma.
- There is a high change (25–40%) that complex hyperplasia with atypia is adenocarcinoma.

8. Endometrial carcinoma (1990)

- Endometrial carcinoma is the most common invasive cancer of female genital tracts.
- Endometrial carcinoma develops in postmenopausal woman (peak: 55–65 yr) presenting with postmenopausal bleeding.
- On the basis of clinicopathologic and molecular basis, two types of endometrial carcinomas are described:

	Type 1	Type 2
Frequency	80%	20%
Age	55–65 yr	65–75 yr
Predisposing factors	• Unopposed estrogen stimulation	• Endometrial atrophy
	• Obesity	• Thin built women

(Contd.)

Endometrial carcinoma (Contd.)

	Type 1	Type 2
	• Hypertension • Diabetes • Infertility • Underlying endometrial hyperplasia	
Morphology	Endometrioid carcinoma (well-differentiated mimicking proliferative endometrium)	• Serus or clear cell type (mimics subtypes of ovarian carcinoma) • Mixed mullerian tumor (poorly differentiated)
Precursor	Endometrial hyperplasia	Endometrial intraepithelial carcinoma
Molecular genetics	• PTEN • PIK3CA • KRAS • MSI • β-catenin • p53	• p53 • Aneuploidy • PIK3CA
Behavior	• Low grade malignant potential • Spread via lymphatics	• Aggressive tumor • Intraperitoneal and lymphatic spread

Morphology

- *Gross*

  Tumor can be either localized polypoid tumor or diffused involving the surface.

  Microscopic examination

  Definitive diagnosis of endometrial carcinoma is made only when invasion of endometrial stroma or myometrium is seen.

  Criteria for stromal invasion

  1. Irregular infiltration by glands including altered fibroblastic stroma (desmoplastic response)
  2. Confluent glands, merging and creating a cribiform pattern with minimal intervening stroma
  3. Extensive papillary formations
  4. Replacement of stroma by masses of squamous epithelium

  Most of the endometrial carcinomas are endometrioid adenocarcinoma. Based on differentiation they have been graded into 3 grades:

  Grade 1 (well-differentiated adenocarcinoma): They have back to back densely arranged well-differentiated glands with minimal atypia (less than 5% of solid growth).

  Grade 2 (moderately differentiated adenocarcinoma): They have glandular as well as solid sheets (less than 50%) of tumor cells.

  Grade 3 (poorly differentiated adenocarcinoma): They have predominantly (more than 50%) solid sheets of tumor cells.

  ### Staging of endometrial carcinoma

  Stage I: Carcinoma is confined to the corpus uteri itself.

  Stage II: Carcinoma involves the corpus and the cervix.

  Stage III: Carcinoma extends outside the uterus, but not outside the true pelvis.

Stage IV: Carcinoma extends outside the true pelvis or involves the mucosa of the bladder or the rectum.

9. Leiomyoma uterus (1989)

- They are commonly called fibroid uterus and are most common tumors of women.
- These are estrogen responsive benign tumors of smooth muscles of uterus occurring during active reproductive life.
- They may regress or even calcify after castration or menopause; on the other hand, its size may increase during pregnancy.
- Women with leiomyoma may be asymptomatic or may present with abnormal bleeding (increased bleeding during menses), compression of bladder (increased frequency), impaired fertility and pain.
- Pregnant women with fibroid may have increased frequency of spontaneous abortion, fetal malpresentation, uterine atony, postpartum hemorrhage.
- Malignant transformation into leiomyosarcoma is extremely rare.
- Few genetic abnormalities like balanced translocation between chromosomes 12 and 14, partial deletion of long arm of chromosome 7 are seen.

- *Gross*
  - They are sharply circumscribed, discrete, round, firm and gray-white tumors varying in size.
  - They can be intramural, submucosal or subserosal in location.
  - Cut section shows whorled pattern of smooth muscle bundle.
  - Leiomyoma may show different types of secondary changes like red degeneration (due to venous thrombosis and congestion), hyaline degeneration, mucinous and cystic degeneration (liquefaction followed by mucinous degeneration), ischemic necrosis, fibrosis and calcification.

- *Microscopy*
  - Acrhitecture resembles to normal myometrium.
  - Whorled bundle of smooth muscle cells
  - Muscle cells are uniform in size and shape, have oval nuclei and long bipolar cytoplasmic processes.
  - Mitotic figures are rare.

10. Classify ovarian tumors (1997)

Surface Epithelial-Stromal Tumors		
Frequency: 65–70%	Proportion of malignant ovarian tumor: 90%	Age group: 20 yr+
Serous tumor	**Mucinous tumors**	
Benign (cystadenoma)	Benign (cystadenoma)	
Borderline (serous borderline tumor)	Borderline (mucinous borderline tumor)	
Malignant (serous adenocarcinoma)	Malignant (mucinous adenocarcinoma)	
Endometrioid tumor	**Clear cell tumor**	
Benign (cystadenoma)	Benign	
Borderline (endometrioid borderline tumor)	Borderline	
Malignant (endometrioid adenocarcinoma)	Malignant (clear cell adenocarcinoma)	
Transitional cell tumors	**Epithelial-stroma**	
Brenner tumor	Adenosarcoma	
Brenner tumor of borderline malignancy	Malignant mixed müllerian tumor	
Malignant Brenner tumor		
Transitional cell carcinoma (non-Brenner type)		

(Contd.)

Classify ovarian tumors (Contd.)

Sex Cord-Stromal Tumors

Frequency: 5–10%   Proportion of malignant ovarian tumor: 2–3%   Age group: All ages

Granulosa tumors	Leydig cell tumors
Fibromas	Sex cord tumors with annular tubules
Fibrothecomas	Gynandroblastoma
Thecomas	Steroid (lipid) cell tumors
Sertoli cell tumors	

Germ Cell Tumors

Frequency: 15–20%   Proportion of malignant ovarian tumor: 3–5%   Age group: 0–25+ yr

Teratoma	Dysgerminoma
Immature	Yolk sac tumor
Mature (cystic, solid)	Mixed germ cell tumor
Monodermal (specialized)	

Malignant, otherwise not specified

Metastatic cancer from nonovarian primary

Frequency: 5%   Proportion of malignant ovarian tumor: 5%   Age group: Variable

Colonic, appendiceal	Gastric
Breast	

11. Hormone producing tumors of ovary (2003)

- Yolk sac tumor (α-fetoprotein, α_1-antitrypsin)
- Choriocarcinoma (HCG)
- Granuloma theca cell tumors (estrogen, rarely androgens)
- Sertoli–Leydig cell tumor or androblastoma (androgens)
- H. mole (HCG)

12. Difference between serous and mucinous ovarian tumors

S. No.	Traits	Serous	Mucinous
1.	Frequency	a. 30% of all ovarian tumors	25% of all ovarian tumors, 10% of
		b. 50% of ovarian epithelial tumor	malignant ovarian tumor, 80% are benign, 15% are malignant
		c. 70% are benign and border-line, 30% are malignant	
		d. Serous carcinoma most common malignant ovarian tumor (40%)	
2.	Age	Benign and borderline: 20–45 yr, malignant: Later age	Middle age; rare before puberty and after menopause
3.	Number of cysts	One/few	Multiple, more
4.	Size of cysts	Small	Large
5.	Surface involvement	Common	Rare

(Contd.)

Difference between serous and mucinous ovarian tumors (*Contd.*)

S. No.	Traits	Serous	Mucinous
6.	Bilateral tumor	Common	Less/rare
7.	Gross	One/few fibrous walled cysts filled with clear serous fluid	Multifocal tumors filled with sticky gelatinous fluid rich in glycoprotein
8.	Cell lining of cyst	Tall, columnar, ciliated epithelial cells	Tall columnar epithelial cells with apical mucin. Cilia are characteristically absent
9.	Papillae	Very common	Less common
10.	Psammoma bodies	Common	Not found
11.	Risk factor	• Nulliparity/low parity • Genetic BRCA1 and BRCA2 mutation	KRAS mutation

13. Teratoma ovary (1988, 08, 11)

Three types:

1. *Mature*
2. *Immature/malignant* and,
3. *Highly specialized or monodermal teratoma:*
   - Always unilateral.
   - Rare, but group of special forms of tumors derived from only one germ layer.
   - Examples are struma ovarii, carcinoid tumor.

- Struma ovarii: Exclusively thyroid tissues, may be functional to produce hyperthyroidism.
- Carcinoid tumor: Arises from argentaffin cells of intestine in teratoma (carcinoid syndrome).
- Struma-carcinoid tumor: Rare combination of two.

14. Mature/benign cystic teratoma ovary/dermoid cyst (1990, 03)

15. Difference between immature and mature teratoma (1994)

S.No.	Traits	Mature teratoma (dermoid cyst)	Immature teratoma
1.	Nature	Benign	Malignant
2.	Age	Young women (active reproductive year)	Adolescent before puberty, young adults before the age of 20
3.	Locations	Bilateral in 10–15% cases	Mostly unilateral
4.	Types	Mostly cystic (dermoid cyst), solid tumor is rare	Almost all are solid tumors
5.	Component tissue	Mature	Immature
6.	Dermoid cyst, gross appearance	Unilocular cyst is lined by very thin wall. Wall is lined by opaque, gray-white, wrinkled epidermis. Cystic wall may have area of calcification or teeth structures in it or hair shafts may protrude from it.	Bulky and smooth external surface. Cut surface shows solid structures. Area of necrosis and hemorrhage are present. Hairs, cartilage, bones, calcification may be present.

(Contd.)

Difference between immature and mature teratoma (Contd.)

S. No.	Traits	Mature teratoma (dermoid cyst)	Immature teratoma
7.	Dermoid cyst, microscopic examination	Cyst wall lined by stratified squamous epithelium. Sebaceous glands, hair shafts, other skin appendages of structures from ectodermal differentiation of totipotent germ cells are found. Structures like cartilage, bones, thyroid tissue or other *organoid structures* derived from other germ cells may also be present.	Immature structure differentiating towards cartilage, glands, muscles, bones, neuroepithelium, etc. resembling fetal or embryonal tissues rather than adult tissues. Proportion of immature neuroepithelium in the tumor is risk factor for its extra ovarian spread
8.	Variant types	Solid mature teratoma is rare, benign looking, tissues and organoid structures from all three germ layers. Dermoid cyst component (1%) may transform into malignant form.	Nor significant
9.	Metastasis and growth rate	No metastasis, slow growing Associated with paraneoplastic syndromes	Penetrates capsule—spread locally or metastasize to distant locations Rapidly growing Not associated

16. Dysgerminoma (= seminoma) (viva) (1997, 2011)

17. Yolk sac tumor of ovary (1992, 94, 2008)

- *See yolk sac tumor of testes for morphology.*
- Second most malignant tumor of germ cell origin.
- *Age:* Children and young women.
- Usually single ovary involved.
- Patient presents with abdominal pain and rapidly developing pelvic mass.
- Rapid growing, aggressive nature.
- Fatal within two years of diagnosis.

18. Choriocarcinoma (read from male genital tract) (1999, 2007)

19. Hydatidiform mole: Gross and microscopic features (1996, 2007)

- H. mole is a subtype of gestational trophoblastic disease, histologically characterized by cystic swelling of the chorionic villi,

accompanied by variable trophoblastic proliferation.
- Ten percent of mole develop into persistent or invasive moles.
- 2–5% of complete moles progress into choriocarcinoma.
- Develops within uterus, but may develop at any site of ectopic pregnancy.
- *Age:* Diagnosed at 4–5 months of pregnancy (now earlier diagnosis due to ultrasound) at any age during active reproductive life, but risk higher in teens or age of 40–50.
- *Clinical features*
  - 4–5th months of pregnancy
  - Vaginal bleeding
  - Passage of thin watery fluid
  - Small grape-like tissue mass in vaginal discharge
  - Uterine enlargement is more than what is anticipated according to period of gestation.

- For diagnosis ultrasonography is very useful.

Morphology (*also see difference*)

- *Gross*
  - Uterine cavity / ectopic site is filled with delicate, friable masses of thin-walled, translucent, cystic and grape-like structures.
  - Amniotic sac is very small and collapsed.
  - No fetal parts seen in complete mole, may be seen in partial mole.

Microscopic examination

- *Complete mole*

- Involve all or most of villous tissues
- Chorionic villi are enlarged, scalloped in shape with central cavitation and lack of adequate vascularity.
- Extensive trophoblast proliferation involving the entire circumference of villi as well as 'extra-villious' proliferation of trophoblast.

- *Partial mole*
  - Villous enlargement and architectural disturbances limited to a few areas of villi.
  - The trophoblastic proliferation is moderate.

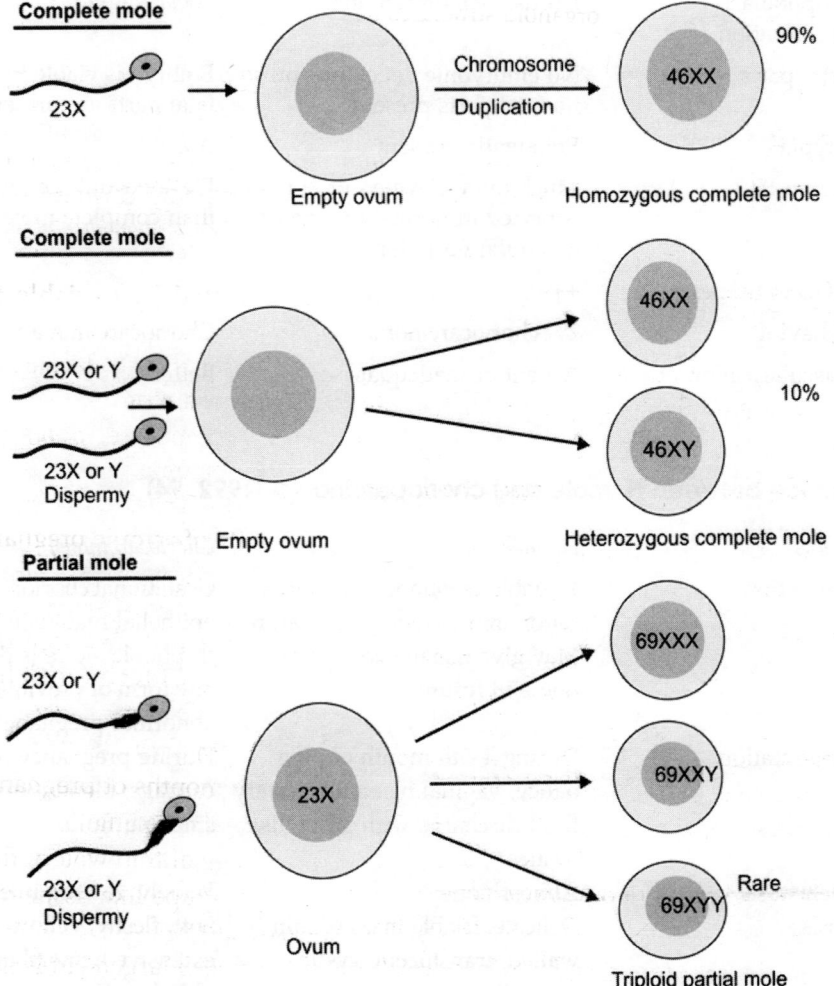

Fig. 21.3: Genetic origin of complete and partial hydatidiform moles

20. Difference between partial and complete H. mole (2000, 08)

S. No.	Traits	Complete/classic mole	Partial mole
1.	Karyotype	46, XX (46, XY)	Triploid (69, XXX or 69, XXY)
2.	Cause	Two sperms fuse with an ovum (without any DNA materials) or one sperm fuses with ovum (without any DNA materials) followed by duplication of sperm DNA.	Fertilization of an egg with DNA material by one diploid or two haploid sperms.
3.	Clinical features		
	• Missed abortion	+	++
	• Heavy bleeding	+++	+
	• Toxemia	+++	+
4.	Villous edema	All chorionic villi are edematous	Only some villi are edematous.
5.	Trophoblast proliferation	Diffuse; circumferential	Focal; slight
6.	Fetal parts	No embryonic development, so no fetal parts present	Embryo is viable for weeks, so fetal parts are present.
7.	Atypia	Frequently present	Absent
8.	Serum HCG	Much more elevated level than expected in normal pregnancy of similar gestation	Elevated, but comparatively lesser than complete mole
9.	HCG in tissues	++++	+
10.	Behavior	2% choriocarcinoma	Choriocarcinoma is rare
11.	Vascularization of villi	Absent or inadequate	Better

21. Difference between H. mole and choriocarcinoma (1992, 94)

S. No.	Traits	H. mole	Choriocarcinoma
1.	Definition	Variable trophoblastic proliferation, mostly benign in nature. May give rise to choriocarcinoma in future	Gestational choriocarcinoma is an epithelial malignant neoplasm of trophoblastic cells derived from any form of previously normal or abnormal pregnancy.
2.	Presentation	During 4–5th month of pregnancy, vaginal bleeding/watery fluid discharge with grape-like tissues	During pregnancy or after miscarriage, bloody, brown, foul smelling fluids
3.	Metastasis	Almost none	Widely; to lung liver, brain
4.	Gross	Delicate, friable mass of thin-walled, translucent, cystic, grape-like structures	Soft, fleshy, yellow-white, extensive hemorrhage, pale area of ischemic necrosis

(Contd.)

Difference between H. mole and choriocarcinoma (*Contd.*)

S. No.	Traits	H. mole	Choriocarcinoma
5.	Microscopy	Villous edema, cytotrophoblast and syncytiotrophoblast cover villi. Epithelial cells produces villi.	Purely epithelial cell malignancy and do not produce chorionic villi; abnormal proliferation of both cytotrophoblast and syncytio-trophoblast
6.	Uterus size	Larger than the expected size for duration of pregnancy	Little abnormal enlargement
7.	HCG level	↑ed	↑↑↑ed
8.	Precedent history	No	H. mole, abortion, normal pregnancy, ectopic pregnancy
9.	Treatment	Curettage, hysterectomy	Curretage and chemotherapy; may be hysterectomy

22. Krukenberg tumor (1989, 98, 2000, 02, 07, 08, 10)

- *Age:* > 45 yr

Morphology

Gross: Bilateral, symmetrical enlarged ovary, but architecture of ovary is maintained.

Microscopically: Signet ring cells (abundant amount of mucin push the nucleus to periphery), diffusely infiltrative growth pattern (not forming glands).

- *Pathogenesis:* It is a diffuse type of gastric tumor, which metastasizes to ovaries.

  Two theories are given for metastasis of tumor from GIT to ovary:
  - *Old theory:* Due to shedding of tumor cells into peritoneum (transcoelomic spread).
  - *New theory:* By the lymphatic spread.

Note: Tumors of breast, uterus, fallopian tube, colon and lung can also metastasize to ovary, which is also called Krukenberg tumor.

22

Breast

1. Classify benign epithelial lesions of breast and their risk of developing breast carcinoma

These lesions have been divided into three groups, according to the subsequent risk of developing breast cancer:

1. Non-proliferative breast changes
2. Proliferative breast disease without atypia
3. Proliferative breast disease with atypia

Risk of developing invasive carcinoma	
Pathologic lesion	*Relative risk (Absolute lifetime risk)*
NON-PROLIFERATIVE BREAST CHANGES • Duct ectasia • Cysts • Apocrine changes • Mild hyperplasia • Adenosis • Fibroadenoma without complex features	1.0 (3%)
PROLIFERATIVE DISEASE WITHOUT ATYPIA • Moderate or florid hyperplasia • Sclerosing adenosis • Papilloma • Complex sclerosing lesion (radial scar) • Fibroadenoma with complex features	0.5 to 2.0 (5–7%)
PROLIFERATIVE DISEASE WITH ATYPIA • Atypical ductal hyperplasia (ADH) • Atypical lobular hyperplasia (ALH)	4.0 to 5.0 (13–17%)
CARCINOMA *IN SITU* • Lobular carcinoma *in situ* (LCIS) • Ductal carcinoma *in situ* (DCIS)	8.0 to 10.0 (25–30%)

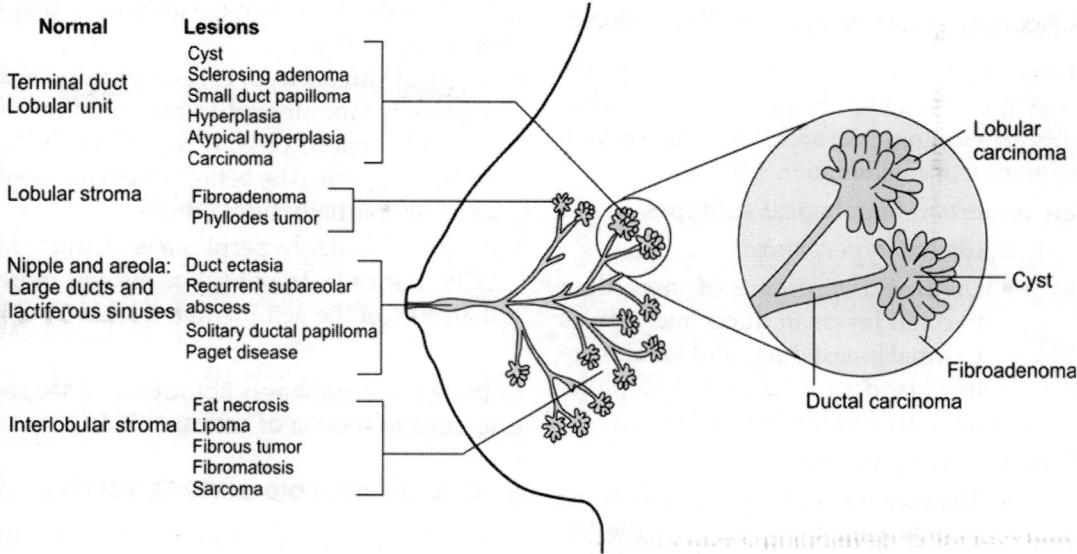

Fig. 22.1: Anatomic origins of some common breast lesions

2. Fibrocystic changes/disease of breast/ benign mammary dysplasia (1989, 90, 93, 98, 99, 2001, 11)

- A large spectrum of very common morphologic alteration (non-proliferative) changes in the female breast involving both components, epithelium and stroma.
- *Age:* 20–40 yr; peak at or just before menopause; rarely after menopause and before adolescence.
- *Etiology:* Hormonal imbalance: increased estrogen and decreased progesterone. Use of oral contraceptive decreases the risk of the disease.
- *Morphology:* Three patterns:
  1. *Cyst formation* with apocrine metaplasia:
     - Multiple and bilateral
     - Small cysts are formed by dilation and unfolding of lobules. These may coalesce to form larger cysts
     - Palpation shows ill defined, diffuse increase in consistency as well as discrete nodularity due to cystic dilation of ducts and lobules
     - Large cysts contain semi-translucent and turbid fluid imparting brown to b'ue color (*blue dome cyst*)

- Calcification of cyst is common (detected by mammography)
- Lining of the cyst is either flattened and atrophic epithelium or metaplastic apocrine cells. Metaplastic apocrine cells have an abundant granular, eosionophilic cytoplasm and round nuclei.
  2. *Fibrosis:* Release of secretory material into stroma causes chronic inflammation and scarring fibrosis: palpable firmness of breast.
  3. *Adenosis:* Increase in number of acini per lobule. Lumens of glands are enlarged (blue duct adenosis) but not distorted. Calcification may be present. The acini are lined by columnar cells, which may appear benign or may show atypia ("flat epithelial atypia")

Clinical features
- Palpable lump, mammographic densities or calcification, nipple discharge.
- No risk of developing cancer.
- Diagnosed by disappearance of the mass after fine needle aspiration of cyst contents.

3. Proliferative breast disease without atypia

These lesions are characterized by proliferation of ductal epithelium and/or stroma without cytologic or architectural features suggestive of carcinoma *in situ*.

Few important histological subtypes

i. Epithelial hyperplasia:
   - Defined as presence of more than two cell layers in ducts and lobules (normal breast ducts and lobules are lined by double layer of myoepithelial cells and luminal cells).

ii. Sclerosing adenosis:
   - The number of acini per terminal duct is increased to at least double the number found in uninvolved lobules.
   - Normal lobular arrangement is maintained, but acini are compressed and distorted in the central portion of lesion and dilated at periphery.
   - Sometimes stromal fibrosis may compress and distorts the lumen to give appearance of cords or sheets.

iii. Complex sclerosing lesion: These lesions have components of sclerosing adenosis, papillomas, and epithelial hyperplasia.

iv. Papilloma:
   - Lesions grow within dilated duct and are composed of fibrovascular cores lined by luminal and myoepithelial cells.
   - Epithelial hyperplasia and apocrine metaplasia are frequent.
   - Large duct papilloma (solitary and located in lactiferous sinuses) and small duct papillomas (multiple and located in the deeper ducts) usually present with nipple discharge.

4. Proliferative breast disease with atypia

These lesions have hyperplasia with atypia resembling carcinoma *in situ*, but lack sufficient qualitative or quantitative features for diagnosis of carcinoma.

- Atypical ductal hyperplasia consits of a relatively monomorphic proliferation of regularly spaced cells. It resembles DCIS, and distinguished by being limited in extent and only partially filling ducts.
- Atypical lobular hyperplasia is identical to LCIS, but cells do not fill or distend more than 50% of the acini within a lobule.

5. Difference between fibrocystic disease and fibroadenoma of breast (1994)

6. Fibroadenoma breast (1993, 2011)

- It is the commonest benign neoplasm of female breast containing both fibrous and glandular tissues, thought to arise as a result of an absolute or relative increase in estrogen activity.
- Multiple and bilateral.
- Due to drug-induced growth stimulation.
- Tumors of stromal origin are clonal, whereas that of epithelial origin are polyclonal.
- Young female presents with a palpable mass, whereas older one with mammographic densities.
- If associated with fibrocystic changes (fibroadenomatoid changes), proliferative breast disease or family history of breast cancer, there is increased risk of breast cancer.
- *Age:* Any time within reproductive period; more common before age of 30.

Morphology

Gross

- Spherical nodule
- Sharply circumscribed
- Freely movable from surrounding substance
- Frequently upper outer quadrant of breast involved
- One to 15 cm (giant fibroadenoma)
- Cut surfaces are gray-white and have slit-like spaces

Microscopic features: Arrangement between fibrous overgrowth and ducts produces two patterns which may coexist in the same tumor:

- Intracanalicular pattern: Stroma compresses ducts to slit-like cleft lined by ductal epithelium or appears as cords of epithelium elements surrounded by abundant fibrous stroma.
- Pericanalicular pattern: Abundant fibrous stroma surrounds patent or dilated ducts.

Mammography: 'Popcorn' calcification.

7. Cystosarcoma phyllodes/phyllode tumor (1989, 92, 97, 2003, 08)

- Name given to uncommon bulky breast tumor with leaf-like gross appearance.
- *Age:* At any age, but more in sixth decade, 10–20 yrs later than the age of fibroadenoma.
  - Arises from intralobular, periductal stroma, and not from a pre-existing fibroadenoma.
  - The term 'cystosarcoma phyllode' is somewhat misnomer because most of these tumors are benign, so phyllode tumor is the appropriate name.
  - *Low-grade tumor:* Recur locally, rare distant metastasis.
  - *High-grade tumor:* Aggressive, local recurrence common; distant hematogenous metastasis present.
  - Lymph node metastasis is rare.

Morphology
Gross

- Few cm to massive involving whole breast;
- Large lesions have bulbous protrusion (leaf-like);
- Cut surface is gray-white with cystic cavities, area of hemorrhage, necrosis and degenerative changes.

Microscopic features

- Differentiated from fibroadenoma on the basis of cellulary, mitotic rate,

nuclear pleomorphism, stromal overgrowth and infiltrative borders;

- Low-grade tumors resemble fibroadenoma, but cellularity and mitotic figures are increased. High-grade tumors are like other soft tissue sarcoma.

8. Intraductal carcinoma breast (2006)

9. Carcinoma breast

10. Medullary carcinoma breast (2006)

Carcinoma breast is the most common non-skin malignancy in women. All breast carcinomas arise from the terminal duct lobular unit.

Age: Fourth decade and onward incidence progressively increase. Rare below age of 25 years, except in familial cases.

Factors

1. Age: Increases with increase in age (> 40 yr)
2. Geography: Six times higher in developed countries.
3. Genetic factors: BRCA1, BRCA2, p53 gene mutation, family history of breast cancer
   - Over expression of HER2/neu proto oncogene
   - Amplification of RAS and MYC gene
4. Hormonal influences: Estrogen excess: Long duration of reproductive life, nulliparity, late age at first child birth, increasing age, exogenous estrogen.
5. Environmental factors: Radiation exposure, dietary fat, coffee, and alcohol.
6. Proliferative breast disease or carcinoma of contralateral breast or endometrium.
7. Breastfeeder: The longer is the duration of breastfeeding, the less is the incidence of breast carcinoma.
8. Age at menarche: Early age of menarche increases risk.
9. Breast density: High breast radiodensity is a strong risk factor for developing cancer.
10. Atypical hyperplasia finding in previous breast lesion increases incidence of cancer.

11. Carcinoma of contralateral breast or endometrium.
12. Diet, obesity, lack of exercise and tobacco use are other factors.

Hereditary breast cancer: Two autosomal dominant genes BRCA1 and BRCA2 are implicated in many familial cancer and some breast cancers.

	BRCA1	BRCA2
Chromosome location	17 q21	13 q12–13
Gene size	Smaller	Larger
Functions	• Tumor suppression • Transcription regulation • DNA repair (double-stranded break)	• Tumor suppression • Transcription regulation • DNA repair (double-stranded DNA break)
Risk of tumors	Breast, prostate, colon, pancreas	Breast, prostate, pancreas, stomach, melanoma, ovarian, gallbladder, bile duct, pharynx
Age of onset of breast cancer	Younger (40–50 yr)	> 50 yr
Pathology of breast cancer	Greater incidence of medullary carcinoma, poorly differentiated carcinoma, ER–PR and HER2/neu-negative (triple negative) carcinoma and carcinoma with p53 mutations	Similar to sporadiac cancer (ER negative cancer)

• *Distribution* of breast carcinoma: Central area (20%), upper outer (50%), upper inner (10%), lower outer (10%), lower inner (10%) quadrants. Left breast is more often involved than right.

11. Classification of breast carcinoma

Non-invasive lesions (lesions that have not penetrated basement membrane) (15–30%)
• Lobular carcinoma *in situ* (LCIS) (80%)
• Ductal carcinoma *in situ* (DCIS) (20%)

Invasive or infiltrative carcinoma [Penetrated the limiting basement membrane (70–85%)]
• Invasive carcinoma. No special type (NST, Invasive ductal carcinoma (79%)
• Invasive lobular carcinoma (10%)
• Medullary carcinoma (2%)
• Colloid (mucinous) carcinoma (2%)
• Tubular carcinoma (6%)
• Papillary carcinoma (1%)
• Metaplastic carcinoma (< 1%)

12. Write briefly on non-invasive carcinoma of breast

• These lesions do not penetrate the limiting basement membrane and are limited to ducts and lobules.
• Despite evidence that all breast carcinomas arise from cells in the terminal duct lobular unit (TDLU), the use of the terms lobular and ductal still persists.
• Earlier use of the terms lobular and ductal was based on the resemblance of the involved spaces to normal ducts or lobules. By current convention, 'lobular' refers to carcinoma of a specific type and 'ductal' is used more generally for adenocarcinomas that have no other designation.

Ductal carcinoma *in situ* (DCIS, intraductal carcinoma)
• Most frequently these lesions present as mammographic calcifications, less frequently as a vaguely palpable mass or nipple discharge.

- The incidence of DCIS has increased from 5 to 15–30% of all breast carcinomas over past few years. It may be attributed to increased use of mammographic screening.
- This lesion may be incidental finding on biopsy.

Morphology
- Consists of malignant cell population limited to the ducts by basement membrane.
- Myoepithelial cells are preserved though may be decreased in number.
- Clonal proliferation of cells usually involve a single ductal system.

  Five architectural subtypes, namely comedo-carcinoma, solid, cribiform, papillary and micropapillary, have been described but majority show a mixture of pattern.

Comedocarcinoma is characterized by solid sheets of pleomorphic cells with central necrosis.
- Necrotic cell membranes frequently calcify and are seen on mammography as speckled micro-calcifications, which may be grouped together or arranged in parallel lines.
- Periductal concentric fibrosis and inflammation is common.

Noncomedo DCIS consists of a monomorphic population of cells completely filling up the duct lumina (solid type), cells may grow into the spaces lining fibrovascular core (papillary DCIS) or project into the spaces without definite fibrovascular cores forming complex intraductal pattern (micropapillary DCIS).

Lobular carcinoma *in situ* (LCIS)
- Always an incidental finding in breast biopsy done for other indication.
- Not associated with clinically apparent mass or a mammographic finding; so is not diagnosed readily.
- Bilateral in up to 40% of patients when both breasts biopsies are taken.
- LSIC is an intraepithelial proliferation of TDLU. The cells of atypical lobular hyperplasia, LSIC, and invasive lobular carcinoma are similar, i.e. loosely cohesive, small

with oval to round nuclei, and small nucleoli. LCIS is diagnosed when the entire lobular unit is replaced by tumor cells.
- Signet ring cells containing mucin are frequently seen.

13. Write briefly on invasive cacinoma of breast

1. Invasive carcinoma. No special type (NST, invasive ductal carcinoma)
   - Most common (70–80%).
   - Has abundant fibrous stroma, and also referred to as scirrhous carcinoma as firm to hard lesion; makes a grating sound on being cut.
   - Irregular borders with small pin-point foci or streaks of chalky-white elastosis/calcification in the centre of the lesion.
   - Well-differentiated tumors consist of tubules lined by minimally atypical cells (typically express hormone receptor and do not express HER 2/neu).
   - Less differentiated lesions are composed of cords and sheets of pleomorphic cells (typically do not express hormone receptors or overexpress HER2/neu).
   - May be accompanied by variable amount of DCIS. Grade of DCIS correlates with the grade of NST.

2. Invasive lobullar carcinoma
   - These lesions present as palpable ill-defined mass or a mammographic density.
   - Incidence increased in post-menopausal females due to usage of hormonal replacement therapy.
   - The histologic hallmark is the presence of dyscohesive infiltrating tumor cells, often arranged in single file or in loose cluster or sheets. Tubule formation is absent. Cytological appearance is similar to the cells of atypical lobular hyperplasia and LCIS. Signet ring cells containing mucin droplets are common. Desmoplasia is minimal or absent.

- Well-differentiated or moderately differentiated lobular carcinomas are usually diploid, express hormone receptors and do not overexpress HER2/neu gene.
- Poorly differentiated tumors are usually aneuploid, lack hormone receptors, and over express HER 2/neu gene.
- Most lobular carcinomas show a loss of a region on chromosome 16 (cluster of eight genes) responsible for cell adhesion.
- Lobular carcinoma metastasizes to unusual sites. Metastases to meninges, serosal surfaces, retroperitoneum, ovaries and GIT are more common than lungs and pleura.

3. Medullary carcinoma
- It is present as a well-circumscribed mass (may be confused with benign lesions).
- Soft, fleshy and lack desmoplasia.
- Solid syncytial arrangement occupying more than 75% tumor, with the tumor cells being large, pleomorphic, having vesicular nuclei with prominent nucleoli and frequent mitoses.
- Lymphoplasmocytic infiltrates are present within the tumor and also surround tumor.
- Margins are not infiltrated.
- DCIS component is minimal or absent.
- Lymphatic or vascular invasion is almost never seen. Lymph node involvement is rare.
- Prognosis is better than NST.
- HER2/neu gene overexpression is absent.

4. Mucinous (colloid) carcinoma
- 1–6% of all breast carcinoma.
- Present as a circumscribed mass in older women and progress slowly.
- Soft in consistency with a pale gray blue gelatinous appearance (due to mucin).
- Large pools of mucin are present, scattered within which are small clusters of malignant cells.

5. Tubular carcinoma
- Two percent of all breast carcinomas.
- Affects women in their late 40s.
- Tumors are generally multifocal and bilateral.
- Histopathologically, tumor consists of well formed tubules lined by malignant cells. There is absence of myoepithelial cells. Tubular pattern should be seen in more than 75% of tumor.
- Apocrine snouts are present and calcification is common.
- A large number of tumor cells are diploid and express hormone receptors.
- Axillary metastasis is seen in less than 10% cases and has excellent prognosis.

6. Invasive papillary carcinoma
- A rare invasive carcinoma of breast
- Papillary architecture
- Clinically present similar to NST, but with better prognosis

14. Paget's disease of breast (1987, 97, 2000, 02, 10)

- Is a rare form of ductal carcinoma *in situ*.
- It presents as an enythematous eruption with scaling and crusting and may be mistaken for eczema. Incidence: 1–4%.
- *Pathogenesis:* Tumor cells from underlying ductal carcinoma migrate up into the lactiferous duct and invade the epidermis producing skin lesion without invading basement membrane.
- *Morphology*
  Gross
  - Skin of nipple and areola is fissured, ulcerated and oozing;
  - Inflammatory edema and hyperemia in surrounding;
  - Underlying palpable mass is present in 50–60% cases of Paget's disease.

Microscopic features: Histologic hallmark is involvement of epidermis by malignant cell (*Paget cell*).

– Paget cells are large with adundant clear or lightly stained cytoplasm and nuclei with prominent nucleoli. Cells contain mucin.

- Cells are positive for epithelial membrane antigens (EMA), *c-erb-B2* and low molecular weight keratins.
- Prognosis depends on the extent of underlying carcinoma.

15. Prognostic or predictive factors for carcinoma of breast (2008, 09)

Major prognostic factors

1. *Invasive carcinoma versus in situ disease:* In *situ* carcinomas are confined to ductal system, while invasive carcinomas invade basement membrane and spread beyond ductal system. So, in general *in situ* carcinoma has better prognosis than invasive.
2. *Distant metastasis:* Once distant metastasis is present, cure is unlikely hence poor prognosis.
3. *Lymph node metastasis:* Axillary lymph node status is the single most important prognostic factor. With no involvement, 10 yrs survival rate is 70–80%, with 1–3 positive node 35–40%, with more than 10 LN positive 10–15%. Size (large) of metastatic

deposits and presence of invasion through the capsule indicate poor prognosis.

4. *Tumor size:* Second most important independent factor. 10 years survival rate for tumor size < 1 cm (node negative) is nearly 90%, whereas survival drops to 77% for cancer > 2 cm.
5. *Locally advanced disease:* Invasion into skin and skeletal muscles indicates poor prognosis.
6. *Inflammatory carcinoma:* Women presenting with a malignant breast disease with redness, oozing, inflamed appearance and skin thickened have poor prognosis.

Minor prognostic factors

1. *Histologic subtype:* Special types of invasive carcinoma (tubular, colloid, medullary, lobular and papillary) have better prognosis than non-special type. Tubular and colloid carcinomas have exceptionally good prognosis.
2. *Histology grade:* The most commonly used grading system (Nottingham). Histologic score (also called Scarff-Bloom-Richardson) combines nuclear grade, tubule formation and mitotic rate to classify invasive carcinoma into three groups that are highly correlated with survival. 10-yr survival for

Stage	T: primary cancer	Lymph nodes (LN)	M: Distant metastasis	5 yr survial (%)
	American Joint Committee on Cancer Staging (AJCC)			
0	DCIS or LCIS	No metastasis	Absent	92%
I	Invasive carcinoma ≤ 2 cm	No metastasis	Absent	87%
II	Invasive carcinoma > 2 cm	No metastasis	Absent	75%
	Invasive carcinoma < 5 cm	1–3 LN positive	Absent	
III	Invasive carcinoma > 5 cm	1–3 LN positive	Absent	
	Any size invasive carcinoma	≥ 4 LN positive	Absent	46%
	Invasive carcinoma with skin or chest wall involvement or inflammatory carcinoma	0 to > 10 positive LN	Absent	
IV	Any size invasive carcinoma	Negative or positive LN	Present	13%

grade I tumor is 85%, grade II 60% and grade III is 15%.

3. *Estrogen and progesterone receptors:* Tumors with high levels of hormone receptors have slightly better prognosis.

4. *HER2/neu:* Over expression of this gene indicates poor prognosis. Herceptin is a monoclonal antibody to HER2/neu which targets tumor cells (targeted therapy).

5. Lymphovascular invasion is associated with poor prognosis.

6. *Proliferative rate:* Tumors with high proliferation rate have a worse prognosis.

7. *DNA content:* Aneuploid tumor with abnormal DNA indices have slightly poor prognosis.

8. *Response to neoadjuvant therapy:* The degree to which tumor responds to this therapy before surgery is an important prognostic factor.

9. Gene expression profiling has been shown to predict survival and recurrence-free interval, and also identifies patients who are most likely to benefit from particular type of chemotherapy.

16. Metastatic tumor of supraclavicular lymph node (Viva)

Carcinoma of: 1. Lung, 2. Breast, 3. Stomach, and 4. Germ cells.

17. Mammographic appearance of breast cancer

(*Rare, read from text*)

23

Endocrine System

1. Hormones secreted by pituitary gland (viva)

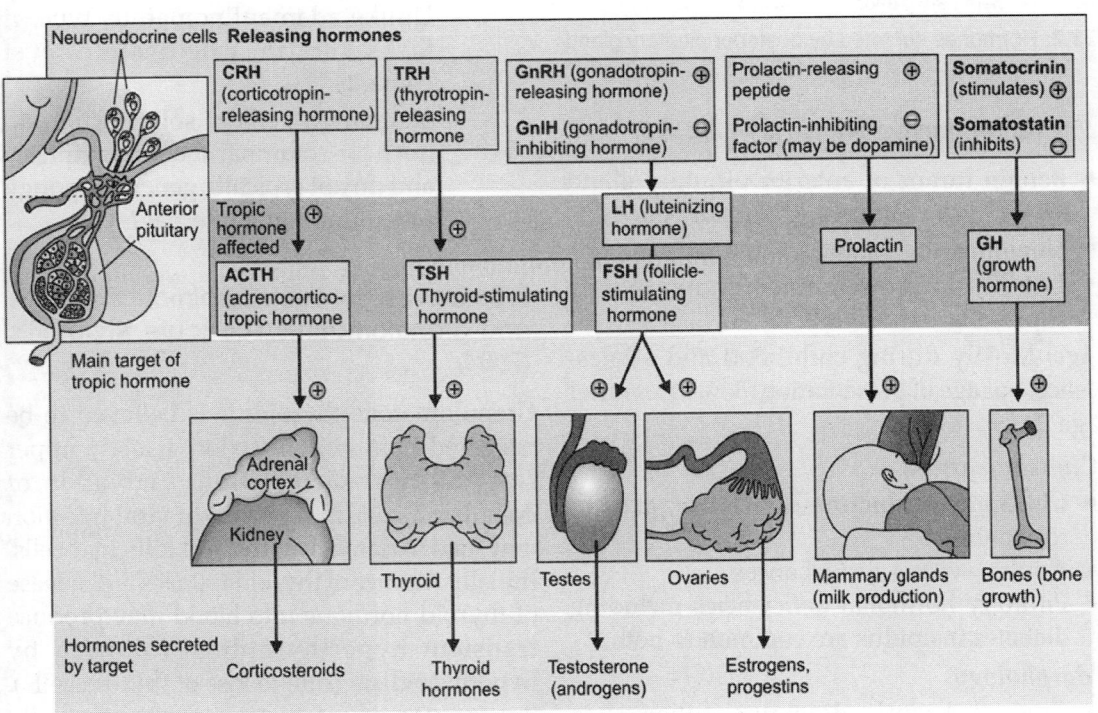

Fig. 23.1: Hormones secreted by anterior pituitary gland and their effect

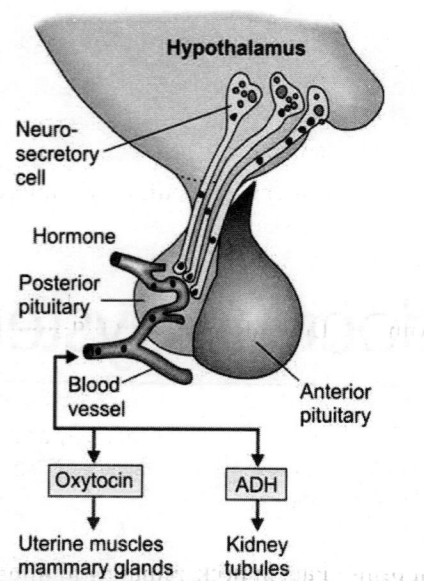

23.2: Hormones secreted by posterior pituitary gland

2. Craniopharyngiomas (1991, 94, 96)

- Benign tumor of anterior pituitary gland arising from remnant of Rathke pouch.
- Slow growing tumor.
- 1 to 5% of intracranial tumors, mostly suprasellar in location.

Age: Mostly during childhood and adolescence; but age of presentation (50% cases) after age 20.

Clinical features
- Children—endocrine deficiency, growth retardation
- Adults—visual disturbances
- Pituitary hormonal deficiencies including diabetes insipidus are common to both.

Morphology
- *Gross:* 3–4 cm in diameter, adherent to surrounding structures and typically cystic

(more common), reddish-gray mass; may be encapsulated and solid. It often encroaches optic chiasma.

- *Microscopic examination:* Two distinct histologic types:
  1. *Adamantinomatous type*
     - Consists of nests or cords of stratified squamous or columnar epithelium embedded in a spongy reticulum often merging into peripheral layer of columnar cell.
     - Keratin formation, cholesterol rich cyst contents, fibrosis, chronic inflammation, and calcification are present (radiologically visualized).
  2. *Papillary type*
     - Unlike adamantinomatous type, it lacks keratin, calcification, cyst contents.
     - Squamouts cells of solid section do not have columnar sheet at periphery and do not typically generate spongy reticulum in the internal layers.

3. Difference between Hashimoto thyroiditis and granulomatous/subacute thyroiditis (2004)

Granulomatous thyroiditis is believed to be triggered by a viral infection, usually upper respiratory tract infection. Activation of cytotoxic T cells in response to viral infection may lead to damage to thyroid follicular cells. Initially rupture of thyroid follicles and release of thyroid hormone into blood may produce transient hyperthyroidism followed by hypothyroidism (due to loss of thyroid cells). But recovery is complete and patient usually becomes euthyroid.

S. No.	Traits	Hashimoto thyroiditis	Granulomatous thyroiditis
1.	Age	45–65 yr	30–50 yr
2.	F: M	10–20:1	3–5:1
3.	Pathology	Autoimmune disease	Viral infection/post-viral inflammation

(Contd.)

S. No.	Traits	Hashimoto thyroiditis	Granulomatous thyroiditis
4.	Recent history	No	Upper respiratory tract infection
5.	Seasonal variation	No	Seasonal incidence, peak at summer
6.	HLA associated	HLA-DR5	HLA B35
7.	Autoantibodies	Present in serum	Absent, antibodies against virus present
8.	Cut surfaces	Pale-gray, firm and somewhat nodular	Firm, yellow-white
9.	Microscopy	Degenerating follicles with variable amount of colloid, mononuclear inflammation cells, like small lymphocytes, plasma cells, and prominent germinal centers. Hürthle cells present	Depends on stage of inflammation. Early: neutrophils forming micro-abscesses. Later: aggregation of lymphocytes, histiocytes, and plasma cells. Hürthle cells absent
10.	Presentation	Diffuse and symmetrical pain-less enlargement of thyroid	Pain in neck, radiating to upper neck, jaws, throat and ear
11.	Risk for B cell lymphoma	Present	Absent
12.	Prognosis	Bad, no recovery, progresses to hypothyroidic state	Good, self-limiting, recovery complete

4. Hashimoto thyroiditis (1989, 90, 92, 95, 2000, 02, 08, 09)

- It is the most common cause of hypothyroidism in areas where iodine level is not deficient.
- There is gradual thyroid failure because of autoimmune destruction of thyroid gland.
- Characterized by:
  1. Diffuse goitereous enlargement of thyroid.
  2. Lymphocytic infiltration of thyroid gland, and
  3. Occurrence of thyroid autoantibodies.
- *Age:* 45 to 65 yrs; but major cause of nonendemic goiter in children.
- *Sex:* female: male = 10:1 to 20:1 (more common in female)
- *Etiopathogenesis*

  First autoimmune disease to be identified.
  1. HLA associated/genetic predisposition: Familial occurrence of disease in associa-tion with HLA-DR5, concordance in monozygotic twins in 40%.
  2. Autoimmune disease association: Associated with Graves' disease, SLE, rheumatoid arthritis, etc.
  3. Iodine intake: Higher the iodine intake higher the incidence.

- *Pathogenesis*

  Both cellular and humoral immunity involved. It is caused by a breakdown of self-tolerance to thyroid autoantigen. T cells recognize processed thyroid antigens in association with specific type of MHC antigen. Diminished suppressor T cells also have role in the pathogenesis. Activated T cells stimulate B cells to secrete antithyroid antibodies and induce the formation of CD8+ cells (cytotoxic cells).

  Autoantibodies are:
  1. Thyroid microsomal/thyroid peroxidase autoantibodies
  2. Thyroglobulin autoantibodies

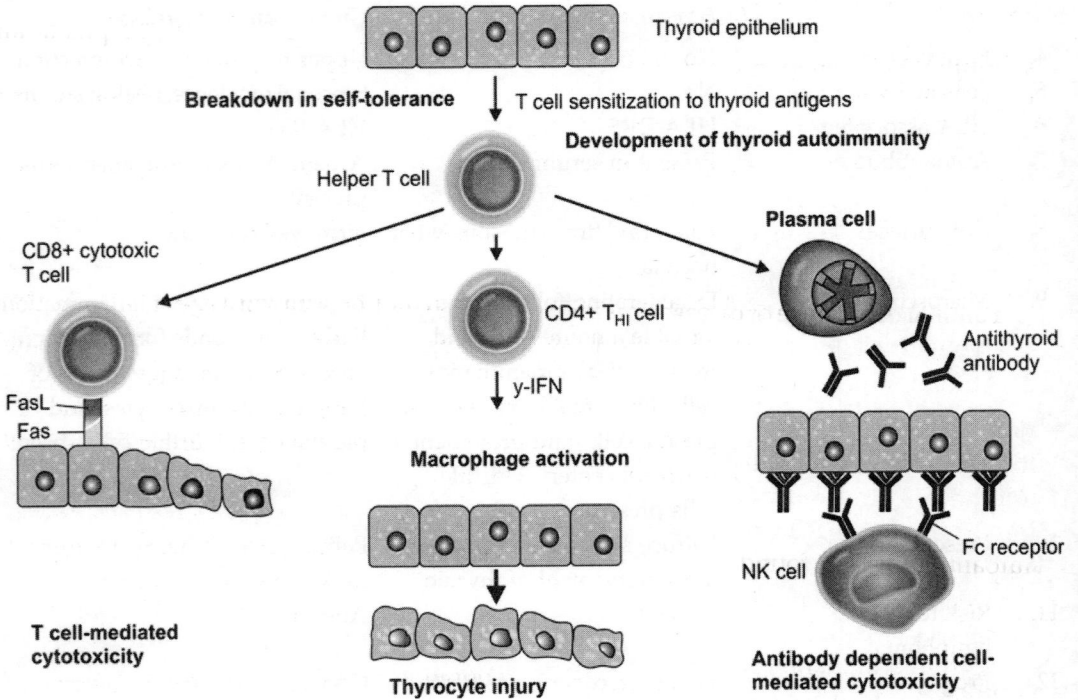

Fig. 23.3: Pathogenesis of Hashimoto thyroiditis

3. TSH receptor autoantibodies
4. Iodine transporter autoantibodies
Destruction of thyroid cells by: 1. Antibody mediated, 2. Cytotoxic T cell mediated, 3. Apoptosis (Fas-FasL mediated).

Morphology
Gross
- Diffuse symmetric, firm and rubbery enlargement of thyroid.
- Cut surface is fleshy with accentuation of normal lobulations, but retained normal shape.
- The capsule is intact, and gland is well demarcated from adjacent structures.

Microscopic examination
- Extensive infiltration by lymphocytes, plasma cells, macrophages and formation of lymphoid follicles with germinal center;
- Decreased number and atrophied thyroid follicles, devoid of colloid;

- Presence of *Hürthle cells* (Askanazy)—epithelial cells of degenerated follicles having abundant eosinophilic and granular cytoplasm due to large number of mitochondria and may contain large nuclei;
- Fibrous thickening of septa.

Clinical features
- Symmetrical, diffuse, *painless enlargement* of thyroid in middle-aged female (mostly).
- Hypothyroidism. T3 and T4 decreased. TSH increased.
- Increased risk for developing B cell lymphoma.

5. Difference between Hashimoto thyroiditis and Graves' disease (2003)

6. Graves' disease (2010)

Most common cause of endogenous hyperthyroidism.
- *Clinical triad characteristics*
  1. Hyperthyroidism

2. Infiltrative ophthalmopathy (exophthalmos)
3. Infiltrative dermapathy (pretibial myxedema)
- *Age:* 20 to 40 yr
- *Sex:* Females are seven times more prone to the disease than males
- *Etiology*
  1. HLA associated/genetic predisposition: Familial occurrence of disease in association with HLA-DR3 and HLA-B8.
  2. Autoimmune disease association.

- *Pathogenesis*
  It is characterized by a breakdown in self-tolerance to thyroid autoantigens, most importantly the TSH receptor. Multiple autoantibodies are found:
  - Thyroid-stimulating immunoglobulin (TSI, also called as LATS-long acting thyroid stimulants): This IgG antibody binds to the TSH receptor and mimics the action of TSH, stimulating adenyl cyclase and increasing the release of thyroid hormones.
  - Thyroid growth-stimulating immunoglobulins: Also directed against the TSH receptor, these have been implicated in the proliferation of thyroid follicular epithelium.
  - TSH-binding inhibitor immunoglobulins: These anti-TSH receptor antibodies prevent TSH from binding normally to its receptor on thyroid epithelial cells. In so doing some forms of TSH-binding inhibitor immunoglobulins mimic the action of TSH, resulting in the stimulation of thyroid epithelial cell activity, whereas other forms may actually inhibit thyroid cell function.

Morphology
Gross
- Diffuse, symmetrically enlarged, increased weight, smooth, soft, intact capsule.
- On cut section parenchyma has soft, meaty appearance resembling normal muscle.

Microscopic examination
- Follicular epithelial hyperplasia and hypertrophy—increased height of follicular lining cells and formation of papillary folding.
- Diminished colloid, light staining.
- Increased vascularity and lymphoid cells in stroma.

Lab finding
Elevated free T3/T4 level, depressed TSH level, radioactive iodine uptake increases; radioiodine scans show a diffuse uptake of iodine.

7. Gross and microscopic features of colloid goiter (2006) or diffuse non-toxic (simple) goiter

It is the diffuse enlargement of thyroid gland without any nodularity. It may be endemic or sporadic.

Because the enlarged follicles are filled with colloid, it is also called colloid goiter.

Endemic
- Occurs in geographical areas where soil, water and food supply are poor in iodine—endemic goiter in Alps, Andes and Himalayas (more than 10% of population is affected)
- Dietary supplements decrease incidence of endemic goiter.
- Goitrogenic foods: Vegetables of Brassicaceae and Cruciferae families (cabbage, cauliflower, brussels sprouts, turnip, and cassava).
- Too much iodine-consuming can also raise the risk of developing goiter.
- Excessive calcium in diet interferes with thyroid hormone synthesis.

Sporadic
- Gender—women are more likely to develop goiter compared to men.
- Seen in young adults.
- Associated with hereditary enzyme defects
  - Iodine transport defect

– Organification defect (Pandred syndrome)
– Dehalogenase defect
– Iodotyrosine coupling defect

Morphology

Two morphological stages are identified:
- Stage of hyperplasia:
  – Diffuse and symmetric enlargement of the thyroid gland
  – Follicles are lined by crowded columnar cells with piling up of epithelium and formation of pseudopapillary projections.
  – The accumulation is not uniform throughout the gland. Some of the follicles are hugely distended, whereas others remain small.
- Stage of colloid involution
  – With decreased demand of thyroid hormone or increased iodine supply, the stimulated follicular epithelium involutes to form an enlarged, colloid rich gland (colloid goiter).
  – The cut surface of thyroid is usually brown, glossy and translucent.
  – Follicular epithelium involutes and become flattened, cuboidal and rich in colloid.

Clinical course

Vast majority of patient are clinically asymptomatic except with an enlarged thyroid gland (neck swelling). Investigation usually reveals normal T3, T4 levels with elevated or at upper normal TSH value.

8. Difference between follicular adenoma and multinodular goiter (1994)

9. Multinodular goiter/adenomatous goiter (1991, 2009, 11)

- It is extreme degree of nodular (multiple nodule) enlargement of the thyroid gland due to recurrent episodes of hyperplasia and involution.
- Almost all long-standing simple goiter will turn into multinodular goiter.
- They produce extreme enlargement so that they can be mistaken for neoplasm.
- They occur as endemic as well as sporadic form with female predominance but in older age group.

Pathogenesis

The main basis of multinodularity is that some of follicular cells are more responsive to TSH

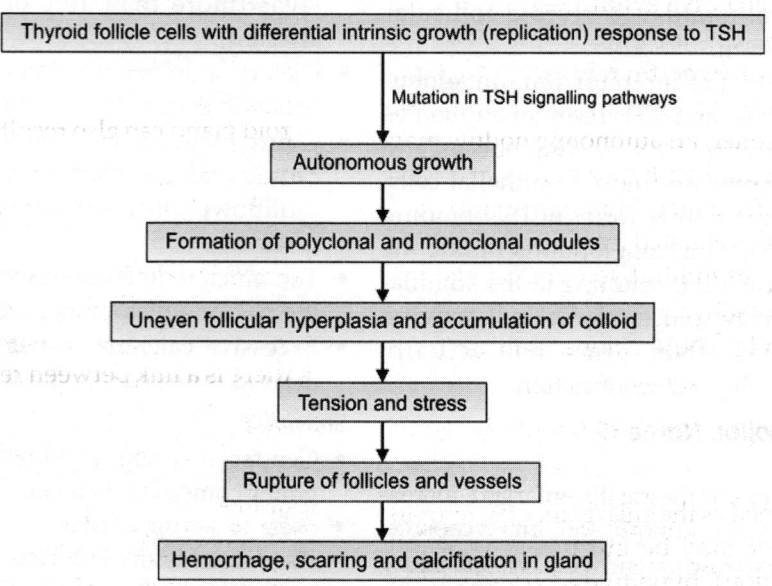

Fig. 23.4: Pathophysiology of multinodular goiter

than other resulting in differential growth of thyroid gland.

Morphology

Gross: Asymmetrical and extreme enlargement of gland showing:

- Nodularity with poor encapsulation
- Fibrous scarring
- Hemorrhage
- Focal calcification
- Cystic degeneration containing brown gelatinous colloids

Microscopic examination

- Colloid rich follicles lined by flattened inactive epithelium
- Follicular epithelial hypertrophy and hyperplasia
- Fibrous scarring with area of focal calcification
- Hemorrhages, hemosiderin laden macrophages
- Microcyst formation

Clinical course

- Major clinical presentation is a large swelling in anterior part of neck and its mass effect, like dyspnoea, dysphagia, and superior vena cava syndrome.
- Most of patients are euthyroid. Some may be subclinical hyperthyroid (normal T3 and T4, with reduced TSH). In few of very long-standing goiter, an autonomic nodule may develop to produce hyperthyroidism (toxic multinodular goiter, Plummer syndrome). It can be differentiated from Graves' disease by absence of infiltrative ophthalmopathy and dermopathy.
- Diagnosed by FNAC, biopsy and USG.

10. Define goiter. Name different causes of goiter

Goiter is defined as the enlargement of thyroid gland. Goiter may be euthyroid (normal thyroid function), hypothyroid or hyperthyroid. Thyroid enlargement may be diffuse, single nodule or multinodular, unilateral or bilateral.

- **Causes of goiter**
  - Endemic goiter and multinodular goiter
  - Autoimmune disease—individuals with a medical history of autoimmune disease, as well as those with a close relative who have/had autoimmune disease have a higher risk of developing goiter.
  - Pregnancy and menopause—goiter is more likely to happen after a woman becomes pregnant, or goes through the menopause.
  - Some medicines—antiretrovirals, immunosuppressants, amiodarone (heart medication), and lithium increase a patient's risk of developing goiter.
  - Radiation—people whose neck or chest areas have been exposed to radiation have a higher risk. This could be due to radiation treatment (radiotherapy), or having worked in a nuclear facility, being involved in a nuclear test or accident.
  - Hyperthyroidism—if the thyroid is overactive, it can become over-stimulated and expand.
  - Hypothyroidism—an under-active thyroid gland can also result in goiter. If the body does not have enough of the hormones produced by the thyroid gland it will stimulate the gland to produce more, which can lead to swelling of the gland.
  - Smoking—some studies suggest that there is a link between regular smoking and goiter risk. A person who smokes and has a low-iodine diet has a significantly higher risk of developing goiter.
  - Some infections—there are some parasites, bacteria and fungi infections which are known to increase goiter risk.

– Thyroid cancer—people who have thyroid cancer have a higher risk of developing goiter.

11. Solitary nodule of thyroid gland

- A solitary nodule is a discrete swelling palpable in thyroid gland.
- A solitary nodule is more likely to be malignant than benign as compared to multinodular thyroid.
- A solitary nodule in younger person and male gender is more likely to be malignant than older and female.
- Nodules that do not take radioactive iodine (cold nodule) are more likely to be malignant.
- FNAC, biopsy and radioactive iodine uptake are a few diagnostic modalities.

12. Adenoma thyroid (1993)

- It is the benign tumor of thyroid typically present as discrete solitary mass. It is derived from follicular epithelium, so sometimes called as follicular adenoma.
- Clinically, it is difficult to differentiate from follicular hyperplasia and follicular carcinoma.

Pathogenesis

Morphology

Gross

- Solitary, spherical, encapsulated
- Average 3 cm in size
- Clearly distinct architecture inside and outside the capsule
- Compression of the thyroid parenchyma outside capsule
- Color gray-white to red-brown
- Intact capsule
- Areas of hemorrhage, fibrosis, calcification and cystic changes are present.

Microscopic examination: Cells forming uniform appearing follicles that contain colloid. Many histological types:

1. *Macrofollicular* (simple colloid): Large colloid filled follicles lined by flattened epithelium.
2. *Microfollicular* (fetal): Numerous, small well-developed follicles lined by flattened epithelium widely separated by abundant loose myxoid stroma.
3. *Embryonal* (trabecular): Small abortive follicles, packed cells forming cords at random and sparse.

   All the above three show little variation in cell and nuclear morphology.
4. *Hürthle cell* (oxyphilic, oncocytic)

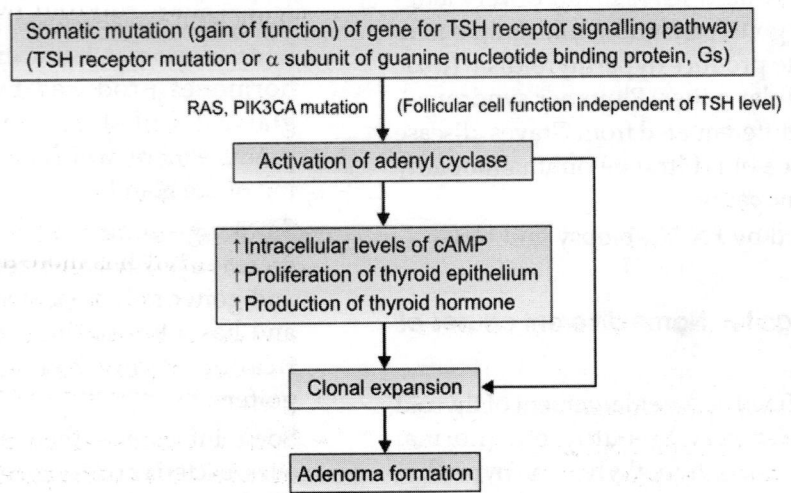

Fig. 23.5: Pathogenesis of adenoma thyroid

5. *Atypical adenoma/spindle cell adenoma:* Follicular adenoma showing some pleomorphism and variation in cell and nuclear size.

6. *Papillary adenoma:* Papillary projection within large follicular or cystic spaces. Encapsulated papillary carcinoma to be suspected.

Clinical features

- Adenoma present as unilateral painless neck mass, mostly discovered during routine check up.
- Progression to malignancy is very rare in adenoma.
- Vast majority of adenomas are non-functional. They take up less radioactive iodine than normal thyroid parenchyma (cold nodule).
- Few adenomas produce excess thyroid hormone (toxic adenoma) independent of TSH stimulation. They take up more radioactive iodine than surrounding tissue (hot nodule).
- USG, and FNAC are helpful but biopsy is usually needed to exclude follicular carcinoma.

13. Papillary carcinoma of thyroid (1990, 93, 99, 2000, 04, 06, 11)

Most common form of thyroid carcinoma (85%).
- *Age:* All ages but 25–50 years more common
- *Sex:* Female: Male = 3:1
- *Cell of origin:* Follicular cells
- *Etiology*
  1. External radiation (most common cause)
  2. Iodine excess
  3. Genetic factor: Association with HLA-DR7
  4. Proto-oncogene RET/PTC

Morphology

Gross
- Solitary or multifocal lesion
- Well circumscribed and even encapsulated to infiltrative and ill-defined
- Fibrosis and calcification
- Cut surface is granular

Microscopic examination
- Pattern: Papillary projection having dense fibrovascular stalk covered by a single to multiple layer of well differentiated uniformly ordered cuboidal cells to anaplastic epithelium;
- Nuclei have finely dispersed chromatin giving optically clear or empty space (*Orphan Annie eye or ground glass nuclei*)—diagnostic feature;
- Eosinophilic intranuclear inclusions or groove, i.e. invagination of cytoplasm (pseudo-inclusion intranuclear grooves or inclusion)
- *Psammoma bodies* (concentrically calcified structures) are seen. If a psammoma body is found within a lymph node or perithyroidal tissues, a hidden papillary carcinoma must be suspected.
- Encapsulated variant, follicular variant (unencapsulated and infiltrative), tall cell variant (large with prominent vascular invasion, local and distant metastasis, poorest prognosis among all papillary carcinoma), diffuse sclerosing and papillary microcarcinoma are to be recognized.
- Lymphatic invasion is common, but involvement of blood vessel is relatively uncommon.

Clinical features

- Asymptomatic thyroid nodule, mass in cervical lymph node (first).
- Single nodule moves freely during swallowing.
- Hoarseness, dysphagia, cough, dyspnea in advanced disease.
- Cold nodule.
- 10 years survival is more than 95%.
- Regional metastasis common, distant metastasis rare.

14. Medullary carcinoma of thyroid (1994, 97, 2000)

- Neuroendocrine neoplasm (5% of thyroid carcinoma).

- *Cell of origin:* Parafollicular cells (C-cells).
- *Sex:* Both sexes are equally affected.
- Secrete calcitonin; may also secrete other polypeptide hormones, like CEA, VIP, somatostatin and serotonin.

Etiology

- *Sporadic* (80%; adulthood—peak 40s to 50s),
- *Familial:* In association with MEN IIA—pheochromocytoma and parathyroid adenoma or with MEN IIB—pheochromocytoma and multiple mucosal neuromas (younger age). RET proto-oncogene mutation plays important role in medullary carcinogenesis.

Morphology

Gross

- Solitary or multiple lesion
- Sporadic neoplasm involves one lobe, but familial cases are bilateral and multicentric;
- Tumor is firm, pale gray to tan, infiltrative;
- Foci of hemorrhage and necrosis in larger lesions are present.

Microscopic examination

- Polygonal to spindle-shaped cells, in some cases anaplastic cells forming nests, trabecular or follicle.
- Acellular amyloid deposits in adjacent stroma (derived from altered calcitonin molecules).

Immunohistochemistry: Calcitonin within the cytoplasm of neoplastic cells.

Electron microscopy: Variable number of membrane bound electron dense granules in cytoplasm of neoplastic cells.

- *Clinical features*
  - *Sporadic cases:* Mass in the neck, local effect—dysphagia or hoarseness, paraneoplastic syndrome.
  - *Familial cases:* Asymptomatic and discovered during screening of affected relatives.
  - Regional metastasis is common (blood), but distant metastasis rare.
  - 10 yrs survival is 60%–70%.

15. Difference between papillary and follicular carcinoma (1994)

S. No.	Traits	Papillary carcinoma	Follicular carcinoma
1.	Incidence	75–85% (most common thyroid malignancy)	10–20% (2nd most common)
2.	Age	All ages, 20–40 yrs most common	Middle to old, more common in 40–50 yrs
3.	Predisposing factors	Previous exposure to ionizing radiations, iodine excess in diet	Dietary iodine deficiency
4.	Number of nodule	Solitary, sometimes multifocal	Solitary nodule
5.	Pattern	Papillary (most common), or irregular follicle with papillae, or entirely follicular	Colloid filled follicles, or trabecular or solid sheets
6.	Diagnostic cell feature	Orphan Annie/ground glass nuclei appearance, psammoma bodies are present	Absent
7.	Blood vessel invasion	Rare	Common
8.	Local invasion	Lesser	Extensive, only sometimes absent
9.	Regional metastasis (LN)	Common	Rare
10.	Distant metastasis	Rare	Common
11.	Growth rate	Slow	Slow, but faster than papillary
12.	Female: Male	3:1	2.5:1
13.	10 yrs survival	80–95%	50–70%

16. Morphology of follicular carcinoma

Gross

- Usually solitary nodule, may be well circumscribed or infiltrative.
- Well-circumscribed nodule difficult to differentiate from adenoma.
- Cut section shows gray to tan to pink surface, somewhat translucent (presence of large colloid-filled follicles).
- Degenerative changes, like central fibrosis, and calcifications, are present.

Microscopic feature

- Most tumors shows follicular pattern with normal type follicular differentiation, others may show trabecular pattern, sheets of polygonal to spindle-shaped cells and Hurthle cells.
- Anaplasia is variable
- Blood vessels are preferentially invaded than lymphatics.

17. Hyperparathyroidism (1990, 96)

Primary hyperparathyroidism: It is caused by over-secretion of parathyroid hormones (PTH) due to disease of the parathyroid gland.

- *Etiology*
  1. Parathyroid adenoma (80% cases)
  2. Carcinoma of parathyroid (2.5–3%)
  3. Primary hyperplasia (15%)
- *Clinical features*
  - Asymptomatic with deranged biochemical findings (↑ serum calcium, ↑ PTH level, ↑ urinary excretion of both calcium and phosphate);
  - Most common nephrolithiasis and (or) nephrocalcinosis;
  - Metastatic calcification in blood vessels, kidney, lungs, stomach, eyes;
  - Generalized osteitis fibrosa cystica due to osteoclastic reabsorption and its replacement by connective tissue;
  - Neuropsychiatric disturbances
  - Bone pain, fracture (pathological)

Secondary hyperparathyroidism: It is caused by any condition, which is associated with chronic hypocalcemia resulting in ↑ PTH level.

- *Etiology*
  1. Chronic renal insufficiency—phosphate retention, impaired intestinal absorption of calcium.
  2. Vitamin D deficiency.
  3. Intestinal malabsorption—deficiency of calcium and vitamin D.
- *Clinical features:* Mild hypocalcemia in contrast to hypercalcemia in primary hyperparathyroidism.

Tertiary hyperparathyroidism: Complication of secondary hyperparathyroidism in which hyperfunction persists even after removal of cause of secondary hyperparathyroidism.

18. Hypercortisolism/Cushing syndrome (1986, 2001, 08)

Elevated level of glucocorticoids *due to*:

- *Iatrogenic Cushing syndrome* (exogenous glucocorticoids; most common cause)— ACTH decreased, glucocorticoid level increased.
- *Pituitary Cushing syndrome/Cushing disease:* Primary hypothalamic-pituitary disease associated with hypersecretion of ACTH, more in females of age 20–30. ACTH increased, glucocorticoid increased.
- *Adrenal Cushing/ACTH independent syndrome:* Hypersecretion of cortisol by an adrenal adenoma, carcinoma or nodular hyperplasia. ACTH decreased, glucocorticoid increased.
- *Paraneoplastic Cushing syndrome:* Ectopic ACTH production by non-endocrine neoplasm (e.g. small cell carcinoma of lung). ACTH increased, glucocorticoid increased.

Morphology

- *Pituitary:* Excess of exogenous cortisol causes Crooke hyaline change (normal granular, basophilic cytoplasm of the ACTH producing cell of anterior pituitary is replaced by homogenous, lightly basophilic material due to deposition of intermediate keratin in cytoplasm).

- Adrenal glands may undergo cortical atrophy, diffuse hyperplasia, nodular hyperplasia or may have adenoma (*yellow tumor*) depending upon cause of the disease.

Clinical features

- Central obesity (about trunk and upper back; buffalo hump)
- Moon facies
- Weakness and fatigability
- Hirsutism
- Hypertension
- Plethora
- Glucose intolerance/diabetes (hyperglycemia, glucosuria, polydipsia)
- Osteoporosis
- Neuropsychiatric abnormality
- Menstrual abnormality
- Skin striae
- Thin fragile and easily bruised skin

Lab diagnosis

- 24-hour free-cortisol level in urine, which is increased;
- Loss of normal diurnal pattern of cortisol secretion;
- Serum ACTH and measurement of urinary steroid excretion after administration of dexamethasone.

19. Pheochromocytoma (1986, 92, 95, 99)

- These are uncommon neoplasms composed of chromaffin cells, which synthesize and secrete catecholamines and cause hypertension.
- Mostly benign.
- *Site:* Adrenal medulla (90%).
- Extra-adrenal pheochromocytomas arising from other paraganglions are called *paragangliomas*.

- *Sporadic type (90%):* Adults between 40 and 50 yr, slight female predominance; familial type (10%): In childhood with strong male predominance associated with MEN syndromes.

Morphology

Gross

- Small, circumscribed lesion confined to adrenal to large hemorrhagic weighing kilograms (well demarcated by either connective tissues or compressed cortical or medullary tissue);
- Cut surfaces of small lesions are yellow tan, whereas larger are hemorrhagic, necrotic and cystic;
- Incubation of fresh tissue into potassium ᵔate solution turns the tumor ᵔ color due to oxidation of ᵔtecholamines thus called (Viva question)

Microscopic examination

- Polygonal to spindle-shaped chromaffin cells with abundant granular amphophilic or basophilic cytoplasm and vesicular nuclei;
- These cluster with supporting cells into small nests or alveoli (zellbalen);
- Abundant fibrovascular supply;
- Tumor cells stain positive for neuron specific enolase and chromogranin.

Clinical features

- Hypertension (abrupt, precipitous, elevation in blood pressure), tachycardia, palpitation, headache, sweating, tremor and sense of apprehension.
- Pain in abdomen or chest.
- Nausea and vomiting.
- Catecholamine cardiomyopathy
- Anginal chest pain

Lab diagnosis: Increased excretion of free catecholamines and their metabolites, like vanillylmandelic acid (VMA) and metanephrines.

20. Addison disease (primary chronic adrenocortical insufficiency)

21. MENS (multiple endocrine neoplasia syndrome)

These are a group of genetically inherited diseases resulting in proliferative lesions (hyperplasia, adenoma and carcinomas) of multiple endocrine organs.

- Tumors occur at a younger age than sporadic tumor.
- They occur in multiple endocrine organs either simultaneously or at different time.
- Tumors are multifocal in a single organ.
- The origin of tumor is usually preceded by hyperplasia phase.
- They are more aggressive and tend to reoccur as compared to sporadic variant.

Condition	MEN 1	MEN 2A	MEN 2B
Eponym	Wermer syndrome	Sipple syndrome	
Parathyroid gland tumors	≥ 90%	10–20%	—
Pancreatic tumors	60–70%	—	—
Pituitary gland tumors	15–42%	—	—
Angiofibroma	64%	—	—
Lipoma	17%	—	—
Medullary carcinoma of thyroid gland	—	> 90%	> 90%
Pheochromocytoma	—	50%	60%
Neuromas on mucous membranes	—	—	Almost 100%
Marfanoid body habitus	—	—	Almost 100%
Genes	MEN1	RET	RET

24

Skin

1. Malignant melanoma or melanocarcinoma

- It is a common skin neoplasm. It is the most rapidly spreading malignant tumor of skin.
- Origin: It originates from melanocytes present in epidermis layer of skin.
- Sites: Tumor involves skin, oral and anogenital mucosal surface, esophageal lining, meninges and eyes. Melanoma most commonly arise on sun-exposed surfaces.
- They affect both sexes equally.
- *Predisposing factors*
  - Sun exposure: Exposure to excessive sunlight at an early age is the single most important predisposing risk factor.
  - Inherited genes mutation in RB genes, p53, PTEN, BRAF.
  - Melanomas are more common in whites than in African Americans, and have a predilection for fair-skinned people.
  - Pre-existing nevus: Dysplastic nevi
  - Hereditary factors: Melanoma in first and second degree relatives is more prone to develop.
  - Exposure to carcinogens
- *Pathogenesis*
  - The pathogenesis of melanoma is a complex process. It involves alteration in genetic expression affecting regulatory pathway of cell survival and proliferation. The final outcome is unregulated excessive growth resulting in melanoma.
- *Clinical features:* Symptoms such as bleeding, itching, ulceration and pain in a pigmented lesion warrant further evaluation. The following signs (ABCDE) are indicative of development of malignancy in earlier benign pigmented lesion:
  - Asymmetry: One-half of the lesion does not match the other half of lesion.
  - Border irregularity: Edges are irregular, ragged, notched, or blurred.
  - Color (variegated): The color of lesion is not uniform and may display shades of brown, black, red, white, gray or blue discoloration.
  - Diameter: A diameter of more than 6 mm is indicative of melanoma.
  - Evolving: Benign lesion evolve over time to melanoma displaying change in shape, size and color in pigmented lesions.
- *Gross:* The lesion has irregular margin. The pigmentation appears in the shades of black, brown, dark blue and gray. Macular areas correlate with the microscopic features of radial growth, while raised areas indicate nodular aggregates of malignant cells in the vertical growth phase.

- *Microscopic features:* The tumor shows initial radial growth, later on vertical growth.

Radial growth

- Radial growth describes the horizontal spread of melanoma within the epidermis and superficial dermis.
- No capacity to metastasize
- Cells fall into several clinicopathologic classes: lentigo maligna (presenting as indolent lesion on the face of older men that may remain in this phase for several decades), superficial spreading (most common type of melanoma, involves sun exposed skin), and acral/mucosal lentiginous (unrelated to sun exposure).
- Tumor cells grow as irregular nest and single cell within epidermis.
- The inflammatory response is present in epidermis as well as dermis.
- Radial growth phase is long and variable.
- With time, growth pattern assumes vertical components.

Vertical growth

- The tumor grows as an expansile mass and invades deeper dermal layers.
- Tumor cells show nodular aggregates of infiltrating cells. The appearance of nodule correlates with the emergence of a clone of cells with metastatic potential.
- The tumor cells lack maturation. They lose the tendency to become smaller as they descend lower and into reticular dermis.
- Metastatic potential is present and is related to the vertical growth, number of mitoses and presence of ulceration.
- Breslow thickness is the distance from the superficial epidermal granular cell layer to the deepest intradermal tumor cells, and it correlates with metastatic potential of melanoma.

  Individual melanoma cells are larger than nevus cells. They are epitheloid (more common) or spindle-shaped. They have large nuclei with irregular contours. Chromatin is clumped at the periphery of the nuclear membrane. There are prominent red (eosinophilic) nucleoli. Melanin pigment may be present or absent. Pigment, if present, tends to be in the form of uniform fine granule, positive for Massons-fontana.

Prognostic factors

1. Tumor depth (Breslow thickness): better prognosis for less than 1.7 mm thickness.
2. Number of mitoses: Less mitoses are better.
3. Evidence of tumor regression due to host immune response: Absence of regression is better.
4. The presence and number of tumor infiltrating lymphocytes: brisk response is better.
5. Gender: Females have better prognosis.
6. Location of tumor: Tumor located on extremity has better prognosis than central.

2. Squamous cell carcinoma

- This is the second most common tumor arising on sun-exposed sites in older people. This may arise in any part of skin or mucus membrane lined by squamous epithelium, but is more prevalent in sun-exposed parts.
- It is more common in men than women.

Risk factors and pathogenesis

- Most important cause is DNA damage induced by exposure to UV light (sunlight).
- Chronic immunosuppression (2nd most common cause) as a result of chemotherapy or organ transplantation.
- Industrial carcinogens (tars and oils)
- Chronic ulcers
- Draining osteomyelitis
- Old burn scars
- Ingestion of arsenicals
- Ionizing radiation
- Tobacco and betel nut chewing (in oral cavity)
- Role of p53 gene, mutation of BCL2 and RAS, alteration in intracellular signal transduction pathways involving epidermal

growth factor receptor (EGFR) and cyclo-oxygenase (CDX) in carcinogenesis have been found.

Morphology

Gross: In situ carcinoma lesion is sharply defined, red scaling plaque. Invasive tumors are nodular, ulcerative and show hyperkeratosis.

Microscopic features

- Squamous cell carcinoma *in situ* (Bowen's disease) is a precursor to invasive SCC. These tumors do not invade through the basement membrane of dermoepidermal junction. Tumor cells with atypical (enlarged and hyperchromatic) nuclei involve all levels of the epidermis.
- Invasive SCC is characterized on invasion of basement membrane by malignant cells. Malignant cells are found in dermis, surrounded by an inflammatory infiltrate.
- Tumors can be divided into three histological grades, based on the degree of nuclear atypia and keratinization.
- A well-differentiated SCC is characterized by cells with near normal appearing nuclei and abundant cytoplasm with extracellular keratin pearls.
- Poorly differentiated SCC is associated with geographic necrosis consisting of highly anaplastic cells that exhibit only abortive, single-cell keratinization (dyskeratosis)
- Moderately differentiated SCC has features between well-differentiated and poorly differentiated lesions.
- Immunohistochemical stains for keratins are useful in diagnosing undifferentiated SCC.
- Histological variants include acantholytic (adenoid) SCC, spindle cell SCC, adenoid SCC, verucous carcinoma, etc.

3. Basal cell carcinoma/rodent ulcers

These are slow growing, locally invasive tumors that rarely metastasize.

- More common in lightly pigmented and prolonged sun-exposed people.
  It occurs exclusively on hairy skin.

- *Gross:* It may present as telangiectatic nodules: Pearly papule often containing prominent dilated subepidermal blood vessels. The advanced or neglected lesion may ulcerate, or may show extensive local invasion of bones or facial sinuses. They usually behave as aggressive tumors forming ulcers, so-called *'rodent ulcers'*.

- *Microscopic features*
  - *Origin:* From epidermis or follicular epithelium.
  - Cells (basaloid) resemble normal basal cell layer of epidermis.
  - These tumors are composed of nests of basaloid cells forming two growth patterns:
    1. *Multifocal growth:* The tumor arises from epidermis and extends over several square centimeters on skin surface.
    2. *Nodular growth:* The tumor grows downward deeply into dermis as cords or islands of cells.
    Tumor cells show variable basophilia and have hyperchromatic nuclei.
    Matrix is mucinous in nature and has abundant fibroblasts and lymphocytes. The cells at the periphery of the tumor cell islands tend to be arranged radially with their long axes in parallel alignment (palisading).

- *Common to both types:* Tumor cells present at the periphery of nests are arranged parallel to each other (palisading) and are separated from stroma by thin, clear looking cleft.

Pathogenesis: Risk is related to skin type and degree of exposure to sun light particularly UV radition.

Genetic syndromes associated with BCC
1. Xeroderma pigmentosa
2. Nevoid basal cell carcinoma (Gorlin syndrome)
3. Epidermodysplasia verruciformis

25

Bones and Joints

1. Osteoporosis

- Is defined as localized or diffused increase in porosity of the skeleton resulting from a reduction in bone mass, predisposing to fracture.
- Generalized osteoporosis may be primary or secondary.
- Osteoporosis is either idiopathic seen in young adults and juvenile though not common; or postmenopausal and senile.
- Secondary osteoporosis may be due to endocrine disorders, neoplasia, gastrointestinal disorders, rheumatological diseases or drug induced.

Pathogenesis: Peak bone mass is achieved during young adulthood depending on:

- Genetic/hereditary factors (vitamin D receptor allele)
- Diet
- Hormonal state
- Sex (female more prone to osteoporosis)
- Race (whites more prone than blacks)
- Physical activity
- Muscle strength

After that bone mass loses at the rate of 0.7% per year in predictable biological phenomenon.

Menopause

- Decreased serum estrogen
- Increased IL-1, INF-α and IL-6
- Increased osteoclast activity

Senile/aging

- Decreased replicative activity of osteoprogenitor cells
- Decreased activity of osteoblasts

Categories of generalized osteoporosis

Primary			Secondary		
	Endocrine disorder	**Neoplasia**	**Gastrointestinal**	**Drugs**	**Miscellaneous**
Post menopausal	Hyperparathyroidism	Multiple myeloma	Malnutrition	Anticoagulants	Organogenesis
Senile	Hyperthyroidism	Carcinomatosis	Malabsorption	Chemotherapy	imperfecta
Idiopathic	Hypothyroidism		Hepatic	Corticosteroids	Immobilization
	Hypogonadism		insufficiency	Anticonvulsants	Anemia
	Pituitary tumors		Vit C, D	Alcohol	
	Type 1 DM		deficiency		
	Addison's disease				

- Decreased biological activity of matrix bound growth factors
- Decreased physical activities

Hormonal disturbances

- Vitamin D calcitonin disturbances
- Parathormone hormone imbalance
- Imbalanced calcium/phosphate metabolism

All of these factors result in deficit in bone formation with every reabsorption and formation cycle of bone; leading to osteoporosis.

Morphology

- Osteoporotic trabeculae are thinned out with loss of their interconnections.
- Cortex thinned out by subperiosteal and endosteal resorption.
- Haversian system widened; sometimes so much that the cortex mimics cancellous bone.

Clinical features: Any bone may show the sign of osteoporosis, but vertebral fracture in thoracic and lumbar region are common and very painful. Multiple fractures in vertebral column may cause lumbar lordosis, kyphoscoliosis and other deformities.

2. Paget's disease (osteitis deformans) (1999)

- This is a skeleton disease characterized by osteoclastic bone reabsorption followed by bone formation, resulting in gain in bone mass. The newly formed bone is disordered and architecturally unsound.

  It was first described by Sir James Paget in 1876.

Age: Predominantly males over 50 years.

Pathogenesis: Slow virus infection by Paramyxovirus or other such viruses; increased IL-6, activation of osteoclastic activity leading to reabsorption of bone.

Morphology

- *Microscopic features:* Mosaic pattern of lamellar bone is pathognomonic to Paget's

disease. Three sequential stages are identified:

1. *Initial osteoclastic stage:* Increased osteoclastic activity producing numerous reabsorption pits. Osteoclasts are abnormally large and number of nuclei increased (normal: nuclei 10–12/cell).

2. *Mixed osteoclastic–osteoblastic stage:* Prominent osteoblasts activity take over forming osteoprogenitor cells, blood vessels, loose connective tissues; newly bone formed that (lamellar or woven) are remodelled into lamellar bone.

3. *Burnt out quiescent osteoclastic stage:* Cell activity decreased, bones larger than normal, coarsely thickened trabeculae. Soft and porous cortices, which lack stability.

- *Radiographic findings:* Lytic stage is seen as close-up; mixed stage reveals central and endosteal cortical reabsorption and replacement by less compact new bone (cotton wool appearance): Sclerotic stage is seen as large bone with irregular thickening of both cortices and trabeculae.

- *Biochemical findings:* Increased serum alkaline phosphatase, normal to high serum calcium level, increased urinary excretion of hydroxyproline.

Clinical features

- Monostotic form (involving single bone) may remain asymptomatic and is discovered incidentally on radiographic examination. Bones involved are tibia, ilium, femur, skull, vertebra and humerus.

- *Polyostotic form:* More widespread involving vertebra, pelvis, femur, skull, sacrum and tibia; may produce pain, fracture, skeleton deformities and occasionally sarcomatous transformations.

- A variety of tumor and tumor-like conditions develop in pagetic bone: Sarcoma occurs in 0.7–0.9% of all individuals with Paget's disease and in (5–10%) of patients with severe polyostotic disease.

3. Pathogenesis of tuberculous (1990) and pyogenic osteomyelitis (1992, 2001, 2004)

4. Difference between tuberculous (1987, 93) and pyogenic osteomyelitis

S. No.	Traits	Pyogenic osteomyelitis	Tubercular osteomyelitis
1.	Cause	Staphylococcus aureus (80–90%), E. coli, Pseudomonas, Klebsiella	Mycobacterium tuberculosis
2.	Spread to bone	Hematogenous spread most common, extension from contiguous sites, direct implantation from outside due to trauma	Hematogenous spread from a foci of active visceral disease, direct spread, lymphatic spread
3.	Onset	Acute	Insidious
4.	Bones	Long bones more involved	Spine (Pott disease, thoracic and lumbar), knee, hip are more involved
5.	Lesion features	Depends on the stage of disease—acute, subacute, and chronic. Suppurative inflammation leading to ischemic necrosis. Subperiosteal and soft tissue abscesses, sequestrum, sinus tract formation, involucrum	Typical TB granuloma with or without caseation
6.	Clinical features	Acute systemic illness with malaise, fever, chills, leukocytosis, marked to intense throbbing pain over affected area	Pain on motion, localized tender, low grade fever, chills, weight loss
7.	Severity	Less	More destructive and resistant to control
8.	Complications	Pathologic fracture, 2° amyloidosis, sepsis, development of squamous cell carcinoma in sinus tract, sarcoma in bone (rare), draining sinus tract, suppurative arthritis. Endocarditis, 2° ankylosis	Scoliosis, kyphosis, neurologic deficit 2° to compression to spinal cord and nerve, tuberculous arthritis, sinus tract formation, amyloidosis, ankylosis, tubercular arthritis

Pyogenic osteomyelitis
Pathogenesis

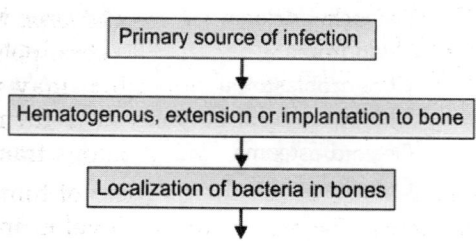

(Contd.)

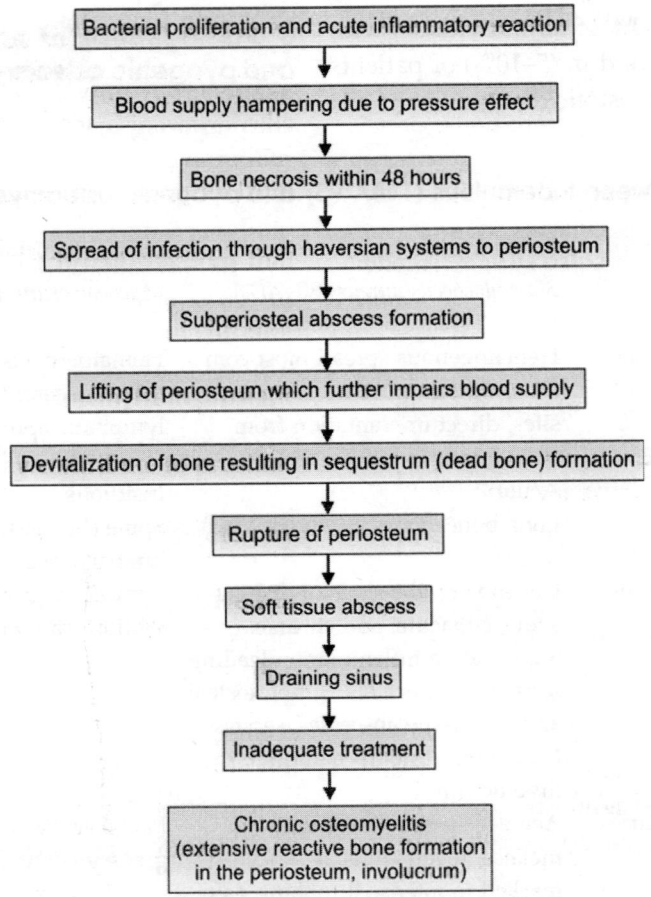

Fig. 25.1: Pathogenesis of pyogenic osteomyelitis

Brodie's abscess (viva): It is a small intra-osseous abscess that frequently involves the cortex and is walled off by reactive bone.

Sclerosing osteomyelitis of Garre: It typically develops in jaw, and is associated with extensive new bone formation that obscures much of the underlying osseous structure.

5. Classify primary bone tumors (1994, 96, 97, 2000)

Histologic type	Benign	Malignant
Hematopoietic (40%)	—	Myeloma
		Malignant lymphoma
Chondrogenic (22%)	Osteochondroma	Chondrosarcoma
	Chondroma	Dedifferentiated chondrosarcoma
	Chondroblastoma	Mesenchymal chondrosarcoma
	Chondromyxoid fibroma	—
Osteogenic (19%)	Osteoid osteoma	Osteosarcoma
	Osteoblastoma	

(Contd.)

Classify primary bone tumors (Contd.)

Histologic type	Benign	Malignant
Fibrogenic	Fibrous cortical defect (fibroma)	Fibrosarcoma
	Non-ossifying fibroma	
	Fibrous histiocytoma	
	Desmoplastic fibroma	
Unknown origin (10%)	Giant cell tumor	—
	Unicameral cyst	
	Aneurysmal bone cyst	
Neuroectodermal	—	Ewing's sarcoma
Notochordal	Benign notochordal cell tumor	Chordoma

6. Osteosarcoma/osteogenic sarcoma: Morphological, radiological and clinical features (1991, 93, 94, 97, 2000, 03, 04, 06, 08, 09, 11)

- Malignant tumor of bone characterized by formation of osteoid or bone or both directly by sarcoma cells.
- *Origin:* Primitive osteoblast forming mesenchyme. It is the most common primary malignant tumor of bone.
- *Sites:* Metaphyseal region of long bones of extremities (mostly). Knee joints (50%), upper end of femur and adjoining pelvis (15%), upper end of humerus (10%) and facial bones (8%).
  - Beyond the age of 25 yr, incidence in flat and long bones are equal.
- *Age:* Biphasic:
  - Primary osteosarcoma <20 yr of age (75% cases).
  - Secondary osteosarcoma in elderly associated with Paget's disease, bone infarct or prior irradiations.
- *Molecular genetics:* Approximately 70% of osteosarcoma have acquired genetic abnormalities such as ploidy changes and chromosomal aberrations.
  - Hereditary osteosarcoma (Rb gene mutation).
  - Sporadic osteosarcoma (p53 gene mutation, over expression of MDM2).

- *Sex:* Female: Male = 1.6:1
- *Morphology:* Two types are medullary or central osteosarcoma and paraosteal or juxtacortical.
  Morphological features of more common *medullary osteosarcoma*
  Gross
  Big, bulky tumors that are gritty, gray-white are often contain areas of hemorrhage and necrosis. Destruction of cortex and soft tissue extension are common. They spread into medullary canal, infiltrate and replace marrow of surrounding preexisting bone, but penetration of epiphyseal plate/entry into joint is infrequent.

Microscopic examination
- *Sarcoma cells:* Undifferentiated mesenchymal stroma cells with marked pleomorphism and polymorphism.
- Anaplastic sarcoma cells form osteoid matrix and bone directly.
- Histological variants are osteoblastic, chondroblastic, fibroblastic, telangiectatic, small cell and giant cells type osteosarcoma.

Radiographic examination
- Large destructive mixed lytic and blastic masses with permeative margins.
- Tumor mass mostly breaks through the cortex and lifts the periosteum resulting in reactive periosteal bone formation.

- The triangular shadow *Codman triangle* which is characteristics (but not diagnostic), is present between the cortex and raised ends of periosteum.

Biochemical tests
- Serum alkaline phosphatase—increased
- Serum calcium and phosphate level—normal

Clinical features
- Painful and progressive enlarging masses
- Sudden fractures
- Compressing symptoms of adjoining structures
- Metastasis to lung, bones and brain (hematogenous spread). Regional lymph nodes are rarely involved.
- Diagnosed by clinical features, radiology, FNAC and open biopsy.
- 5 years survival rate is 60–70% with chemotherapy and limb salvage therapy.

7. Ewing's sarcoma (1998, 2001, 03, 08, 09, 11)

- Primary malignant small round cell (resembling lymphoma, rhabdomyosarcoma, neuroblastoma, and oat cell carcinoma cells) tumor of bones and soft tissues.
- Ewing's sarcoma includes:
  - Classic/skeleton Ewing's sarcoma
  - Soft tissue Ewing's sarcoma
  - Primitive neutroectodermal tumor (PNET)
- *Age:* Children, average age: 10–15 yr; 80% cases below 20 yr (of all bone carcinoma, Ewing's sarcoma has the youngest average age at presentation).
- *Sex:* Male more affected.
- *Race:* Whites more affected.
- *Cell of origin:* Primitive neuroectodermal cells; *neural phenotype.*
- *Site:* Diaphysis of long tubular bones especially femur and the flat bones of pelvis.

Molecular genetics
- Cytogenetic abnormalities present in the form of translocation—t (11; 22) (q24; q12) resulting in fusion genes (EWS-FLI 1) as dominant oncogenes and its chimeric proteins are transcriptional factors playing roles in tumor proliferation.
- *C-myc* oncogene is also present.
- PNET demonstrate neural differentiation by light microscopy, immunohistochemistry, or electron microscopy, while Ewing's sarcoma proper/classic does not.

Morphology (*classic*)
Gross
- Typically located in medullary cavities often extending into the adjacent soft tissues.
- Tumor is gray-white, soft, friable and contains area of hemorrhage and necrosis.

Microscopic examination
- Pattern: Tumor is divided by fibrous septa into irregular lobule of closely packed tumor cells.
- Homer Wright rosette (tumor cells are arranged in a circle about a central fibrillary space), indicative of neural differentiation, may be present.
- Tumor cells: Sheets of uniform small, round cells slightly larger than lymphocytes. Scant cytoplasm, which may appear clear due to high glycogen contents (glycogen gives a granular positivity with PAS stain)
- Stroma—little stroma.
- Area of necrosis may be present.
- Very few mitotic figures.

Radiographic examination: Destructive lytic tumor that has permeative margins, **onion-skin fashion** of reactive bone deposition.

Clinical features
- Painful enlarging mass
- Affected site is tender, warm, swollen
- Fever present
- Anemia present
- ESR is raised

- Leukocytosis
- Metastasizes early by hematogenous routes to lungs, liver, bones and brain
- Use of combined chemotherapy and radiotherapy has improved the clinical outcomes

8. Giant cell tumor of bones (1992, 97, 98, 2001, 02, 03, 04, 10)/osteoclastoma: Morphological, radiological and clinical features (1990, 96)

- It contains a profusion of multinucleated osteoclast type giant cells and mononuclear cells.
- Benign but locally aggressive neoplasm.
- *Age:* 2nd to 4th decades.
- *Cell of origin:* Fusion of mononuclear cells of stroma.
- *Sites:* Adult: Epiphysis and metaphysis. Adolescents: Metaphysis (majority of them around knee joints).

Morphology

Gross

Well circumscribed, dark-tan (red-brown), large often showing cystic degeneration. It is covered by a thin shell of subperiosteal bone.

Microscopic examination: Histologic feature: Presence of *tumor giant cell.*

- Giant cells are multinucleated (more than 100 nuclei per cell) osteoclast like cells scattered throughout the stroma.
- Stromal cells are uniform oval mononuclear cells having indistinct membrane appearing to grow in syncytium. High mitotic rate of these proliferating components of tumor. Nature of these cells determines the biologic behavior of the tumor.
- The stroma is composed of scant collagen, rich blood vessels.
- Hemorrhage is present.
- Macrophages may be seen.

Radiographic examination: It appears as a large, lobulated and osteolytic, mostly solitary lesion at the end of an expanded long bones

having *soap bubble appearance* eroding into subchondral bone plate.

Clinical features

- Arthritic symptoms (involvement of joints)
- Mostly solitary lesion
- Pathologic fractures
- Metastasis to lung

9. Chondrosarcoma (1994)

- Malignant tumor of chondroblasts.
- Slow progression and better prognosis than osteosarcoma.
- *Types:* Two types:
  - *Central/intramedullary chondrosarcoma:*
    1. More common site-medullary cavity of diaphysis or metaphysis.
    2. X-ray shows a lytic lesion with blotchy calcification.
    3. Causes fusiform thickening of shaft and perforation of cortex.
    4. May arise *de novo* (80–90%) or in a preexisting osteochondroma.
  - *Peripheral/juxtacortical chondrosarcoma* in cortex or periosteum of metaphysis, may be primary or secondary.
- *Age:* 3rd to 6th decades
- *Sex:* Male predominance
- *Sites:* More in central skeleton (pelvis, ribs, shoulders) and around knee joints

Morphology

Gross

- Size—a few cm to extreme large
- Lobulated mass.
- Firm consistency, erosion or destruction of cortex is frequent.
- Cut section—translucent, bluish-white, gelatinous or myxoid appearance.
- Foci of calcification are present.

Microscopic examination

- Invasive in nature.
- The tumors vary in degree of cellularity, cytologic atypia and mitotic activity.

Classified into grades I, II and III (low grade to high grade) with increasing cellular and nuclear atypia.

- Two or more nuclei in one cell or two or more cells in one lacuna.
- Abundant mitoses.

Clinical features
- Slow growing tumor.
- Pain and gradual enlargement over the years.
- Higher-grade tumors metastasize to lung, liver, kidney and brain.

10. Fibrous dysplasia of bones

- Benign tumor like lesion of bones characterized by localized developmental arrest, all components of normal bones are present, but they are unable to differentiate into their mature forms.
- Replacement of bone by fibrous connective tissue with a characteristic whorled pattern, and containing trabeculae of woven bone.

Three types
1. *Monostotic fibrous dysplasia (70% of cases):* Single bone affected, Age: 20–30 years, sex: Both male and female equally affected. Bones affected—ribs, craniofacial, femur, tibia and humerus.
2. *Polystotic fibrous dysplasia without endocrine dysfunction:* Several bones, but never all. Bones involved are craniofacial, ribs, vertebrae, and long bones of limbs.
3. *Albright syndrome/McCune-Albright syndrome:* It is a special form of polystotic dysplasia associated with endocrine disorders. More in female; multiple bone lesions, skin pigmentation, sexual precocity, and other endocrinopathies.

Morphology
Gross: Sharply demarcated, localized, present within the cancellous bone, smooth overlying cortex. Tan-white and gritty.

Microscopic examination: Fibroblastic tissues are arranged in loose, whorled pattern. Curvilinear trabeculae of nonlamellar/woven bones surrounded by a moderately cellular fibroblastic proliferation.

- The lesion is readily diagnosed by radiology because of its typical ground glass appearance and well defined margination.
  - Most lesions are asymptomatic, few require orthopedic surgery.
  - A rare complication of polystotic dysplasia is malignant transformation of a lesion into a sarcoma.

11. Rheumatoid arthritis (RA): Pathogenesis (1997)

"A chronic systemic inflammatory disorder that may affect many tissues and organs like skin, blood vessels, heart, lung, and muscles; but involves mainly joints, producing a nonsuppurative proliferative synovitis that often progresses to destruction of the articular cartilage and ankylosis of the joints."

Age: 20–40 years of life.

Sex: Female 4–5 times more prone.

Pathogenesis: "RA is triggered by exposure of an immunogenetically susceptible host to an arthritogenic microbial antigens."

Factors
1. Genetic factors: HLA-DR4 or HLA-DR2.
2. Microbial agents (initiator of the disease): Epstein-Barr virus, retroviruses, parvoviruses, mycobacteria, borrelia, mycoplasma, etc.
3. Autoimmunity: Once inflammatory synovitis is triggered by exogenous factors, autoimmunity (T cell mediate immunity) causes chronic destruction in RA (*see* Fig. 25.2).

Morphology
Microscopic examination
- Diffuse proliferative synovitis (multilayering of synovial cells)
- Number of folds of large villi increases.
- Thickening of synovial membrane—edema, congestion, increases in number of synoviocytes.

Pathogenesis

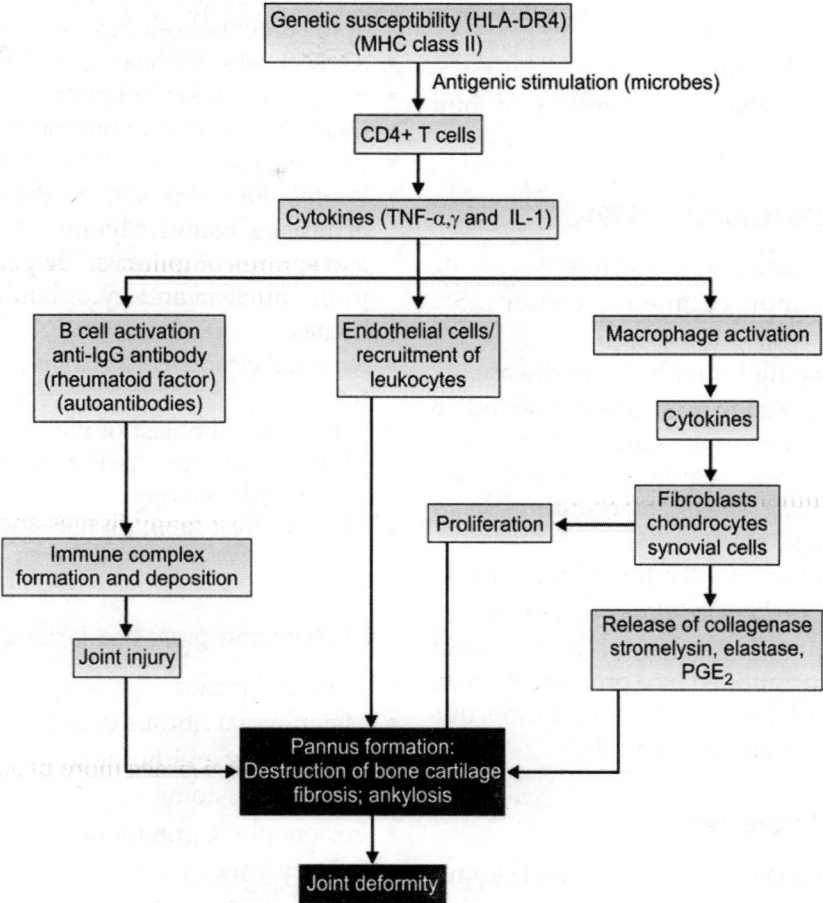

Fig. 25.2: Pathogenesis of rheumatoid arthritis

- Inflammatory cell infiltrate—lymphocytes, plasma cells, macrophages, etc.
- Fibrin deposition in synovium and accumulation of neutrophils in synovial fluid.
- Osteoclastic activity in underlying bone.

Clinical features

Commonly affected joints include metacarpophalangeal and proximal interphalangeal joints. Small joints of hands and feet are first invovled followed by symmetrical involvement of wrist, elbow, ankle, and knees.

X-ray

- Joint effusion

- Juxta-articular osteopenia with bone erosions
- Narrowing of joint spaces due to loss of articular cartilage

Diagnosis

Four of the following features should be present:

1. Morning stiffness of more than 1 hour for at least 6 weeks.
2. Arthritis and soft tissue swelling of more than 3 joints, present for at least 6 weeks.
3. Arthritis of hand joints, present for at least 6 weeks.

4. Symmetric arthritis, present for at least 6 weeks.
5. Rheumatoid nodule.
6. Rheumatoid factor.
7. Radiological changes suggestive of joint erosion.

12. Rheumatoid nodule (1999)

- Present in rheumatoid arthritis.
- Most common cutaneous lesion (25% patients).
- Present in patients with severe disease.
- Parts of the skin that are subjected to pressure like ulnar aspect of forearm, elbow, occipital region, etc. or less commonly in lung, spleen, myocardium, heart valves, aorta, etc.
- Nodule is firm, nontender, round to oval.
- Skin arise in the subcutaneous tissues.
- *Microscopic:* Central zone of fibrinoid necrosis surrounded by a prominent rim of epithelioid histiocytes and numerous lymphocytes and plasma cells.

13. Types of giant cells

- *Foreign body giant cell* (*see* acute and chronic inflammation)
- *Langhans' giant cells* (*see* acute and chronic inflammation)
- Tumor giant cell (*see* neoplasm)

- *Touton giant cell:* These are multinucleated cells having vacuolated cytoplasm due to lipid contents, seen in xanthoma.
- *Aschoff cells* (*see* heart and blood vessel)
- *RS cells:* Hodgkin lymphoma (*see* WBC)
- *Osteoclasts:* Found in normal bone
- *Giant cells of giant cell tumor of bone* (bones)
- *Warthin-Finkeldey giant cell:* Pathognomonic of measles. Found in lymphoid organ, lung, and sputum of patients. They have eosinophilic nuclear and cytoplamic inclusion bodies.
- *Syncytial giant cell of seminoma:* Male genital tract
- Syncytiotrophoblast of placenta
- *Multinucleate giant cells of subacute thyroiditis:* Endocrinology
- *Giant cells of myocarditis* (*see* heart and blood vessel)

14. Enumerate giant cell lesions of bone

- Giant cell tumor
- Metaphyseal fibrous defect
- Chondromyxoid fibroma
- Chondroblastoma
- Eosionophilic granuloma
- Solitary bone cyst
- Osteitis fibrosa cystica
- Aneurysmal bone cyst
- Osteoid osteoma
- Osteoblastoma

26

Central Nervous System and Eye

1. Hydrocephalus (1993)

It refers to the accumulation of excess of CSF within the ventricular system of brain producing dilatation of ventricular cavities and increased intracranial pressure.

Normal physiology: CSF is produced by the choroids plexus within the lateral, third and fourth ventricles; and is absorbed into blood by the arachnoid villi present along the dural venous sinuses. Total volume of CSF in adult is 90–150 ml.

Clinical features: If hydrocephalus develops before closure of cranial sutures in early infancy: Enlargement of head.

If it develops after closure of cranial sutures—later ages: Expansion of ventricles; increased intracranial pressure, but no change in head circumference. In both cases, headache is the chief complaint.

Findings: Autopsy shows large brain, dilated ventricle(s) with thinning of walls of cerebral hemispheres, atrophy of central white matter. Sulci are narrow and gyri flattened.

Compression of adjacent structures may be seen.

Types
1. Non-communicating type: *Some obstruction* (e.g. tumors) to flow of CSF leading to dilatation of ventricular system proximal to the block.
2. Communicating type: No obstruction to flow of CSF, all ventricles are involved. Due to *decreased* reabsorption of CSF (most common cause) or overproduction of CSF (rare; choroid plexus tumors).

2. Laboratory diagnosis of tubercular meningitis (2008)

3. Difference between acute pyogenic and tubercular meningitis (1992, 97, 99, 2000, 01, 03)

4. CSF findings in pyogenic meningitis (2012)

5. Difference between CSF findings in viral and tubercular meningitis (2011)

6. CSF in viral meningitis (1990)

Traits (CSF)	Normal	Acute pyogenic	Viral	Tubercular
Pressure	50–180 mm water	Normal/↑ed	Normal	Normal/↑ed
Color	Clear, colorless, no coagulum	Turbid, cloudy, coagulum present	Clear	Clear, colorless, cobweb coagulum on keeping

(Contd.)

CSF in viral meningitis (Contd.)

Traits (CSF)	Normal	Acute pyogenic	Viral	Tubercular
RBC (mm³)	0–4	Normal	Normal	Normal
WBC (mm³)	0–4	1000–5000	10–2000	50–5000
Predominant		polymorphs	lymphocytes	lymphocytes
Glucose	>60% of blood level (50–80 mg/dl)	↓↓ed	Normal	↓ed
Protein	<0.45 g/L	↑ed	Normal/↑ed	↑↑↑ed
Chloride	720–750 g/100 ml	600–700 mg/100 ml	Normal	450–600 mg/100 ml (↓ed)
Microbiology	Sterile	Organism on Gram stain/culture	Sterile/virus detected	ZN stain—AFB
Oligoclonal band	Negative	Can be positive	Can be positive	Can be positive
Organisms	No	See below	See below	Mycobacterium tuberculosis

- *Meningitis*
  - Meningitis refers to inflammation of leptomeninges and CSF within the subarachnoid space.
  - Meningoencephalitis includes inflammation of meninges and brain parenchyma.
  - Meningitis is usually caused by an infection, but it may also occur in response to a nonbacterial irritant introduced into the subarachnoid space (chemical meningitis).
  - Infection may reach through hematogenous route, direct implantation (trauma) or local extension from adjacent structures (air sinuses, infected tooth, cranial or spinal osteomyelitis).

Acute pyogenic (bacterial) meningitis

Causes

Neonates
- Gram-negative bacilli (*E. coli*, *Proteus*, etc.)
- Gr B streptococci

Preschool
- *H. influenzae*
- *N. meningitidis*
- *S. pneumoniae*

Older children and adults
- *N. meningitidis*
- *S. pneumoniae*

Pathology

Gross: When CSF tap is done, CSF comes out with increased pressure (flow). CSF becomes turbid or frankly purulent due to pus accumulation in the subarachnoid space.

Microscopic feature: CSF shows numerous polymorphonuclear leukocytes, Gram staining will show specific bacteria.

- *Clinical features*
  - It is a medical emergency. Patient presents with fever, severe headache, vomiting, drowsiness, stupor, coma and convulsions.
  - Neck stiffness, positive Kernig's sign, and Brudzinski's sign suggest meningitis.

- *Complications*
  - Cerebral abscess formation
  - Obstructive hydrocephalus
  - Subdural empyema
  - Cerebral infarction
  - Epilepsy

Acute aseptic (viral) meningitis

It is a clinical term referring to the absence of recognizable organism in a patient with meningeal irritation, fever and alterations of consciousness of relatively acute onset.

- *Causes*
  - Enteroviruses (polio, coxsackie)
  - Influenza
  - Mumps
  - Herpes simplex
- *Clinical features*
  - Clinical course is less severe than bacterial meningitis.
  - It is benign and self-limiting and usually ends in complete recovery.

7. Prion diseaes (transmissible spongiform encephalopathies) (2000)

- Prions are abnormal forms of a cellular protein that cause transmissible neurodegenerative disorders
- It *includes*
  - In human Creutzfeldt-Jakob disease (CJD), Gerstmann-Straussler-Scheinker syndrome (GSS), fatal familial insomnia and kuru
  - Scrapie in sheep and goat
  - Mink transmissible encephalopathy
  - Bovine spongiform encephalopathy (mad cow disease)
- *Characterized by*
  - Spongiform change in neuronal cells of cerebral cortex and often, deep gray mater.
  - Microscopic vacuoles of varying sizes are noted in neuropil and parykaryon of neurons. In advanced cases, there is severe neuronal loss, reactive gliosis and expansion of vacuolated areas into cyst like spaces (status spongiosus).
  - Absence of immune response, or an immune response that does not arrest the disease, but may actually contribute to pathogenesis.

- Kuru plaques are extracellular deposits of aggregated abnormal proteins. These proteins are Congo red and PAS positive and usually occur in cerebellum.
- In all cases, immunohistochemical staining shows presence of proteinase k-resistant PrP in tissue.
- Genetic predisposition
- Incubation period ranging from months to years.
- Progressive dementia
- Invariable fatal termination

- *Pathogenesis:* PrP (prion protein) presents in normal neuron cells are in α-helix isoform (PrP-c). Prion proteins are both infectious and transmissible. Whenever there is conformational change to abnormal β-pleated sheet isoform (PrP-*sc*: *Scrapie*; PrP-*res*: *Protease resistant*) disease occurs.

This conformational change may be spontaneous at an extremely low rate (in sporadic cases) or at higher rate (inherited case; may be transmitted to person-inoculation, infection by abnormal prion protein).

In both cases, *PrP-res* resists protease digestion and facilitates transformation of other *PrP-c* to *PrP-res*. Accumulation of *PrP-res* in neural tissue causes development of cytoplasmic vacuoles and thus spongiform changes, followed by neuronal death by an unknown mechanism.

8. Classify brain tumor

Primary tumors

1. Tumors of neuroepithelial origin (gliomas)
   i. Astrocytomas
      - Infiltrating astrocytoma (diffuse astrocytoma, anaplastic, gemistocytic astrocytoma, glioblastoma)
      - Non-infiltrating (pilocytic astrocytoma)
      - Pleomorphic xanthoastrocytoma
      - Brainstem glioma

   ii. Oligodendroglioma
   iii. Ependymomas
   iv. Subependymomas
   v. Choroid plexus papillomas
2. *Neuronal tumors*
   i. Ganglioneuromas and ganliogliomas
   ii. Neuroblastomas
   iii. Dysembryoplasticneuroepithelial tumor
   iv. Central neurocytoma
3. *Poorly differentiated neoplasm*
   i. Medulloblastoma (embryonal origin)
   ii. Atypical teratoid (rhabdoid tumor)
4. *Other parenchymal tumors*
   i. Primary CNS lymphoma
   ii. Germ cell tumors
   iii. Pineal parenchymal tumors
5. *Meningiomas*

Metastatic (secondary) tumors

Most commonly from lung, breast, skin (melanoma), kidney, and gastrointestinal tract: Accounting for 80% of metastatic brain tumor.

9. Astrocytoma (1991, 92, 95)

- Astrocytomas are derived from glial cells. It may be divided into infiltrating astrocytomas and non-infiltrating astrocytomas.
- These tumor types have characteristic histologic features, distribution within the brain, age groups and clinical course.

Infiltrating astrocytomas
- It includes diffuse astrocytoma, anaplastic astrocytoma, gemistocytic astrocytoma and glioblastoma.
- These accounts for 80% of adult primary brain tumor.
- *Sites:* Usually occurs in cerebral hemisphere; may also occur in cerebellum, brainstem or spinal cord.
- *Age:* 40–60 yr.

Diffuse astrocytoma
Gross
- Poorly defined gray infiltrating mass that expands and distorts the infiltrated part of the brain.

- *Size:* Few centimeter to large enough to replace the entire hemisphere.
- Cut surface of tumor is either firm or soft, gelatinous cystic degeneration may be present.
- Sometime, tumor may appear well demarcated from the surrounding brain tissue, but infiltration beyond the outer margin (into normal looking brain) is almost always present.

Microscopic features
- Mild to moderate increase in number of glial cells.
- Variable nuclear polymorphism is present.
- Fibrillary appearance of GFAP positive astrocytic processes.
- Transition between neoplastic and normal tissue is indistinct.

Anaplastic astrocytomas
- They show more cellular and nuclear pleomorphism, more mitotic figures.
- Gemistocytic astrocytoma is a type of tumor in which neoplastic astrocyte cells show brightly eosinophilic cell body from which abundant, stout processes emanate.
- *Pathology of infiltrating astrocytoma*
  Molecular genetics

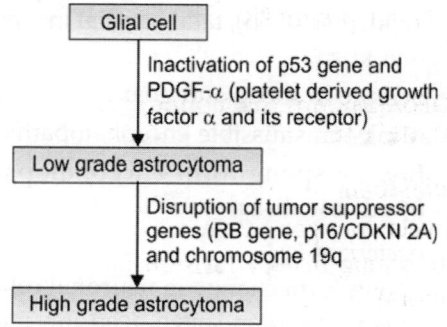

Clinical presentation
- It depends on the location of tumor, its size, rate of growth and metastasis (through CSF).
- Patient may present with headache, seizure, features of increased intracranial pressure, and focal neurological deficit.
- *Non-infiltrating astrocytoma*
  Pilocytic astrocytoma
    – They usually occur in children and young adults.

- Usually located in cerebellum, but may also involve floor and walls of third ventricle, the optic nerves and cerebral hemisphere.
- They have usually benign behaviour than other astrocytomas.

Gross: Usually cystic lesion, may be well circumscribed (rarely infiltrative) solid lesion.

- **Microscopic feature**
  - The tumor mass is composed of bipolar cells with long thin hair-like processes that are GFAP positive and form dense fibrillary meshwork.
  - 'Rosenthal fibers' (amorphous aggregates of GFAP) and eosinophilic granular bodies are often present.
  - Increased number of blood vessels with thick walls are present.
  - Necrosis and mitoses are not common.

- **Clinical features**
  - These are slow growing tumors. They rarely have p53 gene mutation.
  - They are usually resectable and has better prognosis.

10. Glioblastoma multiforme/glioblastoma (2001, 04, 06)

Glioblastoma
- Affects younger patients
- Has a long history (arise from low grade tumors)
- It was previously called as glioblastoma multiforme

Morphology
Gross
- Size and appearance varies according to the site and is characteristic.
- Large firm and white to soft and yellow (due to tissue necrosis).
- Cystic degeneration and hemorrhage may be present.

- Tumor may appear demarcated, but infiltration beyond margin is always present.

Microscopic examination
- Similar to anaplastic astrocytoma with additional features of necrosis and vascular or endothelial cell proliferation.
- Highly cellular appearance.
- Greater nuclear pleomorphism than diffuse astrocytoma.
- Mitotic activity prominent.
- Endothelial proliferation—tufts of pilled up vascular cells that bulge into the vascular lumen (ball-like structure *glomeruloid body*).
- Necrosis present in serpentine manner in areas of hypercellularity with highly malignant cells crowded along the edge of the necrotic regions—*pseudopalisading* appearance.

11. Medulloblastoma

- 20% of brain tumor of children.
- Exclusively in cerebellum—mostly midline in children; lateral in adults.
- Poorly differentiated; neuronal and glial markers may be expressed.
- Highly malignant.
- Prognosis is poor for untreated patients, but tumor is highly radiosensitive.
- With total excision and radiation therapy 5 years survival rate is as high as 75%.

Morphology
- *Gross:* Well circumscribed, gray, friable mass.
- *Microscopic examination*
  - Tumor is extremely cellular.
  - Sheets of anaplastic cells.
  - Tumor cells are small; have little cytoplasm; hyperchromatic; elongated or crescent shaped nuclei.
  - Mitoses are high and many cells are positive for cellular proliferation marker as ki-67.

- They may express neurosecretory granules or Homer Wright rosettes and glial (GFAP+) phenotype.
- Desmoplastic variant has stromal response with areas of collagen and reticulin deposition.
- Dissemination through CSF is common (drop metastases to cauda equina)
- Most common genetic finding is loss of material from the short arm of chromosome 17.

12. Meningiomas (1997, 2002, 07, 08, 11)

They are usually attached to dura and arise from the meningothelial cell of the arachnoid.

- Benign tumor of adults, uncommon in children. They are usually slow growing lesion.
- *Sex:* Female: Male = 3:2.
- *Origin:* Meningiothelial cell of the arachnoids.
- *Sites:* Along the external surface of brain; and within the ventricular system (here it arises from stromal arachnoid cells of choroids plexus). *Mostly midline.*

Morphology

- *Gross:* Usual patterns are:
  - Found as masses within well-defined dural base that compresses underlying brain, but are easily separable from it.
  - Encapsulated with thin fibrous tissue and may have a bosselated polypoid appearance.
- Variant growth pattern (en plaque):
  - Sheet-like fashion along the surface of dura.
  - Lesion may be firm and fibrous to finely gritty or extremely calcified with Psammoma bodies.
  - There is no gross necrosis or hemorrhage.

Microscopic examination: Several histologic growth patterns without any prognostic significance:

1. *Syncytial (meningothelial):* Whorled cluster of cells in tight groups without visible cell membranes.
2. *Fibroblastic:* Elongated cells, abundant collagen matrix.
3. *Transition:* Features of syncytial and fibroblastic.
4. *Psammomatous:* Psammoma bodies, formed from calcification of syncytial nests of meningiothelial cells.
5. *Secretory:* PAS positive intracytoplasmic droplets; keratin and CEA positive.
6. *Microcystic:* Loose spongy appearance with microcyst formation.
7. Atypical meningiomas and anaplastic (malignant) meningiomas are more aggregasive.
8. *Papillary:* Pleomorphic cells; frequency of recurrence is high.

- Meningiomas are positive for epithelial membrane antigens.
- *Molecular genetics:* Loss of chromosome 22 or its long arm (NF2 gene).

13. Ependymoma

- *Sites and origin:* Glial cell origin; cells forming the ependymal lining of ventricular system in brain and central canal or spinal cord.

  Up to age of 20, tumor arises near fourth ventricle; 5–10% or primary brain tumor in this age group.
- *Adult:* Spinal cord is most commonly involved.

Morphology

- *Gross*
  - Solid or papillary masses extending from the floor of ventricle or canal of spinal cord distorting, compressing, and infiltrating surrounding structures.
  - Demarcation is present, but not very sharp in ventricular system as compared to spine, where demarcation is sharp.

- *Microscopic examination*
  - Mostly well differentiated tumor cells with regular, round to oval nuclei and abundant granular chromatin;
  - Variable dense fibrillar background is present between nuclei;
  - Tumor cells may form gland like or elongated structure (rosette)—more frequently perivascular pseudorosette with a blood vessel in the center and tumor cells (thin epidymal process directed towards the wall of blood vessel) present in periphery.
- *Clinical features*
  - Headache
  - Increased intracranial pressure
  - Secondary hydrocephalus due to posterior fossa ependymoma
  - CSF dissemination is common
  - Poor prognosis despite slow growth rate and absence of anaplasia

14. Retinoblastoma (1996, 2008, 11)

- Most common malignant eye tumor of childhood.
- *Age:* < 15 years; 90% less than 7 years of age.
- *Sex:* Both sexes are equally affected.
- *Molecular genetics*
  - Loss of heterozygosity of tumor suppressor gene (Rb) allele.
  - *Cell origin:* Neuroepithelial origin in retina.
- *Types:* Two types:
  1. *Hereditary*
     - Bilateral (both eyes are affected);
     - Associated with other tumors like osteosarcoma later on;
     - One of the two alleles of RB gene has undergone mutation in germ line itselt and is inherited as germ line mutation in all cells. Mutation of normal allele of RB gene produces retinoblastoma;
     - Most patients do not have previous family history, as they have a new germ line mutation.

  2. *Non-hereditary:* Initially there is acquired mutation in one allele of RB gene in somatic retinal cells/somatic cells (precursor of the developing retina). It is followed by "second hit" giving rise to tumor.

Mostly only one tumor in one eye, not associated with or no increased risk for other tumors.

Morphology

Gross: Nodular, poorly cohesive masses with often satellite seedling.

Microscopic examination

1. *Undifferentiated areas:* Cells resembling normal retinoblasts—small round cells with hyperchromatic nuclei and scant cytoplasm.
2. *Differentiated areas: Flexner-Wintersteiner rosette* (true rosette):
   - Clusters of cuboidal and short columnar cells arranged around a central lumen.
   - The nuclei (appear having limiting membrane similar to external limiting membrane of retinal) are displaced away from the lumen.
   - Photoreceptors like elements protrude through membrane and tapers into fine filaments.
3. Homer Wright rosettes and fleurette types are found less commonly.

Metastasis

- Local invasion into nearby organs; distant metastasis to CNS, skull, distal bones and lymph nodes.
- It is usually fatal once it has spread outside eye and orbit.

Clinical features

- Median age at presentation is two years.
- Presenting finding includes poor vision, strabismus, a whitish hue to the pupil (cat's eye reflex) and pain in eye.
- With enucleation, chemotherapy and radiotherapy, survival rate is high.

27

Miscellaneous Questions for Paper II

1. Etiopathogenesis and morphology of fibrocongestive spleen (2002)

2. Classify and give pathogenesis of HD (1996, 2004)

3. Hodgkin's disease (1990, 1995, 1999, 2004)

4. Nodular sclerosis type of Hodgkin's lymphoma (2001, 04)

5. Mixed cellularity HD (1994, 97)

6. Difference between lymphocyte predominant and lymphocytic depletion HD (1997)

7. Difference between microscopic features of mixed cellularity and nodular sclerosis HD (2003)

8. Difference between low grade and high grade non-Hodgkin's lymphoma

9. Lesions caused by EBV (1995)

10. Burkitt lymphoma (1990, 95, 99, 2004)

11. Enumerate the causes of splenomegaly. Give gross and microscopic picture of fibrocongestive spleen

12. HLA and disease association (2004)

13. Fat necrosis (2004)

PART III: Practicals

28

Hematology Practical

Hemoglobin Estimation

Sahli's method

Principle: Blood is added to N/10HCl, which converts Hb into acid hematin. Brown color of acid hematin is matched against the brown color of the comparator.

Apparatus
1. Hemoglobinometer
2. Dropper
3. N/10 HCl
4. Stirrer
5. Hb pipette
6. Distilled water

Procedure
1. Add N/10 HCl with the help of dropper into Hb meter tube up to mark 3 g%.
2. Blood sample should be mixed well. Add 0.002 ml of blood into Hb meter tube, mix well.
3. Allow acid to act on the RBCs for 10 minutes to lyse the red cells and convert Hb to acid hematin.
4. Add distilled water with the help of a dropper to Hb meter tube and stir the solution. Dilute the solution till the color of the solution matches the comparator color.
5. During color matching process, stirrer should be out of solution, but not of Hb meter tube (to avoid spilling of solution).
6. Take the reading from the upper, meniscus in g% (g/dl).

Normal values
Male: 13.5–17.5 g/dl
Female: 12.0–16.0 g/dl

Sources of errors/disadvantages
1. If stored blood sample is not mixed properly, reading may be high or low depending on whether the plasma or the sedimented RBCs are taken in the pipette.
2. After 10 minutes, color of acid hematin starts fading; so lower value will be obtained if reading is delayed.
3. Acid does not convert all Hb into acid hematin, so Hb value obtained is slightly lower than the actual Hb level.

Advantages
1. Simple technique
2. Fast method
3. Cost effective

1. Why is N/10 HCl is used in Sahli's method?

Brown color of the comparator glass is equivalent to the color of acid hematin produced using N/10 HCl for a blood sample of 14.8 g%. Test solution is compared against it. So, no other strength of HCl can be used.

Other methods of hemoglobin estimation
1. *Cyanmethemoglobin:* HiCN method (using Drabkin solution):

Principle: Hb is oxidized to methemoglobin by potassium ferricyanide. MetHb gets converted to a stable compound cyanmethemoglobin by potassium cyanide.

Color of this solution is compared against a standard (known) Hb value by colorimetry.

2. *Alkali hematin method:* Strong alkali (N/10 NaOH) converts Hb into alkali hematin. Color of alkaline hematin is compared against a standard.

3. *Oxyhemoglobin method:* NH$_4$OH is used. It lyses the red cells. Optical density of oxyhemoglobin solution so obtained is taken by colorimetry.

4. *Haldane method:* RBCs are laysed and carbon monoxide is added to convert Hb to carboxyhemoglobin whose color is compared with that of a standard.

- *Advantages of cyanmethemoglobin method over Sahli's method:*
  1. No personal visual errors (as it is colorimetric method).
  2. Cyanmethemoglobin Hb is a stable compound. Its color does not change with time.
  3. In cyanmethemoglobin method, all Hb axcept sulfhemoglobin are converted into cyanmeth Hb. In Sahli's method carboxy Hb, carbamino Hb and sulfhemoglobin are not converted into acid hematin with resultant lower Hb value.

WHO classification of anemia

Group	Gram/dl (venous blood)	MCHC (percent)
Males (>15 yr age)	<13	34
Adult females, non-pregnant (>15 yr)	<12	34
Adult female, pergnant	<11	34
Children, 6 months to 5 yr	<11	34
Children 5 – 11 yr	<11.5	34
Children 12–14 yr	<12	34

2. Causes of anemia (*see* disorders of RBC)

3. Causes of polycythemia (*see* disorders of RBC)

Total leukocyte count (TLC)

Principle: Whole blood is diluted with WBC fluid that hemolyses red cells. Nucleated cells—WBCs stained by gentian violet are counted in a Neubauer chamber.

Apparatus
1. WBC pipette
2. Improved Neubauer chamber
3. Coverslip
4. WBC fluid (Turk's fluid)

Turk's fluid
1. Glacial acetic acid: Lyse RBCs

2. Gentian violet: Stain WBC nuclei
3. Water

Procedure
1. Mix the blood sample by shaking the vial.
2. Fill blood in WBC pipette up to mark 0.5 and wipe off excess blood on the sides of the pipette nozzle.
3. Fill the pipette with Turk's fluid up to mark 11.
4. Mix blood and fluid thoroughly in the bulb of pipette by rotating the pipette slowly.
5. Discard 1–2 drops of fluid (as fluid up to mark 1 has not been mixed with blood).
6. Put coverslip on the ruled area of cleaned Neubauer chamber.
7. Charge the chamber with solution. Take care of over filling and under filling.

8. Wait for approximately 5 minutes for cells to settle.
9. Count cells in 4 ruled areas (squares) for WBCs under low power (10X).

Calculation

1. Let, total number of leukocytes in four ruled areas (squares) = N
2. Volume of each WBC square = length × breath × depth = 1 × 1 × 0.1 mm = 0.1 mm^3
3. So, volume of four WBC squares = 4 × 0.1 mm^3 = 0.4 mm^3
4. Since 0.4 mm^3 of diluted blood contains N number of leukocytes, so 1 mm^3 of diluted blood will contain (N/0.4) leukocytes.
5. Dilution factor is 20, so 1 mm^3 of undiluted blood will have (N/0.4) × 20 leukocytes.
6. Leukocyte count = N × 50/mm^3.

Normal value: 4.5 – 11.0 × 10^9/L (4.5 – 11.0 × 10^3/mm^3)

Sources of errors

1. Sample not properly mixed.
2. Improper charging of chamber.
3. Overflowing of chamber.
4. Presence of nucleated RBCs. If nRBCs are more than 4/100 WBCs in DLC, a correction for nRBCs should be made.
Corrected TLC

$$= \frac{TLC \times 100}{100 + \text{number of nRBCs}/100 \text{ WBCs}}$$

4. Causes of leukocytosis and leukopenia

5. Leukemoid reaction

6. Leukemia

7. Difference between WBC pipette and RBC pipette

1. Markings are 0.5, 1 and 11 in WBC pipette; 0.5, 1 and 101 in RBC pipette.
2. Dilution is 1 in 20 in WBC pipette; 1 in 200 in RBC pipette.
3. White bead in WBC pipette; red bead in RBC pipette.

8. Other uses of WBC pipette

1. Eosinophil count
2. Platelet count
3. Sperm count
4. Cell counts of CSF, pleural/ascitic tap
5. For RBC count when patient has a severe anemia.

When TLC is very high—RBC pipette method should be used.

Differential Leukocyte Count (DLC)

Stains used: (Romanowsky stains)
1. Wright's stain
2. Leishman stain
3. Giemsa stain
4. Jenner's stain
5. Jenner-Giemsa stain

These stains consists of mixture of methylene blue, eosin and methylene blue oxidation products (azures)—which are formed by interaction and chemical treatment of the stain.

These products are responsible for different shades of staining, e.g. red blood cells—pink; eosinophilic granules—red-orange; basophilic granules—red-orange; neutrophilic granules—lilac; nuclear chromatin—purple-black; white cell cytoplasm—faint purple.

Composition

1. *Eosin:* It is negatively charged (acidic dye) and stains positively charged (basic) particles like RBCs and granules of eosinophils.
2. *Methylene blue:* It is positively charged (basic) dye and stains negatively charged (acidic) particles like cytoplasm, nuclei of WBCs and granules of basophils.
3. *Acetone free methyl alcohol:* It acts as fixative, i.e. it preserves the cells in whatever chemical and metabolic state they are at the time of staining; and the blood smear also gets fixed to the slide, so that it cannot be washed off (due to precipitation of protein by alcohol).

Note: Methanol should not have traces of acetone as it causes shrinkage of cells (crenation and cell lysis). Also it should be completely water free because water favors rouleaux formation.

Procedure

Smear making

1. Take a smooth edged slide as spreader.
2. Put a drop of blood at one end of other slide. Spread the blood with the spreader making angle of 45°. Smear should be tongue shaped.
3. Smear should not be too thick or too thin. Avoid air-bubbles and scratch marks in the smear during smear making.

Staining

1. Put the smear on the staining rack.
2. Pour the stain on the slide to cover whole slide with the stain. Count number of drops of stain (fixing of smear occurs; no staining taker place).
3. After 2 minutes, pour double the number of drops of buffer water on the slide and mix buffer water with stain, using air blow by the dropper.
4. Leave the slide for 10 minute (time may vary—look for instruction given by teachers). Staining takes place.
5. Pour running water from one side till no more stain comes out.
6. Dry the slide. First examine in low power (10X) and then focus in oil immersion (100X).

Counting of cells: Count 100 cells by moving slides in continous *tally-bar method/* like fashion.

Area for DLC: DLC should be carried out in thin part of the smear next to tail. Tail and edges of smear should be avoided, since

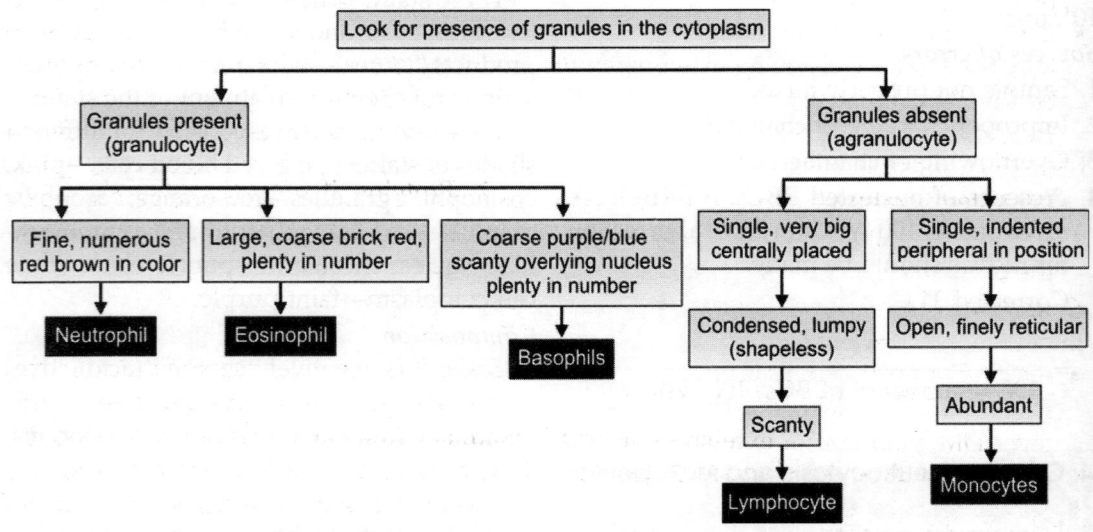

Fig. 28.1: Working rules for identification of leukocytes

monocytes and neutrophils predominate in these areas (being heavier).

Other uses of DLC slides: Information about red cells, platelets, white blood cells, abnormal cells, hemoparasites like malaria, microfilaria (tail area preferred).

9. Causes of cytopenia and cytosis (like neutrophilia and neutropenia) (*see* disorders of WBC)

10. Normal value of DLC (*see* disorders of RBC)

29

Urine Practical

Urinometer (viva)

- Normal specific gravity of a 24-hour urine sample is 1.016 to 1.030.
- Urinometer is used for the measuring specific gravity of urine.
- It is calibrated for a temperature correction also. For every 3°C rise in room temperature beyond the calibration temperature (usually 20°C), 0.001 is added to the recorded reading; and 0.001 substracted for every 3°C fall in temperature.
- Urinometer should not touch the walls of the container.

Conditions in which specific gravity of urine increases and decreases.

- *Specific gravity increased:* Dehydration, restricted fluid intake, diarrhea, vomiting, fever, DM, albuminuria, excessive sweating, acute glomerulonephritis.
- *Specific gravity decreased:* Excessive fluid intake, diabetes insipidus, end stage kidney (chronic glomerulonephritis), etc.

Examination of Urine for Abnormal Constituents

Test for Proteinuria

- If urine is alkaline, urine should be acidified with a few drops of glacial acetic acid.

Methods

1. Heat coagulation method
2. Sulfosalicylic acid test

3. Heller's test (concentrated nitric acid test)
4. Esbach's reagent test (quantitative estimation of protein for 24-hour urine sample)
5. Dipstick method

Heat coagulation method

- *Procedure*
  1. Fill three-fourths of a test tube with urine and heat the upper part of the urine on Bunsen burner.
  2. Proteins, if present, coagulate. Lower part of the urine acts as control for checking turbidity in the heated upper part.
  3. Add a few drops of 10% glacial acetic acid. Phosphates, if present, dissolve, while proteins persists in coagulated form.

Interpretation

Proteins present in urine are reported as negative, trace, +, ++, +++, and ++++

1. White cloudiness + (<0.10%)
2. Granular white precipitate ++ (0.1–0.25%)
3. Floccular precipitate +++ (0.25–0.50%)
4. Thick opaque precipitate ++++ (>0.5%)

Detection of albumin and Bence-Jones protein in urine

If both proteins are suspected, boil the urine and filter. Precipitated albumin will be filtered out. Take the filtrate and heat it to 45–60°C when Bence-Jones proteins precipitate. These dissolves on boiling.

Test for Proteins

- Heat coagulation test:

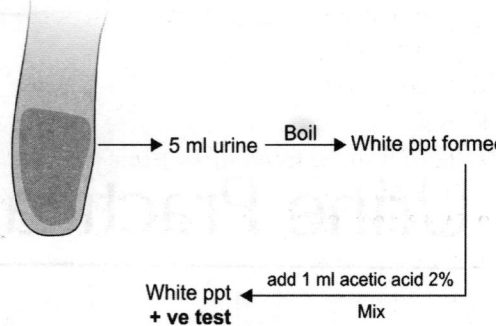

Fig. 29.1

- Sulfo-salicylic acid test:

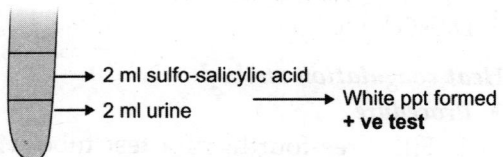

Fig. 29.2

Test for Glycosuria

Methods
1. Benedict's test
2. Glucose oxidase test

Benedict's test (semi-quantitative test)
- *Composition:* Cupric sulfate, sodium carbonate, sodium citrate.
- *Principle:* Reducing substances, like glucose, present in urine reduce Cu^{2+} to Cu^+ present in Benedict's solution. Cu^+ produces Cu_2O, which gives color to the solution.

$$Cu^{2+} (CuSO_4) \xrightarrow[\text{High temperature}]{\text{Reducing sugar}}$$

$$Cu^+ \xrightarrow{OH^-} Cu_2O$$

- *Procedure*
  1. Take 5 ml of Benedict's reagent in a test tube (take care of amount).

2. Add 8 drops of urine (take care of amount).
3. Boil the mixture for 5 min. Note the color after cooling.

Interpretation
1. Blue color of solution: Negative
2. No precipitate: Negative
3. Greenish solution: Trace (<0.5 g/dl)
4. Yellow precipitate: ++ (1.0–1.5%)
5. Orange precipitate: +++ (1.5–2%)
6. Brick red precipitate: ++++ (>2%)

Test for Glucose

- Benedict test:

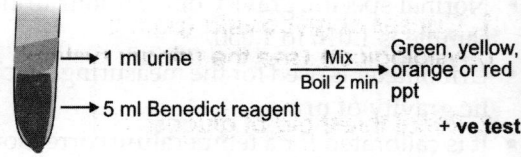

Fig. 29.3

- Fehling test:

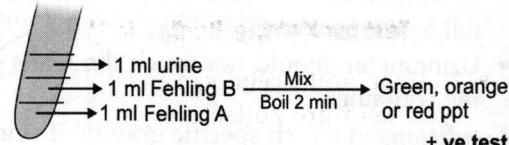

Fig. 29.4

Substances giving false positive test
- *Sugars*
  - Fructose
  - Pentose
  - Galactose
- *Non-sugars*
  - Ascorbic acid
  - Glucuronides
  - Phenol
  - Uric acid
  - Salicylates
  - PAS
  - Urates
  - Streptomycin

Glucose Oxidase Test

Reagents present in ready-made strips (diastix/multistix/dipstix) are:

1. Glucose oxidase
2. Peroxidase
3. Chromogen (O-toluidine, potassium iodine)

If urine sample contains glucose, following reactions occur:

$$\text{Glucose} + H_2O + O_2 \xrightarrow{\text{Glucose oxidase}}$$
$$\text{Gluconic acid} + H_2O_2$$

$$H_2O_2 + \text{Chromogen} \xrightarrow{\text{Peroxidase}} H_2O + \text{oxidized chromogen (color)}$$

1. Causes of glycosuria (pathological and physiological) (*see* the urinary system)

2. Renal threshold of glucose (170 mg/dl)

3. Blood sugar level and diabetes (*see* the pancreas, GTT)

Test for Ketone Bodies in Urine

- Acetone, acetoacetic acid and β-hydroxybutyric acid are collectively called ketone bodies.

Methods

1. Rothera's test (positive for acetone/acetoacetic acid)
2. Gerhardt's test (positive for acetoacetic acid and β-hydroxybutyric acid)
3. Heat test (positive for β-hydroxybutyric acid)
4. Dipstick method (positive for acetone/acetoacetic acid)

- *Rothera's test*
- *Procedure*
  1. Take 4 ml of urine in a test tube.
  2. Add a few drops of freshly prepared sodium nitroprusside to it. Saturate the urine solution with ammonium sulfate crystals. Mix well to dissolve the crystal.

3. Add a few drops of liquor ammonia along the wall of the tube.
4. Development of purple ring indicates the presence of acetone/acetoacetic acid or both.

Gerhardt's test

Procedure

1. Take 5 ml of fresh urine sample to a clean test tube.
2. Add 10% $FeCl_3$ solution dropwise.
3. Observe for formation of any red-brown precipitate.

Test for Ketone Bodies

- Rothera test (nitroprusside test):

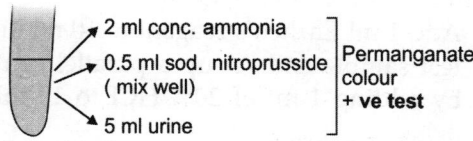

2 ml conc. ammonia
0.5 ml sod. nitroprusside (mix well)
5 ml urine
Permanganate colour + ve test

Fig. 29.5

- Iodo-form test:

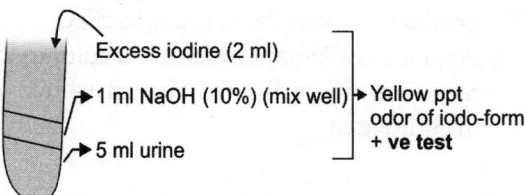

Excess iodine (2 ml)
1 ml NaOH (10%) (mix well) → Yellow ppt odor of iodo-form + ve test
5 ml urine

Fig. 29.6

Test for Bilirubin Pigment in Urine

Normally there is no detectable bilirubin in urine, but whenever there is increased serum level of direct (conjugated, soluble) bilirubin as in obstructive jaundice or late in hepatocellular jaundice: It appears in urine. It is absent in case of hemolytic jaundice from urine.

Methods

1. Fouchet's test
2. Dipstick method

Fouchet's method

Principle: Fouchet's reagent having trichloroacetic acid and ferric chloride oxidize bilirubin to biliverdin, which gives a dark green color.

Procedure

1. Take 5 ml of urine in a test tube, add equal amount of 10% barium chloride, mix.
2. Filter the mixture through filter paper. Bilirubin along with barium salts remains on filter paper.
3. Keep the filter paper to dry to some extent; add a few drops of Fouchet's reagent on the filter paper.
4. Green color appears if bilirubin is present in the sample. Darkness of color indicates amount of bilirubin in urine.

Ehrlich's test for urobilinogen

1. Add 1 ml Ehrlich's reagent to 10 ml urine test sample and set up a parallel control by adding 1 ml of 20% HCl to 10 ml of urine.
2. Mix the contents of both the tubes by inverting then and leave for 3–5 minutes at room temperature. If no pink color is produced warm the content to 50°C.
3. Appearance of pink or faint red color in the test sample indicates the presence of urobilinogen.

Test for Bile Salts in Urine

Normally bile salts (sodium and potassium salts of glucocholates and taurocholates) are absent from urine. It is present in urine in case of obstructive and hepatocellular jaundice.

Hay's surface tension test

Principle: Normal urine has enough surface tension to prevent sinking of sulfur powder. But presence of bile salts decreases the surface tension and hence sulfur powder sinks.

Procedure

1. Take 5 ml of test urine in a test tube. Also set up a positive (known bile salts containing urine) and negative (known normal urine) controls, if possible.
2. Sprinkle sulfur powder over the surface of urine sample and control samples.
3. Sinking of sulfur powder indicates positive test, i.e. presence of bile salts in urine sample.

Test for Blood in Urine

Hematuria is defined as the presence of blood as a whole in urine, whereas the presence of only blood pigments without corpuscles is called hemoglobinuria.

Benzidine Test

Principle: In benzidine test, benzidine reagent is oxidized to give a blue colored solution that result from the oxygen released when hemoglobin peroxidase acts on the hydrogen peroxide present in the reagent:

$$2H_2O_2 \xrightarrow{\text{Hb peroxidase}} 2H_2O_2 + O_2$$
$$\text{Benzidine} + O_2 \qquad \text{Blue color}$$

Procedure

1. Add 3 ml of urine sample to 3 ml of benzidine (saturated solution of benzidine in glacial acetic acid) followed by 1 ml of H_2O_2
2. Look for the presence of a green or blue color within a few minutes, which indicates the presence of blood in urine.

- Benzidine test:

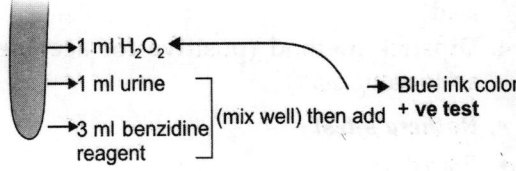

Fig. 29.7

Note: Interpret your finding/s and give provisional diagnosis (name one/more disease/s where your finding/s are present).

Proteinuria	Glycosuria	Ketonuria

• Kidney diseases:
  – Nephrotic syndrome
  – Acute glomerulonephritis
  – TB of kidney
  – Renal cell carcinoma
  – Renal vein thrombosis
  – Diabetic nephropathy
  – Hypertensive nephrosclerosis
• Muscular exertion
• High grade fever/heat injury
• Heavy metal poisoning
• Orthostatic albuminuria (only when patient is active on his feet)
• Toxemia of pregnancy
	• Diabetes mellitus
	• Pregnancy
	• Hyperthyroidism
	• Liver disease
	• Renal glycosuria (renal disease)
	• Alimentary glycosuria
	• IV infusion of glucose
	• ↑ed intracranial pressure
	• Patients receiving total parenteral nutrition (TPN)
		• Uncontrolled DM
		• Starvation
		• Fasting/anorexia
		• Glycogen storage disease
		• High protein diet
		• Low carbohydrate diet
		• Frequent vomiting
		• Hyperthyroidism
		• Fever
		• Acute and severe illness
		• Burn
		• Pregnancy/lactation
		• Dehydration

Bilirubin in urine	Bile salts in urine
• Biliary tract disease • Cirrhosis • Gallstones in biliary tract • Hepatitis • Liver disease • Tumors of liver, gall bladder/pancreas: Obstructive jaundice	Biliary obstruction due to gallstone/pancreatic tumor or gallstone

30

Gross Specimen

1. Identify the organ.
2. How did you identify the organ?
3. Describe the specimens (gross features, whatever you can appreciate from that particular specimen. Do not speak the gross features remembered from book; rather be selective, pick up those points that you can see in that specimens).
4. Identify the lesion/disease.
5. Related theory viva depending upon what you have answered in above questions.

Some selected specimens that are most frequently asked are given below, but it may vary from college to college. So, select or add other specimens list according to your requirements.

The heart and blood vessels

1. Atherosclerosis of aorta (atheroma)
2. MI
3. Fibrous pericarditis

Lungs

1. Ghon focus
2. TB lung
3. CVC lung
4. Bronchiectasis
5. Pneumonia
6. Bronchogenic carcinoma

GIT

1. Pleomorphic adenoma
2. TB ulcer
3. Typhoid ulcer
4. Benign peptic ulcer
5. Malignant peptic ulcer
6. Benign polyps
7. Carcinoma colon

Liver and biliary system

1. Fatty liver
2. Cirrhosis
3. CVC liver
4. Metastatic cancer of liver
5. Hepatocellular carcinoma
6. Gallstones (most are cholesterol stones)

Kidney

1. Hydronephrosis
2. Tuberculous pyelonephritis
3. Pyelonephritis
4. Amyloidosis
5. Renal cell carcinoma
6. Wilms' tumor
7. Transitional cell carcinoma
8. Renal infarct

Male genital tract

1. Seminoma
2. Teratoma
3. Nodular hyperplasia of prostate

Female genital tract and breast
1. Squamous cell carcinoma of cervix
2. Hydatidiform mole
3. Leiomyoma
4. Teratoma
5. Granulosa cell tumor (yellow tumor)
6. Krukenberg tumor
7. Carcinoma breast (mostly infiltrative ductal cell carcinoma)
8. Fibroadenoma

Endocrinology
1. Pheochromocytoma (yellow tumor)

2. Secondary tumor of adrenal gland (adenoma; rare)
3. Multiple nodular goiter
4. Adenoma thyroid

Bones
1. Osteosarcoma
2. Chondrosarcoma

Others
1. TB lymph node
2. CVC spleen
3. Splenic infarct

31

Histopathology Slides

General pathology

1. Coagulation necrosis
2. Liquefactive necrosis
3. Caseous necrosis
4. Fat necrosis
5. Fibrinoid necrosis
6. Granulation tissue
7. Monckeberg's medial calcification of uterus
8. Recanalization of thrombus
9. Allergic rhinitis
10. Hemangioma
11. Lipoma
12. Rhabdomyosarcoma
13. Tumor emboli
14. Hydatid cyst with scolices
15. Cysticercus cellulosae (parasite calcification)
16. Tubercular leprosy
17. Lepromatous leprosy
18. Borderline leprosy
19. Hyaline changes
20. Pus cells in urine (spotting)
21. Red cell cast in urine (spotting)

The heart and blood vessels

1. MI
2. Fibrinous pericarditis
3. TB pericarditis
4. Rheumatoid pancarditis
5. Aschoff's nodule
6. Atherosclerosis

Disorders of RBC

1. Normal peripheral blood smears (PBS)
2. PBS microcytic hypochromic anemia
3. PBS thalassemia major
4. PBS thalassemia trait
5. PBS anemia of chronic disease
6. PBS sickle cell anemia
7. PBS reticulocyte (spotting)
8. Normal BM
9. BM megaloblastic anemia
10. PBS macrocytic anemia

Disorders of WBC

1. Neutrophilia
2. Neutropenia
3. Eosinophilia
4. Basophilia
5. Lymphocytosis
6. Monocytosis
7. Hodgkin's lymphoma
8. Non-Hodgkin's lymphoma
9. ALL
10. CLL
11. AML
12. CML

Lymph node and spleen
1. TB lymph node
2. Reactive lymph node
3. Metastatic carcinoma of lymph node
4. Normal spleen
5. Splenic infarct
6. CVC spleen
7. Fibrocongestive spleen

Lung
1. Bronchopneumonia
2. Lobar pneumonia
3. Bronchitis
4. Bronchiectasis
5. Emphysema
6. Lung abscess
7. TB lung
8. CVC lung
9. Bronchial carcinoid
10. Bronchogenic carcinoma

GIT
1. Carcinoma tongue
2. Pleomorphic adenoma
3. Carcinoma esophagus
4. Gastric ulcer/peptic ulcer
5. Adenocarcinoma stomach
6. Amoebic colitis
7. Amoebic ulcer
8. Typhoid ulcer
9. TB ulcer
10. TB intestine (granuloma)
11. Acute appendicitis
12. Adenocarcinoma colon

The liver and biliary system
1. Normal liver
2. Viral hepatitis
3. Fatty liver
4. Cirrhosis
5. Post-necrotic cirrhosis
6. Micronodular cirrhosis
7. Amyloidosis liver
8. Granulomatous hepatitis (TB)
9. Hepatocellular carcinoma
10. Chronic cholecystitis
11. Carcinoma gallbladder

The urinary system
1. Normal kidney
2. Acute progressive glomerulonephritis
3. RPGN
4. Chronic glomerulonephritis
5. Chronic pyelonephritis
6. Diabetic nephropathy
7. Benign nephrosclerosis
8. Malignant nephrosclerosis
9. Amyloidosis of kidney
10. Wilms' tumor
11. RCC
12. TCC (transitional cell carcinoma)
13. TB kidney

Male genital tract
1. Seminoma
2. Atrophy testes
3. BPH (benign prostatic hyperplasia)
4. Carcinoma prostate

Female genital tract
1. Carcinoma cervix (scc)
2. Chronic cervicitis
3. Proliferative endometrium
4. Secretory endometrium
5. Hyperplasia endometrium
6. Leiomyoma uterus
7. Cystic teratoma (dermoid cyst)
8. Papillary cystadenoma ovary
9. Mucinous cystadenoma ovary
10. Serous cystadenoma ovary
11. Hydatidiform mole

The breast
1. Fibroadenoma breast
2. Carcinoma breast

The endocrine system
1. Colloid goiter
2. Hashimoto's thyroiditis
3. Adenoma thyroid
4. Carcinoma thyroid
5. Papillary carcinoma thyroid
6. Adenoma parathyroid

Skin
1. Melanin pigment of skin
2. Basal cell carcinoma
3. Malignant melanoma
4. Squamous cell carcinoma of skin

CNS
1. TB meningitis
2. Pyogenic meningitis
3. Astrocytoma
4. Meningioma
5. Neurilemoma

Bones
1. Osteogenic sarcoma
2. Chronic osteomyelitis
3. TB osteomyelitis
4. Giant cell tumor

Reader's Notes

Reader's Notes